Drug Metabolism and Transport

METHODS IN PHARMACOLOGY AND TOXICOLOGY

Y. James Kang, DVM, PhD, SERIES EDITOR

Drug Metabolism and Transport: Molecular Methods and Mechanisms,
    edited by **Lawrence Lash**, 2005
Optimization in Drug Discovery: In Vitro Methods
    edited by **Zhengyin Yan** and **Gary W. Caldwell**, 2004
In Vitro Neurotoxicology: Principles and Challenges
    edited by **Evelyn Tiffany-Castiglioni**, 2004
Cardiac Drug Development Guide
    edited by **Michael K. Pugsley**, 2003
Methods in Biological Oxidative Stress
    edited by **Kenneth Hensley** and **Robert A. Floyd**, 2003
Apoptosis Methods in Pharmacology and Toxicology:
  Approaches to Measurement and Quantification
    edited by **Myrtle A. Davis**, 2002
Ion Channel Localization: Methods and Protocols
    edited by **Anatoli N. Lopatin** and **Colin G. Nichols**, 2001

METHODS IN PHARMACOLOGY AND TOXICOLOGY

Drug Metabolism and Transport

Molecular Methods and Mechanisms

Edited by

Lawrence H. Lash

*Department of Pharmacology
Wayne State University School of Medicine
Detroit, MI*

HUMANA PRESS ✳ TOTOWA, NEW JERSEY

© 2005 Humana Press Inc.
999 Riverview Drive, Suite 208
Totowa, NJ 07512

www.humanapress.com

All rights reserved. No part of this book may be reproduced, stored in a retrieval system, or transmitted in any form or by any means, electronic, mechanical, photocopying, microfilming, recording, or otherwise without written permission from the Publisher.

The content and opinions expressed in this book are the sole work of the authors and editors, who have warranted due diligence in the creation and issuance of their work. The publisher, editors, and authors are not responsible for errors or omissions or for any consequences arising from the information or opinions presented in this book and make no warranty, express or implied, with respect to its contents.

This publication is printed on acid-free paper. ∞
ANSI Z39.48-1984 (American National Standards Institute) Permanence of Paper for Printed Library Materials.

Cover design by Patricia F. Cleary

Cover illustrations: Ribbon representation of a human GSTZ subunit (*foreground;* Fig. 3, Chapter 4; *see* full caption and discussion on p. 92). Immunohistochemical localization of p65/RelA subunit of NF-κB transcription factor in sections from acetaminophen-treated liver tissue (*background;* Fig. 5, Chapter 8; *see* full caption on p. 212 and discussion on p. 211).

For additional copies, pricing for bulk purchases, and/or information about other Humana titles, contact Humana at the above address or at any of the following numbers: Tel.: 973-256-1699; Fax: 973-256-8341; E-mail: humana@humanapr.com or visit our website: http://humanapress.com

Photocopy Authorization Policy:
Authorization to photocopy items for internal or personal use, or the internal or personal use of specific clients, is granted by Humana Press Inc., provided that the base fee of US $25.00 per copy is paid directly to the Copyright Clearance Center at 222 Rosewood Drive, Danvers, MA 01923. For those organizations that have been granted a photocopy license from the CCC, a separate system of payment has been arranged and is acceptable to Humana Press Inc. The fee code for users of the Transactional Reporting Service is: [0-58829-324-6/05 $25.00].

Printed in the United States of America. 10 9 8 7 6 5 4 3 2 1

eISBN 1-59259-832-3

Library of Congress Cataloging-in-Publication Data
Drug metabolism and transport : molecular methods and mechanisms / edited by Lawrence H. Lash.
   p. ; cm. — (Methods in pharmacology and toxicology)
 Includes bibliographical references and index.
 ISBN 1-58829-324-6 (hardcover : alk. paper)
 1. Drugs—Metabolism. 2. Drugs—Physiological transport.
 [DNLM: 1. Pharmaceutical Preparations—metabolism. 2. Biological Transport—drug effects. 3. Drug Delivery Systems—methods. QV 38 D79363 2005] I. Lash, Lawrence H. II. Series.
 RM301.55.D7625 2005
 615'.7—dc22
                                                                                           2004013419

Preface

Two key aspects of how the body handles drugs and other chemicals are metabolism and transport. Metabolism is critical because it enables the body to process highly lipophilic molecules for further metabolism and eventual excretion, inactivates biologically active molecules, or detoxifies potentially toxic chemicals. Transport processes are critical because they determine the ability of drugs and other chemicals to gain access to sites of metabolism or to physiological or toxicological targets within tissues. The remarkable advances in molecular and cell biology and the development of novel in vitro model systems to study the various processes involved in metabolism and transport have expanded our knowledge and led to numerous, new therapeutic approaches to treatment of chemically induced toxicity and disease.

Drug Metabolism and Transport: Molecular Methods and Mechanisms, which is part of the *Methods in Pharmacology and Toxicology* series, presents a collection of chapters on selected aspects of metabolism and transport. The general approach of the chapters is to first present background on the topic to define the state of the science, to summarize key experimental models and methods that are used in the study of the process, and then to evaluate the utility of the various approaches and methods. Along the way, the various authors have endeavored to provide insight into why each model or approach is advantageous and discuss limitations and cautions in the application of these models or approaches. The goal here is not to provide step-by-step recipes for how to conduct specific assays, although selected procedures are outlined in some detail. Rather, the goal is to present some rationale for why certain models or approaches are used and to describe insight into how they are used to address various issues in drug metabolism and transport.

No single volume can address all the major metabolic and transport systems that handle drugs and other chemicals. However, this volume has selected several of the major drug metabolizing systems, including the cytochrome P450 family, flavin-containing monooxygenases, glutathione *S*-transferases, glucuronidation, *N*-acetylation, and sulfotransferases. Additional chapters present approaches to the study of signaling pathways in the regulation of drug metabolism enzymes, how modulation of thiols and other low-molecular-weight cofactors can alter drug metabolism, how one studies metabolism and toxicity of a prototypical toxicant, acetaminophen, and how modulation of drug metabolism pathways can influence antiviral therapy. Three chapters on transport are included to cover other very diverse processes: the multidrug-resistance proteins, the reduced folate carrier, and the plasma membrane and mitochondrial glutathione transporters. Many of the principles enunciated in these chapters can be applied to numerous other transport systems, so the present chapters serve as examples and prototypes.

Overall, the aim of *Drug Metabolism and Transport: Molecular Methods and Mechanisms*—by necessity only a partial survey of the drug metabolism enzymes and transporters—is to make clear the general principles and illustrate those approaches with wider application. Moreover, this compact reference is intended as a ready resource to investigators in their immediate work on either the specific processes the book describes or on other systems.

Lawrence H. Lash

Contents

Preface v

Contributors ix

1 Renal Cytochrome P450s and Flavin-Containing Monooxygenases:
   *Potential Roles in Metabolism and Toxicity of 1,3-Butadiene,
   Trichloroethylene, and Tetrachloroethylene*
   Adnan A. Elfarra 1

2 Experimental Approaches for the Study of Cytochrome P450
   Gene Regulation
   *Hollie I. Swanson, Susan D. Kraner, Soma S. Ray,
   Martin Hoagland, Earl D. Thompson, Xinyu Zheng,
   and Yanan Tian* 19

3 Insulin and Growth Factor Signaling:
   Effects on Drug-Metabolizing Enzymes
   *Sang K. Kim, Kimberley J. Woodcroft,
   and Raymond F. Novak* 45

4 Catalytic Function and Expression of Glutathione
   Transferase Zeta
   Philip G. Board, M. W. Anders, and Anneke C. Blackburn 85

5 Glucuronidation of Fatty Acids and Prostaglandins
   by Human UDP-Glucuronosyltransferases
   *Anna Radominska-Pandya, Joanna M. Little,
   and Arthur Bull* 109

6 Transcriptional Regulation of UDP-
   Glucuronosyltransferases
   *Anna Radominska-Pandya, Peter I. Mackenzie,
   and Wen Xie* 133

7 Phenotypic and Genotypic Characterization
   of N-Acetylation
   Craig K. Svensson and David W. Hein 173

8 Methods and Approaches to Study Metabolism
   and Toxicity of Acetaminophen
   Sam A. Bruschi 197

9 Modulation of Drug Metabolism and Antiviral Therapies
   Bernhard H. Lauterburg 233
10 Modulation of Thiols and Other Low-Molecular-Weight
   Cofactors: *Effects on Drug Metabolism
   and Disease Susceptibility*
   Charles V. Smith 253
11 Multidrug Resistance Proteins and Hepatic Transport
   of Endo- and Xenobiotics
   Phillip M. Gerk and Mary Vore 273
12 Structural Determinants of Folate and Antifolate
   Membrane Transport by the Reduced Folate Carrier
   Wei Cao and Larry H. Matherly 291
13 Glutathione Transport in the Kidneys:
   Experimental Models, Mechanisms, and Methods
   Lawrence H. Lash 319
14 Human Cytosolic Sulfotransferases:
   Properties, Physiological Functions, and Toxicology
   Charles N. Falany 341

Index 379

Contributors

M. W. ANDERS • *Department of Pharmacology and Physiology, University of Rochester, Rochester, NY*

ANNEKE C. BLACKBURN • *Molecular Genetics, Division of Molecular Bioscience, Institute of Advanced Studies, The John Curtin School of Medical Research, Australian National University, Canberra, Australia*

PHILIP G. BOARD • *Molecular Genetics, Division of Molecular Bioscience, Institute of Advanced Studies, The John Curtin School of Medical Research, Australian National University, Canberra, Australia*

SAM A. BRUSCHI • *Department of Medicinal Chemistry, University of Washington, Seattle, WA*

ARTHUR BULL • *Department of Chemistry, Oakland University, Rochester, MN*

WEI CAO • *Developmental Therapeutics, Karmanos Cancer Institute and Department of Pharmacology, Wayne State University School of Medicine, Detroit, MI*

ADNAN A. ELFARRA • *Department of Comparative Biosciences, University of Wisconsin, Madison, WI*

CHARLES N. FALANY • *Department of Pharmacology and Toxicology, University of Alabama at Birmingham, Birmingham, AL*

PHILLIP M. GERK • *Graduate Center for Toxicology, University of Kentucky Medical Center, Lexington, KY*

DAVID W. HEIN • *Department of Pharmacology and Toxicology, University of Louisville, Louisville, KY*

MARTIN HOAGLAND • *University of Kentucky Medical Center, Lexington, KY*

SANG K. KIM • *Institute of Environmental Health Sciences, Wayne State University, Detroit, MI*

SUSAN D. KRANER • *Department of Molecular and Biomedical Pharmacology, University of Kentucky Medical Center, Lexington, KY*

LAWRENCE H. LASH • *Department of Pharmacology, Wayne State University, Detroit, MI*

BERNHARD H. LAUTERBURG • *Department of Clinical Pharmacology, University of Bern, Bern, Switzerland*

JOANNA M. LITTLE • *Department of Biochemistry and Molecular Biology, University of Arkansas for Medical Sciences, Little Rock, AR*

PETER I. MACKENZIE • *Department of Clinical Pharmacology, Flinders University, Bedford Park, Australia*

LARRY H. MATHERLY • *Developmental Therapeutics, Karmanos Cancer Institute and Department of Pharmacology, Wayne State University School of Medicine, Detroit, MI*

RAYMOND F. NOVAK • *Institute of Environmental Health Sciences, Wayne State University, Detroit, MI*

ANNA RADOMINSKA-PANDYA • *Department of Biochemistry and Molecular Biology, University of Arkansas for Medical Sciences, Little Rock, AR*

SOMA S. RAY • *University of Kentucky Medical Center, Lexington, KY*

CHARLES V. SMITH • *Center for Developmental Toxicology, Columbus Children's Research Institute, Columbus Children's Hospital; Department of Pediatrics, The Ohio State University, Columbus, OH*

CRAIG K. SVENSSON • *Division of Pharmaceutics, University of Iowa, Iowa City, IA*

HOLLIE I. SWANSON • *Department of Molecular and Biomedical Pharmacology, University of Kentucky Medical Center, Lexington, KY*

EARL D. THOMPSON • *Department of Molecular and Biomedical Pharmacology, University of Kentucky Medical Center, Lexington, KY*

YANAN TIAN • *Department of Veterinary Physiology and Pharmacology, Texas A & M University, College Station, TX*

MARY VORE • *Graduate Center for Toxicology, University of Kentucky Medical Center, Lexington, KY*

KIMBERLEY J. WOODCROFT • *Institute of Environmental Health Sciences, Wayne State University, Detroit, MI*

WEN XIE • *Center for Pharmacogenetics and Department of Pharmaceutical Sciences, University of Pittsburgh, Pittsburgh, PA*

XINYU ZHENG • *Department of Molecular and Biomedical Pharmacology, University of Kentucky Medical Center, Lexington, KY*

1

Renal Cytochrome P450s and Flavin-Containing Monooxygenases

Potential Roles in Metabolism and Toxicity of 1,3-Butadiene, Trichloroethylene, and Tetrachloroethylene

Adnan A. Elfarra

Summary

It is widely recognized that the kidneys contain several enzymes capable of catalyzing the metabolism of drugs and toxicants to yield chemically reactive metabolites that can cause nephrotoxicity. Reactive metabolites generated in the kidneys, and metabolites translocated to the kidneys via the circulation after being formed in the liver, can also be detoxified in the kidneys. The kinetics of these bioactivation and detoxification reactions, which vary between chemicals and depend on the age, sex, renal cell type, and species involved, are important determinants of nephrotoxicity. This chapter reviews current knowledge and experimental approaches used to investigate the potential roles of renal cytochrome P450s (P450s) and flavin-containing monooxygenases (FMOs) in the metabolism and toxicity of three important industrial chemicals—1,3-butadiene (BD), trichloroethylene (TRI), and tetrachloroethylene (TETRA; also known as perchloroethylene)—as model compounds. The chapter illustrates examples of significant species-, tissue-, and sex-related differences in specific metabolic reactions. Because metabolic differences can be both qualitative and quantitative, depending on the chemical nature of the substrate, extrapolating data from one chemical to another, and among different genders and/or species can lead to inaccurate conclusions.

Key Words

Apoptosis; blood urea nitrogen; 1,3-butadiene; butadiene monoxide; cysteine conjugate β-lyase; cytochrome P450s; diepoxybutane; flavin-containing monooxygenases; GSH conjugation; kidney; liver; mercapturates; National Toxicology Program (NTP); necrosis; reactive metabolites; renal organic anion transporters; species extrapolation; sulfoxides; target organ toxicity; tetrachloroethylene; trichloroethylene; US Environmental Protection Agency.

From: *Methods in Pharmacology and Toxicology,*
Drug Metabolism and Transport: Molecular Methods and Mechanisms
Edited by: L. Lash © Humana Press Inc., Totowa, NJ

1. INTRODUCTION

The kidneys can be exposed to high concentrations of drugs and toxicants present in the blood because they receive nearly 25% of the cardiac output, have the ability to concentrate tubular fluids, and have several active transport systems that can cause the accumulation of organic acids, organic bases, and other chemicals into kidney cells. Because the kidneys also contain a wide variety of biotransformation enzymes, kidney cells can play an important role in the metabolism and disposition of drugs and toxicants. Indeed, it is now widely recognized that the kidneys contain several enzymes capable of catalyzing the metabolism of drugs and toxicants to yield chemically reactive metabolites that can cause nephrotoxicity. Reactive metabolites generated in the kidneys, and metabolites translocated to the kidneys via the circulation after being formed in the liver, can also be detoxified in the kidneys. The kinetics of these bioactivation and detoxification reactions, which vary between chemicals and depend on the age, sex, renal cell type, and species involved, are important determinants of nephrotoxicity. They are also important determinants of the relative contribution of the kidneys to overall drug and toxicant metabolism and disposition after systemic exposure. Because several aspects of renal drug metabolism have recently been reviewed *(1–4)*, this chapter focuses on reviewing current knowledge regarding the potential roles of renal cytochrome P450s (P450s) and flavin-containing monooxygenases (FMOs) in the metabolism and toxicity of three important industrial chemicals—1,3-butadiene (BD), trichloroethylene (TRI), and tetrachloroethylene (TETRA; also known as perchloroethylene)—as model compounds.

2. BD

BD, a petrochemical used in the manufacture of synthetic rubber and plastic and commonly detected in urban air, gasoline vapors, and cigarette smoke, has been associated with development of lymphohematopoietic cancers among exposed workers. The US Department of Health and Human Services—National Toxicology Program (NTP) and US Environmental Protection Agency have recently upgraded BD to the classification of "known to be a human carcinogen" based on epidemiological data and experimental results obtained using rats and mice *(5–7)*. Mice were significantly more susceptible to BD-induced carcinogenicity compared to rats; sites of tumor formation in mice included the hematopoietic system, lung, liver, and kidneys *(7)*.

P450-mediated oxidation of BD to yield the mutagenic metabolites, butadiene monoxide and diepoxybutane (Fig. 1), has been suggested to play a significant role in the mechanisms of BD carcinogenicity *(8–12)*. The rates of BD

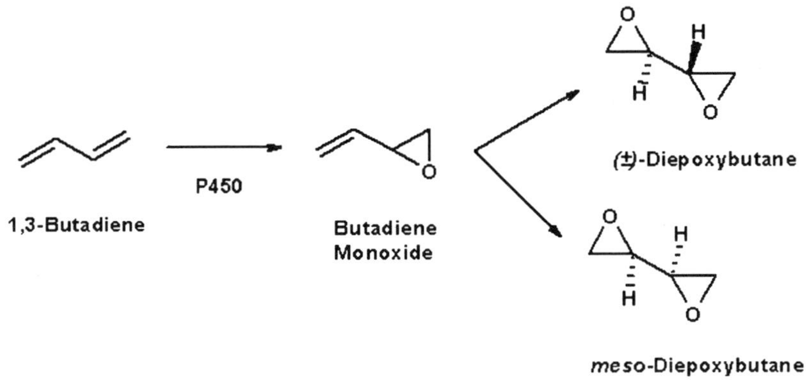

Fig. 1. Oxidation of 1,3-butadiene (BD) to butadiene monoxide and further oxidation of butadiene monoxide to meso- and (±)-diepoxybutane by cytochrome P450s.

oxidation to butadiene monoxide by male mouse liver, lung, and kidney microsomes were nearly 2-, 4-, and 50-fold higher than those of male rat liver, lung, and kidney microsomes, respectively *(13)*. These results, and the finding that male mouse liver and kidney microsomes were also much more efficient in their metabolism of BD to the known carcinogen crotonaldehyde, are consistent with the high sensitivity of the mouse tissues to BD-induced carcinogenicity. The findings that rates of detoxification of butadiene monoxide by epoxide hydrolase and glutathione *S*-transferases in the male mouse kidney were much lower than the corresponding rates in the male mouse liver *(9,10,13,14)* suggest a role for the butadiene monoxide formed in the kidneys in the renal carcinogenicity of BD in male mice, and may also be contributing to the much higher blood concentrations of butadiene monoxide and diepoxybutane in mice after BD exposure in comparison with the corresponding rat blood levels *(11)*.

Male mouse kidney microsomes, which contain much less cytochrome P450s than male mouse liver microsomes, were more effective in catalyzing BD oxidation to butadiene monoxide than male mouse liver microsomes (Fig. 2) and BD metabolism in male mouse kidney microsomes was also more sensitive to inhibition by inclusion of 1-benzylimidazole, a nonspecific P450 inhibitor, than male mouse liver microsomes (Fig. 3; *13*). These results suggest the involvement of multiple P450s in BD bioactivation. Interestingly, preliminary results from our laboratory using a monoclonal antibody specific for mouse CYP4B1 suggest CYP4B1 is the major catalyst of BD bioactivation in the male mouse kidney *(15)*, whereas CYP2E1 and CYP2A5 are the major catalysts of BD oxidation in male and female mouse liver *(10,12)*.

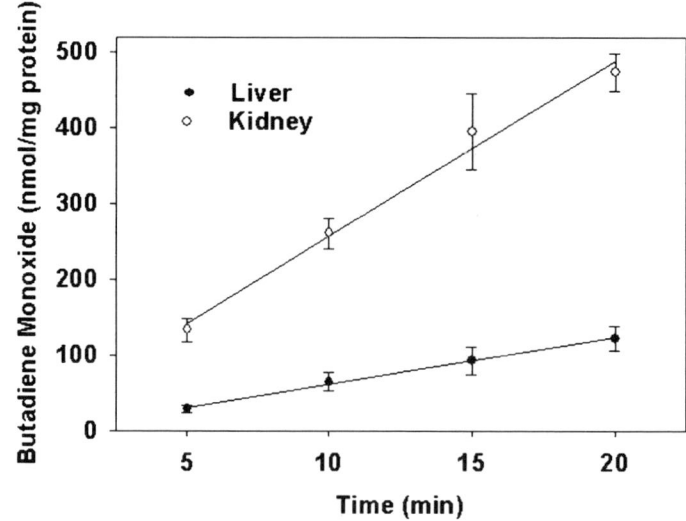

Fig. 2. NADPH- and time-dependent formation of butadiene monoxide from 1,3-butadiene (BD) by male B6C3F1 mouse liver and kidney microsomes. (Data were taken from ref. *13*.)

3. TRI AND TETRA

TRI and TETRA, hazardous air pollutants and major surface and ground water contaminants, are commonly used in industry as solvents and as metal degreasing and dry cleaning agents *(16)*. The NTP has listed both compounds as "reasonably anticipated to be a human carcinogen" *(16)*. Although the liver and kidneys are the two prominent target organs of toxicity in humans and in experimental animals *(17–19)*, considerable species- and sex-dependent differences have been observed in TRI and TETRA target organ toxicity. For example, TRI and TETRA are nephrotoxic to both rats and mice and are kidney carcinogens in rats. In addition, male rats are more susceptible to the nephrotoxic effects of TETRA than female rats *(17–19* and references therein).

The toxic effects of TRI and TETRA are dependent on their bioactivation to reactive metabolites. This bioactivation occurs predominantly via two pathways, the P450-mediated pathway and the glutathione (GSH)-conjugation pathway *(4,20–25)*. Because both TRI and TETRA are substrates for both pathways, the same or similar types of metabolites are formed after exposure to both compounds. However, the kinetics of individual steps are different, and thus the flux through each step and the importance of each metabolite differ between the two compounds. For example, TRI is the better substrate for the

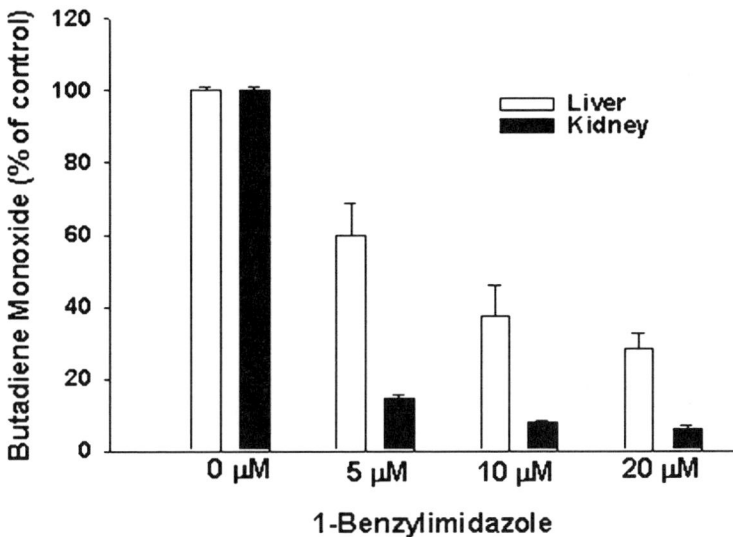

Fig. 3. Effect of inclusion of 1-benzylimidazole on 1,3-butadiene (BD) oxidation to butadiene monoxide by male B6C3F1 mouse liver and kidney microsomes. (Data were taken from ref *13*.)

P450-mediated oxidative pathway whereas TETRA is the better substrate for the GSH-conjugation pathway.

P450-mediated oxidation is a major pathway of TRI and TETRA metabolism (Fig. 4). The initial oxidation of TRI and TETRA is catalyzed primarily by CYP2E1 but additional isoforms have also been suggested to play a role *(17,22,23)*. Further metabolism, hydrolysis, and/or decomposition of the initial oxidation products result in the formation of several metabolites *(17,21,23)*. Known metabolites of TRI and/or TETRA include trichloroacetic acid, dichloroacetic acid, chloral, trichloroacetyl chloride, trichloroethanol and trichloroethanol glucuronide, oxalate dichloride, and oxalic acid (Fig. 4). Of these metabolites, trichloroacetic acid and dichloroacetic acid are considered the most important liver toxicants. The liver is quantitatively the most important tissue in the oxidative metabolism of TRI and TETRA, because of the high expression levels of P450s in the liver and because of its size. P450-mediated metabolism of TRI and TETRA may also occur in the kidney, although at a rate lower than that in the liver. However, the significance of oxidation of TRI and TETRA in the kidney is unclear because, whereas CYP2E1 is expressed in the rat kidney, it has not been found in the human kidney *(22)*. Thus, considerable species differences exist in the oxidative metabolism of TRI and TETRA between humans and rodents.

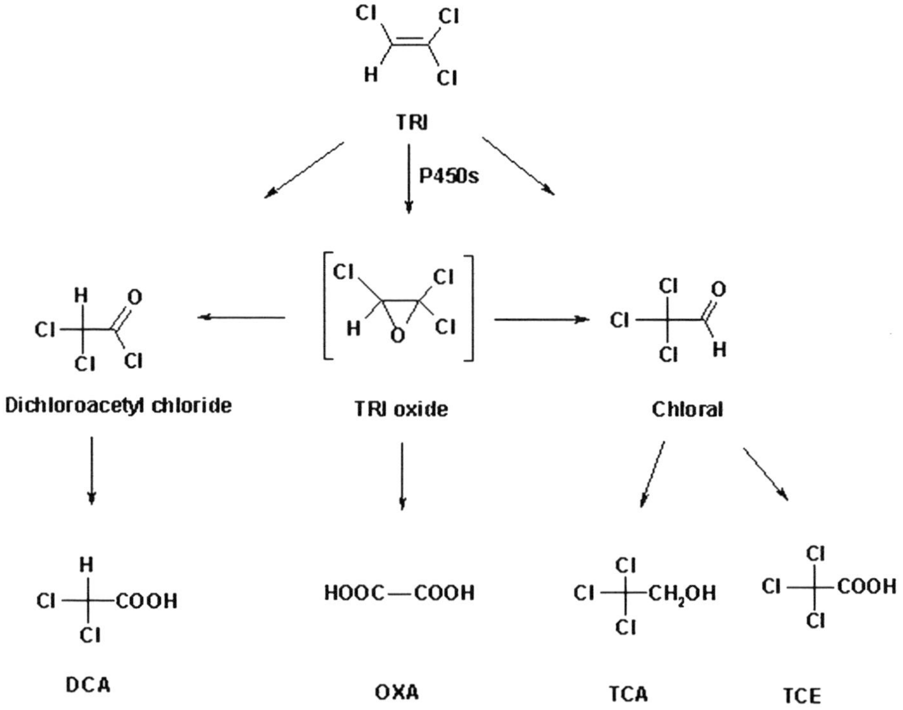

Fig. 4. Cytochrome P450-dependent oxidative metabolism of trichloroethylene (TRI) in liver microsomes and further metabolites and/or hydrolysis or decomposition products. DCA, Dichloroacetic acid; OXA, oxalic acid; TCA, trichloroacetic acid; TCE, trichloroethanol.

Whereas P450-mediated oxidation is a major metabolic pathway for TRI and TETRA, the nephrotoxicity of these compounds is associated with the GSH-conjugation pathway (Fig. 5). The initial step in this pathway is the glutathione S-transferase (GST)-mediated conjugation of GSH with TRI or TETRA to form S-(1,2-dichlorovinyl)glutathione (DCVG) or S-(1,2,2-trichloro-vinyl)glutathione (TCVG), respectively *(20,24,25)*. This step takes place predominantly in the liver but can also occur in the kidneys. It is also possible that DCVG and TCVG formed in the liver can be translocated to the kidneys. The further metabolism of DCVG and TCVG by γ-glutamyltransferase and dipeptidases to yield the metabolites S-(1,2-dichlorovinyl)-L-cysteine (DCVC) and S-(1,2,2-trichlorovinyl)-L-cysteine (TCVC) occurs primarily in the kidney *(4,17)*. DCVC and TCVC are critical metabolites in TRI- and TETRA-induced nephrotoxicity because they are substrates for multiple bioactivation and detoxification pathways. In addition, DCVC and TCVC are substrates for renal

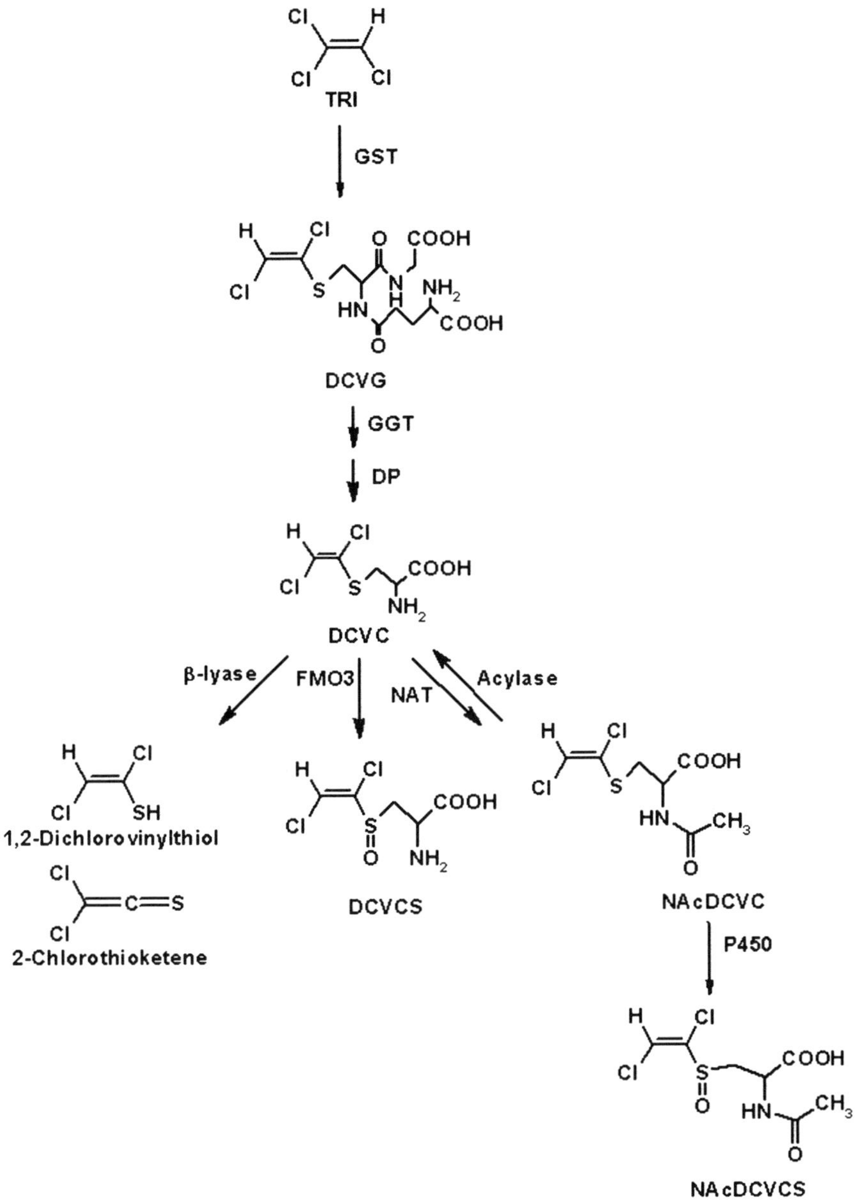

Fig. 5. Glutathione (GSH)-dependent metabolism of trichloroethylene (TRI). DCVC, S-(1,2-Dichlorovinyl)-L-cysteine; DCVCS, S-(1,2-dichlorovinyl)-L-cysteine sulfoxide; DCVG, S-(1,2-dichlorovinyl)glutathione; DP, dipeptidase; FMO3, flavin-containing monooxygenase 3; GGT, γ-glutamyltransferase; GST, glutathione S-transferase; β-lyase, cysteine conjugate β-lyase; NAcDCVC, N-acetyl-S-(1,2-dichlorovinyl)-L-cysteine; NAcDCVCS, N-acetyl-S-(1,2-dichlorovinyl)-L-cysteine sulfoxide; NAT, N-acetyltransferase.

organic anion transporters and are selectively taken up and accumulated in the kidney *(4,17,20)*. Thus, the concentrations of DCVC and TCVC in the kidney can be significantly higher than in other tissues.

One of the important bioactivation reactions of DCVC and TCVC is the formation of 1,2-dichlorovinylthiol and 1,2,2-trichlorovinylthiol, respectively, catalyzed by one of the cysteine S-conjugate β-lyases found in many tissues, including the kidneys *(3,4,17,23)*. The halothiols formed in this β-lyase-mediated bioactivation of DCVC and TCVC are unstable compounds that spontaneously rearrange to form thioketenes that can form adducts with proteins and DNA. These findings are in agreement with the observation that DCVC was mutagenic in some forms of the Ames test. This mutagenicity was decreased by preincubation with the β-lyase inhibitor aminooxyacetic acid, demonstrating the role of β-lyases in the generation of the mutagenic species.

Another important bioactivation reaction of DCVC and TCVC is the oxidation of the sulfur moiety to form DCVC sulfoxide (DCVCS; Fig. 5) and TCVC sulfoxide (TCVCS), respectively. Experiments with recombinant rabbit and human FMOs and with intact and solubilized rabbit and human liver and kidney microsomes provided strong evidence that the oxidation of DCVC to yield DCVCS is primarily catalyzed by FMO3, whereas TCVC oxidation to TCVCS can be catalyzed by both FMO3 and P450s *(26,27)*. DCVCS and TCVCS are Michael acceptors and thus react rapidly with cellular thiols such as GSH and thiol groups in proteins *(26,28)*. The half-life of DCVCS when incubated with 3.3 equivalents (Eq) of GSH in buffer at pH 7.4 and 37°C was only 1.2 min whereas the half-life of TCVCS under the same conditions was approx 20 min (Fig. 6; *26*). In accordance with this rapid rate of reaction of DCVCS and TCVCS with thiols, treatment of renal cells with DCVCS results in depletion of cellular GSH *(29,30)*. Furthermore, DCVCS and TCVCS selectively depleted kidney GSH levels after in vivo treatment *(28,31)*.

DCVCS and TCVCS are much more potent nephrotoxicants than DCVC and TCVC, respectively *(29,31)*. Blood urea nitrogen (BUN) levels in rats treated with 230 µmol/kg of DCVC were comparable to those of rats treated with saline only, and only a 2.5-fold increase in BUN levels compared with controls was observed in rats treated with 460 µmol/kg of DCVC (Fig. 7). In contrast, rats treated with 230 and 460 µmol/kg DCVCS had approx 7-fold increases in BUN levels compared with controls. DCVC and DCVCS induce necrosis in human proximal tubular cells *(30)*. Necrosis, as measured by lactate dehydrogenase (LDH) release, was dose- and time-dependent but fairly high doses of DCVCS and long incubation times (200 μM for 48 h or 500 μM for 2 h for DCVCS) were required to increase LDH release significantly as compared with controls. In contrast, DCVCS induced apoptosis in renal proximal tubular cells at fairly low concentrations and short time points; treatment of renal proximal tubular

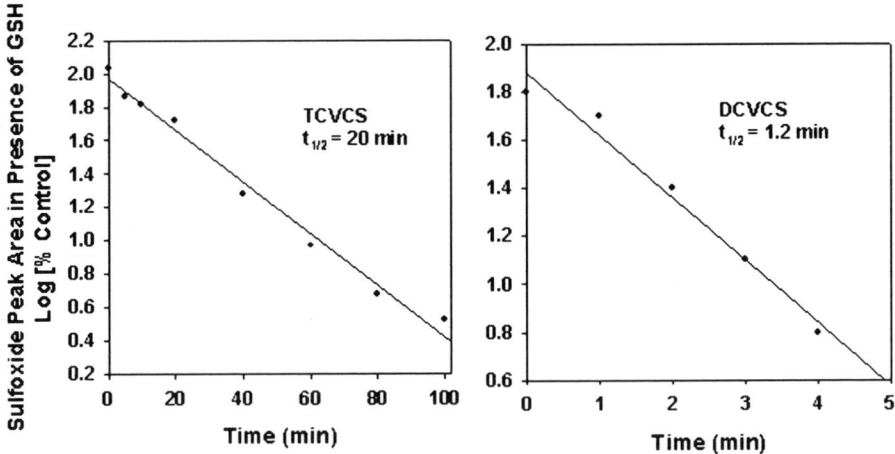

Fig. 6. Stabililty of S-(1,2,2-trichlorovinyl)-L-cysteine sulfoxide (TCVCS) and S-(1,2-dichlorovinyl)-L-cysteine sulfoxide (DCVCS) in the presence of glutathione (GSH). (Data were taken from ref. 26.)

cells with DCVCS at concentrations as low as 10 μM for only 2 h significantly increased the number of cells undergoing apoptosis (Fig. 8; 30). Recent evidence suggest that the mitochondria may be especially sensitive toward the toxic effects of DCVCS (29,30). Treatment of isolated human renal proximal tubular cells with as little as 10 μM DCVCS for 1 h decreased the cellular ATP concentration by approx 60% compared with untreated cells (Fig. 9; 30). This decrease in ATP concentration was both dose- and time-dependent.

Detoxification of DCVC and TCVC occurs by N-acetylation by cysteine conjugate N-acetyltransferase found in the endoplasmic reticulum, to form mercapturates that are readily excreted into urine (3,4). However, these mercapturates can be deacetylated by acylase I to reform DCVC and TCVC that may either be reacetylated or enter the bioactivation pathways. Moreover, N-acetyl-DCVC and N-acetyl-TCVC may be S-oxidized to form N-acetyl-DCVCS and N-acetyl-TCVCS (32), respectively, in reactions catalyzed by P450s, but the toxicological significance of these reactions is unclear at present because of the low rates of these reactions in liver or kidney microsomes in comparison with the corresponding deacetylation reactions. Recently, the rate of S-allyl-L-cysteine (SAC) sulfoxidation in rat liver microsomes was found to be nearly 20-fold higher than the corresponding rate measured with the SAC mercapturic acid, N-acetyl-S-allyl-L-cysteine (33). The latter results suggest mercapturic acids are not effective substrates for the oxidative enzymes present in rat liver microsomes in comparison with their corresponding

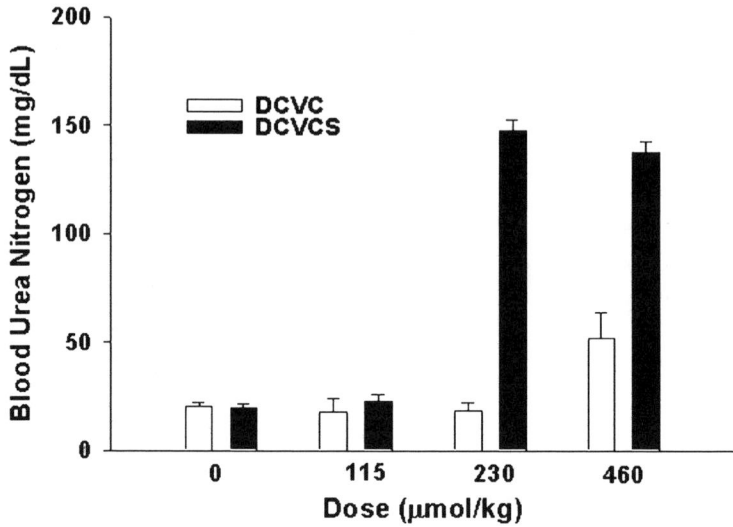

Fig. 7. Blood urea nitrogen concentrations of male rats after treatment with S-(1,2-dichlorovinyl)-L-cysteine (DCVC) and S-(1,2-dichlorovinyl)-L-cysteine sulfoxide (DCVCS). (Data were taken from ref. 29.)

cysteine S-conjugates. DCVCS and TCVCS, which can be formed from DCVC and TCVC, respectively, may also be substrates for N-acetyltransferases, acylases, and β-lyases, but the significance of these pathways in DCVCS and TCVCS metabolism is at present questionable, especially because of the high reactivity of these sulfoxides in the presence of biological nucleophiles *(26,28,31)*.

4. PERSPECTIVES

The preceding discussion highlights the importance of renal P450s and/or FMOs in the metabolism and toxicity of BD, TRI, and TETRA and provides examples of significant species-, tissue-, and sex-related differences in specific metabolic reactions. Because metabolic differences can be both qualitative and quantitative, depending on the chemical nature of the substrate, extrapolating data from one chemical to another, and among different genders and/or species can lead to inaccurate conclusions.

Our data on BD bioactivation by CYP4B1 in the male mouse kidney should not be extrapolated to the male mouse liver or the female mouse kidney because CYP4B1 is not expressed in these tissues. Until CYP4B1 expression and function in human kidneys are characterized, the male mouse kidney data should also not be extrapolated to the human kidneys. As indicated earlier, the

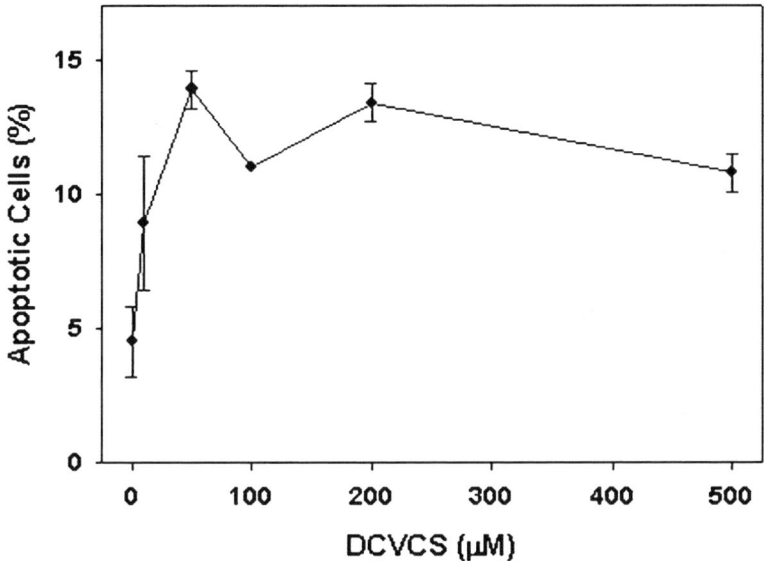

Fig. 8. Apoptosis in primary cultures of human proximal tubular cells induced by a 2-h treatment of S-(1,2-dichlorovinyl)-L-cysteine sulfoxide (DCVCS). (Data were taken from ref. 30.)

human kidneys seem not to express CYP2E1, one of the major P450s involved in BD bioactivation in male mouse and male and female human liver.

Mercapturic acid formation is a major metabolic pathway by which many drugs, industrial chemicals, and environmental pollutants are detoxified in liver and kidney cells before excretion into urine. However, for many widely used halogenated hydrocarbons, including TRI and TETRA, formation of cysteine S-conjugates has been implicated in mutagenicity, carcinogenicity, and nephrotoxicity of these chemicals (3,4,17). Recently, evidence implicating FMOs in bioactivation and cytotoxicity of DCVC and TCVC has been obtained (26–31). Although FMO-mediated oxidations of many sulfur- and nitrogen-containing chemicals, such as methimazole, chlorpromazine, nicotine, parathion, and thiourea have long been recognized (34–36), the role of FMOs in the metabolism and toxicity of metabolites formed by the mercapturic acid pathway has not been recognized until we provided clear evidence for the involvement of FMOs in the oxidative metabolism of S-benzyl-L-cysteine (SBC), a model cysteine S-conjugate in rat liver and kidney microsomes (37). Further characterization of this SBC S-oxidase activity revealed it to be mediated by FMO1 (38). FMO1 is highly expressed in the kidneys of mice, rats, and humans, and in the liver of mice and rats, but not in the adult human liver (38–41). Studies with human liver and kidney microsomes have shown DCVCS formation only with

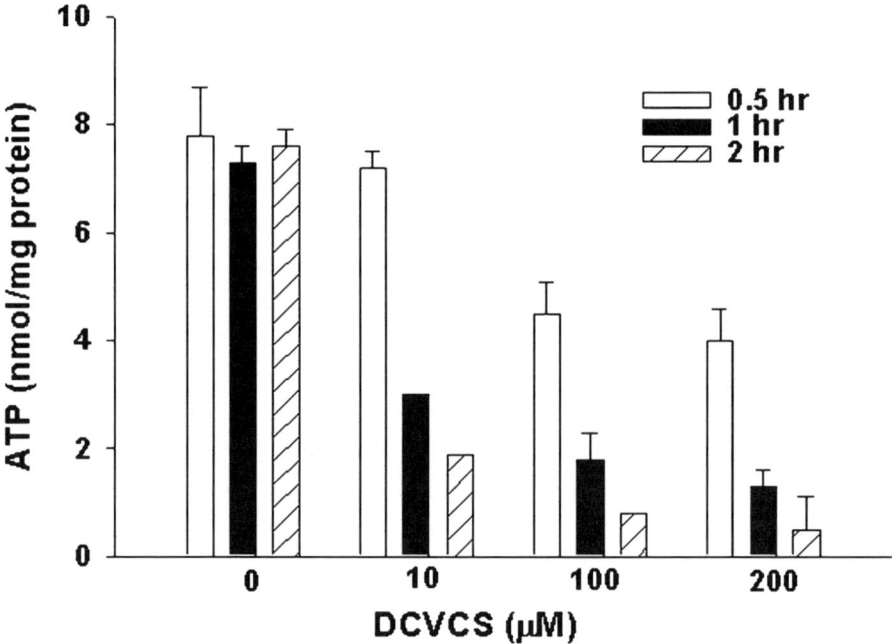

Fig. 9. Effect of S-(1,2-dichlorovinyl)-L-cysteine sulfoxide (DCVCS) on ATP levels in human proximal tubular cells. (Data were taken from ref. 30.)

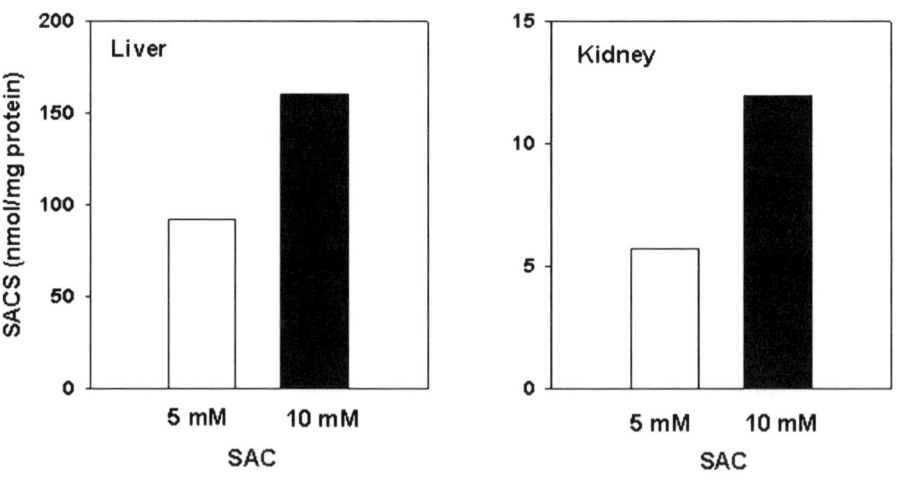

Fig. 10. NADPH-dependent S-allyl-L-cysteine (SAC) metabolism to its corresponding sulfoxide by human liver and kidney microsomes. (Data were taken from ref. 27.)

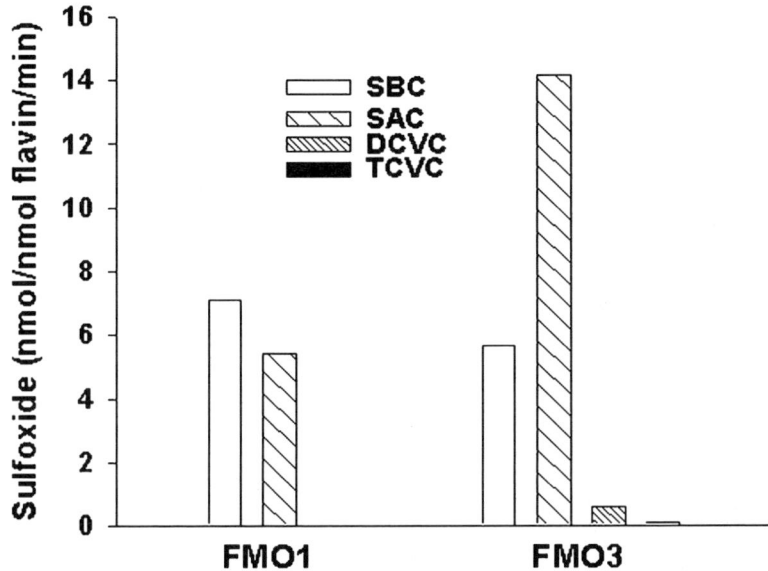

Fig. 11. Cysteine conjugate S-oxidase activities of cDNA-expressed rabbit FMO1 and FMO3. (Data were taken from ref. 26.)

the liver microsomes whereas SAC sulfoxidation can be quantitated in both the liver and kidney microsomes (27). An approx 10-fold higher amount of SACS was formed in liver microsomes compared with kidney microsomes (Fig. 10).

Because five active mammalian FMO isoforms are now recognized (different isoforms share approx 50% sequence identity whereas orthologs [same isoform from different species] share more than 80% identity) (34), we examined the substrate selectivity of rabbit and human cDNA-expressed FMOs using SBC, SAC, DCVC, and TCVC as substrates (26,42,43). The results showed that SBC was oxidized primarily by FMO1 and FMO3 (Fig. 11). SACS formation was catalyzed by FMOs 1, 2, 3, and 4, with FMO3 being the major active isoform. DCVCS and TCVCS formations were observed only in incubations containing FMO3; however, the specific activities of these reactions were much lower than those observed using SBC and SAC as substrates (Fig. 11). FMO5 did not produce any detectable sulfoxide for any of the substrates tested. Additional studies with rat, rabbit, and human liver and kidney microsomes and purified rat liver FMO3, and studies using an antirabbit FMO3 monoclonal antibody showed that FMO3 is a major enzyme involved in the oxidation of methionine, and that the methionine S-oxidase activity is a good biomarker of FMO3 expression levels in these tissues (44,45).

Table 1
Sex- and Race-Related Expression of Flavin Monooxygenases in Human Kidney Samples

Group	N	Age (yr)	FMO1	FMO3 (pmol/mg protein)	FMO5
All	26	61 ± 17	5.8 ± 2.3	0.5 ± 0.4	2.4 ± 1.4
Males	14	58 ± 21	5.5 ± 2.4	0.4 ± 0.3	2.0 ± 1.3
Females	12	64 ± 11	6.1 ± 2.2	0.7 ± 0.4	2.8 ± 1.5
African American	8	66 ± 15	7.7 ± 2.4*	0.7 ± 0.5	1.6 ± 1.2
Caucasian	17	58 ± 19	5.0 ± 1.7	0.5 ± 0.3	2.7 ± 1.5

The value marked with the asterisk is significantly different from the corresponding Caucasian group ($p < 0.05$). Values listed are means ±SD. Data were taken from ref. 27.

Recently, we quantitated the expression of FMO1, FMO3, and FMO5 in 26 human kidney microsomal samples using immunoblotting (Table 1; 27). Because antibodies recognizing human FMO4 are currently unavailable, we were unable to quantitate the expression of FMO4 in the human kidney. FMO1 was the major isoform in all but one of the samples examined. The expression levels of FMO1 ranged from 3.2 to 11.5 pmol/mg of protein with a mean value of 5.8 ± 2.3 pmol/mg of protein. In contrast, not all samples had quantifiable levels of FMO3 and FMO5. The expression levels of FMO3 ranged from trace amounts up to 1.3 pmol/mg of protein with a mean value of 0.5 ± 0.4 pmol/mg of protein, whereas FMO5 expression ranged from trace amounts up to 5.8 pmol/mg of protein with a mean value of 2.4 ± 1.4 pmol/mg of protein. Comparison of expression levels between samples from males and females did not reveal any sex-related differences. In contrast, samples from African-Americans had significantly higher levels of FMO1 compared with samples from Caucasians (Table 1). These race-related differences in expression were not observed for FMO3 and FMO5.

The studies just described provide significant insights into the potential roles of renal FMOs in the metabolism and toxicity of cysteine S-conjugates. However, more studies are needed to characterize the regional distributions of these FMOs within the kidneys to determine more fully the extent to which these enzymes play a role in the nephrotoxicity of DCVC and TCVC. Although FMO3 expression in the human kidneys is much smaller than the levels present in the liver, renal FMO3-mediated oxidations of DCVC and TCVC may still play significant roles in the nephrotoxicity of TRI and TETRA because of possible variations in FMO3 expression among different renal cells and because of the potency of the sulfoxides as renal toxins. It is recognized, however, that

DCVC sulfoxidation may be occurring primarily in the liver with subsequent translocation of DCVCS via the circulation to the kidneys. Consistent with this hypothesis, rats given DCVCS developed severe nephrotoxicity *(29)*. On the other hand, other cysteine S-conjugates that are good substrates for multiple FMOs may be metabolized in the human kidney much more than DCVC.

ACKNOWLEDGMENTS

Research conducted in the author's laboratory was made possible primarily by Grants ES06841 and DK44295 from the National Institute of Environmental Health Sciences and the National Institute of Diabetes and Digestive and Kidney Diseases, respectively.

REFERENCES

1. Lohr JW, Willsky GR, Acara MA. Renal drug metabolism. Pharmacol Rev 1998; 50:107–141.
2. Mugford CA, Kedderis GL. Sex-dependent metabolism of xenobiotics. Drug Metab Rev 1998;30:441–498.
3. Lock EA, Reed CJ. Renal xenobiotic metabolism. In: Goldstein RS, ed., Sipes IG, McQueen CA, Gandolfi AJ, eds.-in-chief. Comprehensive Toxicology, Vol. 7: Renal Toxicology. New York: Elsevier, 1997:77–97.
4. Elfarra AA. Halogenated hydrocarbons. In: Goldstein RS, ed., Sipes IG, McQueen CA, Gandolfi AJ, eds.-in-chief. Comprehensive Toxicology, Vol. 7: Renal Toxicology. New York: Elsevier, 1997:601–616.
5. US Environmental Protection Agency. Health Assessment of 1,3-butadiene. Washington, DC, 2000.
6. National Toxicology Program. The Ninth Report on Carcinogens, National Toxicology Program, US Department of Health and Human Services, Public Health Services, Research Triangle Park, NC, 2000.
7. Melnick RL, Huff J, Chou BJ, Miller RA. Carcinogenicity of 1,3-butadiene in C57BL/6 × C3HF1 mice at low exposure concentrations. Cancer Res 1990;50: 6592–6599.
8. Elfarra AA, Moll TS, Krause RJ, Kemper RA, Selzer RR. Reactive metabolites of 1,3-butadiene: DNA and hemoglobin adduct formation and potential roles in carcinogenicity. In: Dansette PM, Snyder RR, Monles TJ, et al., eds. Biological Reactive Intermediates, VI. New York: Kluwer Academic/Plenum, 2001:93–103.
9. Kemper RA, Krause RJ, Elfarra AA. Metabolism of butadiene monoxide by freshly isolated hepatocytes from mice and rats: different partitioning between oxidative, hydrolytic, and conjugation pathways. Drug Metab Dispos 2001;29:830–836.
10. Krause RJ, Elfarra AA. Oxidation of butadiene monoxide to meso- and (±)-diepoxybutane by cDNA-expressed human cytochrome P450s and by mouse, rat, and human liver microsomes: evidence for preferential hydration of meso-diepoxybutane in rat and human liver microsomes. Arch Biochem Biophys 1997; 337:176–184.

11. Thorton-Manning JR, Dahl AR, Bechtold WE, Griffith WC, Henderson RF. Comparison of the disposition of butadiene epoxides in Sprague-Dawley rats and B6C3F1 mice following a single and repeated exposures to 1,3-butadiene via inhalation. Toxicology 1997;123:125–134.
12. Duescher RJ, Elfarra AA. Human liver microsomes are efficient catalysts of 1,3-butadiene oxidation: evidence for major roles by cytochromes P450 2A6 and 2E1. Arch Biochem Biophys 1994;311:342–349.
13. Sharer JE, Duescher RJ, Elfarra AA. Species and tissue differences in the microsomal oxidation of 1,3-butadiene and the glutathione conjugation of butadiene monoxide in mice and rats: possible role in 1,3-butadiene toxicity. Drug Metab Dispos 1992;20:658–664.
14. Krause RJ, Sharer JE, Elfarra AA. Epoxide hydrolase-dependent metabolism of butadiene monoxide to yield 3-butene-1,2-diol in mouse, rat, and human liver. Drug Metab Dispos 1997;25:1013–1015.
15. Krause RJ, Philpot RM, Elfarra AA. Role of cytochrome P450 4B1 in 1,3-butadiene oxidation in lung microsomes of humans, rats, and rabbits. Toxicol Sci (Suppl) 1999;48:411.
16. National Toxicology Program. The Tenth Report on Carcinogens, U.S. Department of Health and Human Services, Public Health Service, National Toxicology Program, Research Triangle Park, NC, 2002.
17. Lash LH, Parker JC. Hepatic and renal toxicities associated with perchloroethylene. Pharmacol Rev 2001;53:177–208.
18. Lash LH, Qian W, Putt DA, et al. Renal toxicity of perchloroethylene and S-(1,2,2-trichlorovinyl)glutathione in rats and mice: sex- and species-dependent differences. Toxicol Appl Pharmacol 2002;179:163–171.
19. Lash LH, Qian W, Putt DA, et al. Renal and hepatic toxicity of trichloroethylene and its glutathione-derived metabolites in rats and mice: sex-, species-, and tissue-dependent differences. J Pharmacol Exp Ther 2001;297:155–164.
20. Lash, LH, Xu Y, Elfarra AA, Duescher RJ, Parker JC. Glutathione-dependent metabolism of trichloroethylene in isolated liver and kidney cells of rats and its role in mitochondrial and cellular toxicity. Drug Metab Dispos 1995;23:846–853.
21. Elfarra AA, Krause RJ, Last AR, Lash, LH, Parker JC. Species- and sex-related differences in metabolism of trichloroethylene to yield chloral and tetrachloroethanol in mouse, rat, and human liver microsomes. Drug Metab Dispos 1998;26:779–785.
22. Cummings BS, Lasker JM, Lash LH. Expression of glutathione-dependent and cytochrome P450s in freshly isolated and primary cultures of proximal tubular cells from human kidneys. J Pharmacol Exp Ther 2000;293:677–685.
23. Lash LH, Fisher JW, Lipscomb JC, Parker JC. Metabolism of trichloroethylene. Environ Hlth Perspect 2000;108:177–200.
24. Lash LH, Qian W, Putt DA, et al. Glutathione conjugation of trichloroethylene in rats and mice: sex-, species-, and tissue-dependent differences. Drug Metab Dispos 1998;26:12–19.

25. Lash LH, Qian W, Putt DA, et al. Glutathione conjugation of perchloroethylene in rats and mice in vitro: sex-, species-, and tissue-dependent differences. Toxicol Appl Pharmacol 1998;150:49–57.
26. Ripp SL, Overby LH, Philpot RM, Elfarra AA. Oxidation of cysteine S-conjugates by rabbit liver microsomes and cDNA-expressed flavin-containing monooxygenases: studies with S-(1,2-dichlorovinyl)-L-cysteine, S-(1,2,2-trichlorovinyl)-L-cysteine, S-allyl-L-cysteine, and S-benzyl-L-cysteine. Mol Pharmacol 1997;51:507–515.
27. Krause RJ, Lash LH, Elfarra AA. Human kidney flavin-containing monooxygenases and their potential roles in cysteine S-conjugate metabolism and nephrotoxicity. J Pharmacol Exp Ther 2003;304:185–191.
28. Sausen PJ, Elfarra AA. Reactivity of cysteine S-conjugate sulfoxides: formation of S-[1-chloro-2-(S-glutathionyl)vinyl]-L-cysteine sulfoxide by the reaction of S-(1,2-dichlorovinyl)-L-cysteine sulfoxide with glutathione. Chem Res Toxicol 1991;4: 655–660.
29. Lash LH, Sausen PJ, Duescher RJ, Cooley AJ, Elfarra AA. Roles of cysteine conjugate β-lyase and S-oxidase in nephrotoxicity: studies with S-(1,2-dichlorovinyl)-L-cysteine and S-(1,2-dichlorovinyl)-L-cysteine sulfoxide. J Pharmacol Exp Ther 1994;269:374–383.
30. Lash LH, Putt DA, Hueni, SE, Krause RJ, Elfarra AA. Roles of necrosis, apoptosis, and mitochondrial dysfunction in S-(1,2-dichlorovinyl)-L-cysteine sulfoxide-induced cytotoxicity in primary cultures of human renal proximal tubular cells. J Pharmacol Exp Ther 2003;305:1163–1172.
31. Elfarra AA, Laboy JI, Cooley AJ. S-(1,2,2-trichlorovinyl)-L-cysteine sulfoxide is a potent nephrotoxin. Toxicol Sci (Suppl) 1999;48:28.
32. Werner M, Birner G, Dekant W. Sulfoxidation of mercapturic acids derived from tri- and tetrachloroethene by cytochrome P450 3A: a bioactivation reaction in addition to deacetylation and cysteine conjugate β-lyase mediated cleavage. Chem Res Toxicol 1996;9:41–49.
33. Krause RJ, Glocke SC, Elfarra AA. Sulfoxides as urinary metabolites of S-allyl-L-cysteine in rats: evidence for the involvement of flavin-containing monooxygenases. Drug Metab Dispos 2002;30:1137–1142.
34. Lawton MP, Cashman JR, Cresteil T, et al. A nomenclature for the mammalian flavin-containing monooxygenase gene family based on amino acid sequence identities. Arch Biochem Biophys 1994;308:254–257.
35. Overby LH, Carver GC, Philpot RM. Quantitation and kinetic properties of hepatic microsomal and recombinant flavin-containing monooxygenase 3 and 5 from humans. Chem Biol Interact 1997;106:29–45.
36. Cashman JR, Yang Z, Yang L, Wrighton SA. Role of hepatic flavin-containing monooxygenase 3 in drug and chemical metabolism in adult humans. Chem Biol Interact 1995;96:33–46.
37. Sausen PJ, Elfarra AA. Cysteine conjugate S-oxidase: characterization of a novel enzymatic activity in rat hepatic and renal microsomes. J Biol Chem 1990;265: 6139–6145.

38. Sausen PJ, Duescher RJ, Elfarra AA. Further characterization and purification of the flavin-dependent S-benzyl-L-cysteine S-oxidase activities of rat liver and kidney microsomes. Mol Pharmacol 1993;43:388–396.
39. Phillips IR, Dolphin CT, Clair P, et al. The molecular biology of the flavin-containing monooxygenases of man. Chem Biol Interact 1995;96:17–32.
40. Itagaki K, Carver GT, Philpot RM. Expression and characterization of a modified flavin-containing monooxygenase 4 from humans. J Biol Chem 1996;271: 20102–20107.
41. Lattard V, Longin-Sauvageon C, Benoit E. Cloning, sequencing and tissue distribution of rat flavin-containing monooxygenase 4: two different forms are produced by tissue-specific alternative splicing. Mol Pharmacol 2003;63:253–261.
42. Duescher RJ, Lawton MP, Philpot RM, Elfarra AA. Flavin-containing monooxygenase (FMO)-dependent metabolism of methionine and evidence for FMO3 being the major FMO involved in methionine sulfoxidation in rabbit liver and kidney microsomes. J Biol Chem 1994;269:17525–17530.
43. Ripp SL, Itagaki K, Philpot RM, Elfarra AA. Methionine S-oxidation in human and rabbit liver microsomes: evidence for a high-affinity methionine S-oxidase activity that is distinct from flavin-containing monooxygenase 3. Arch Biochem Biophys 1999;367:322–332.
44. Krause RJ, Ripp SL, Sausen PJ, Overby LH, Philpot RM, Elfarra AA. Characterization of the methionine S-oxidase activity of rat liver and kidney microsomes: immunochemical and kinetic evidence for FMO3 being the major catalyst. Arch Biochem Biophys 1996;333:109–116.
45. Ripp, SL, Itagaki K, Philpot RM, Elfarra AA. Species and sex differences in expression of flavin-containing monooxygenase form 3 in liver and kidney microsomes. Drug Metab Dispos 1999;27:46–52.

2

Experimental Approaches for the Study of Cytochrome P450 Gene Regulation

Hollie I. Swanson, Susan D. Kraner, Soma S. Ray, Martin Hoagland, Earl D. Thompson, Xinyu Zheng, and Yanan Tian

Summary

This chapter uses cytochrome P450 1A1 (CYP1A1) as a model "xenobiotic inducible" gene and the aryl hydrocarbon receptor (AHR) as a regulator of this gene product to illustrate how studies may be performed to understand the relationships between the regulator protein and its target genes. The methodology described was developed to study transcriptional activation. Because transcriptional repression occurs nearly as frequently as activation, the assays described may require modifications to accommodate both mechanisms. Approaches typically used to determine whether changes in gene expression induced by a particular drug or xenobiotic are a result of an increase in gene transcription mediated by specific protein/DNA interactions are described. These approaches and assays include the use of inhibitors of transcription and translation, nuclear runoffs, promoter analysis, and reporter assays to determine the role of specific DNA sequences, determination of specific DNA–protein interactions both in vitro and in vivo using electrophoretic gel mobility shift assays, UV-crosslinking, Southwestern blotting, yeast one-hybrid screening, DNA footprinting, site affinity amplification binding, and the chromatin immunoprecipitation (ChIP) assay, and studies to determine functional roles for specific transcription factors.

Key Words

Aryl hydrocarbon receptor; aryl hydrocarbon receptor nuclear translocator; chromatin immunoprecipitation assay; CYP1A1; cytochrome P450; dioxin responsive element; DNA footprinting; DNA microarrays; electromobility shift assays; gene regulation; luciferase activity; nuclear runoff; promoter analysis; protein–DNA interactions; reporter analysis; reverse transcription-polymerase chain reaction; site-affinity amplification binding; small inhibitory RNA; Southwestern blot, 2,3,7,8-tetrachlorodibenzo-p-dioxin; transfection; transient; transfection, stable; transfection, viral; UV-crosslinking; yeast one-hybrid screening.

From: *Methods in Pharmacology and Toxicology,*
Drug Metabolism and Transport: Molecular Methods and Mechanisms
Edited by: L. Lash © Humana Press Inc., Totowa, NJ

1. INTRODUCTION

The regulation of cytochrome P450s (CYPs), like most gene products, is complex, involving pre- and posttranscriptional events, receptors, and other nuclear transcription factors and signaling mechanisms that are initiated both within the cellular environment and within the cellular milieu. Given the historical focus of CYP1A1 as a model "xenobiotic inducible" gene and the role of the aryl hydrocarbon receptor (AHR) in regulating this gene product, we will use these two players as an example of how studies may be performed to understand the relationships between the regulator protein and its target genes. It should also be noted that the methodology described in this subheading was developed to study transcriptional activation. With the use of DNA microarrays, it has become clear that transcriptional repression occurs nearly as frequently as that of activation. Thus, in some cases the assays described may require modifications to accommodate both mechanisms. For example, a higher sensitivity in the detection levels in assays such as nuclear runoffs may be required for conditions in which an agent inhibits synthesis of newly transcribed mRNA as compared to those conditions in which an agent increases mRNA levels. Here, we describe approaches typically used to determine whether changes in gene expression induced by a particular drug or xenobiotic are a result of an increase in gene transcription mediated by specific protein–DNA interactions.

2. DISCRIMINATION BETWEEN TRANSCRIPTIONAL VS POSTTRANSCRIPTIONAL GENE REGULATION

2.1. Use of Transcription and Translation Inhibitors

After first observing that exposure to a particular pharmacological or xenobiotic agent results in corresponding alterations (i.e., either increases or decreases) in the protein and mRNA levels of a gene of interest, the first question to be addressed is whether this event occurs at the pre- or posttranscriptional level. When using DNA microarrays, this question may be approached either via limiting the exposure to 4 h prior to harvesting the mRNA or cotreatment with cycloheximide *(1)*. However, it should be noted that there are concerns that use of cycloheximide may lead to complications owing to the unknown nature of its nonspecific effects.

The initial experiments require pharmacological approaches that inhibit transcription, elongation, or translation and are performed in a time-dependent manner. Reagents typically used to inhibit transcription include α-Amanitin, actinomycin D, and 5,6-dichloro-1-β-D-ribofuranosyl benzimidazole. α-Amanitin is a specific inhibitor of polymerase II that blocks both transcriptional initiation and elongation *(2)* and is typically used at concentrations

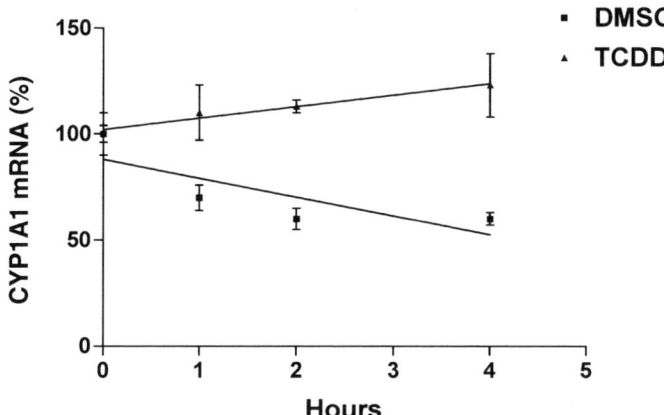

Fig. 1. Use of actinomycin D to determine the role of mRNA stability in TCDD-induced increases in CYP1A1 mRNA levels. Normal human keratinocytes were treated with either 1 nM TCDD or 0.01% DMSO (control) for 4 h, followed by treatment with actinomycin D (5 µg/mL). Samples were taken at 0, 0.5, 1, 2, and 4 h following actinomycin D treatment. Comparisons are made to mRNA levels at time 0 for each respective treatment.

of 1–5 µg/mL. Although the precise mode of action of actinomycin D is unknown, it is thought to stall the RNA polymerase via DNA intercalation *(3)* and is used at concentrations of 0.1–10 µg/mL. 5,6-Dichloro-1-β-D-ribofuranosyl benzimidazole, on the other hand, inhibits elongation *(4)* and is used at concentrations of 50–100 µM. A time-dependent experiment using these agents typically involves a 30- to 60-min pretreatment with the transcriptional/elongation inhibitor followed by a 1- to 24-h incubation with the pharmacological or xenobiotic agent of interest. A significant change in the half-life of the mRNA that is revealed by plotting the mRNA levels as a percent of the control at time 0 indicates that the effect involves mRNA stability *(5)*. Occasionally, it has been found that the mechanism involves both transcriptional and posttranscriptional events *(6,7)*.

An example of this type of analysis is shown in Fig. 1. Here, cells were treated with either dimethyl sulfoxide (DMSO) or 2,3,7,8-tetrachlorodibenozo-*p*-dioxin (TCDD), in the presence of actinomycin D. The mRNA levels of either the DMSO or TCDD-treated cells are expressed as a percentage of the time 0 point. The mRNA half-life is represented by the slope of each linear regression line. Given that TCDD significantly alters the slope of this line, we have concluded that the effects of TCDD on CYP1A1 in this cell type involves an increase in mRNA stability. These data, in addition to those performed using reporter assays (not shown), have led us to conclude that in human keratinocytes, TCDD increases expression of CYP1A1 both by increasing its promoter activity and increasing its mRNA stability.

If mRNA stability is found to be altered, the approaches to be taken involve identification of *cis*-acting sequences typically found within the 5'- and 3'-untranslated region (UTR) and the *trans*-acting factors that interact with these sequences *(7)*.

2.2. Nuclear Runoffs

A final test of whether the observed event involves newly synthesized mRNA is performed using nuclear runoffs *(8)*. In this assay, isolated nuclei obtained from cells treated with the agent of interest (typically for 3–4 h) are incubated with ^{32}P-nucleotides to allow for the in vitro synthesis of nascent, radiolabeled RNA that is detected following hybridization with immobilized CYP cDNA. For a more sensitive approach, the incubation may be performed using unlabeled nucleotides and the newly synthesized mRNA is detected using an RNase protection protocol that requires hybridization with the ^{32}P-labeled antisense transcript *(9)*. Achieving maximum sensitivity requires the use of the reverse transcription polymerase chain reaction (RT-PCR), in which the newly synthesized hnRNA is detected following amplification using primers that recognize sequences within an exon and an intron, preferably those near the 5'-end *(8,10)*. Besides the enhanced sensitivity of this approach, an additional advantage is that only mRNA is subjected to the analysis and thus isolation of nuclear extracts is not required. This poses an advantage given that in some cell types (e.g., keratinocytes) or in vivo analyses, isolation of high-quality nuclear extracts may be a limiting factor. As with most approaches that rely on RT-PCR, care must be taken to ensure that genomic DNA is not amplified. This can be accomplished by adding DNase to the RNA-containing samples prior to the reverse transcription reaction and subjecting a sample of the RNA (that has not been converted to cDNA) to the amplification step. An additional consideration is that in some cases, the stability of the hnRNA, but not the mature form, may be altered by the treatment of interest *(8)*.

Even if the nuclear runoff assay implicates a direct transcriptional regulatory mechanism, it is important to discriminate whether the event is primary (i.e., acts directly on the gene of interest) or secondary (requires the synthesis of an effector molecule that then acts on the gene of interest). Toward this end, experiments similar to those described in the preceding are performed, that is, time-dependent experiments in the absence or presence of the protein synthesis inhibitor, cycloheximide (1–10 µg/mL) *(5,11)*.

3. DETERMINING THE ROLE OF SPECIFIC DNA SEQUENCES USING PROMOTER ANALYSIS AND REPORTER ASSAYS

Once it has been determined that the pharmacological or xenobiotic agent exerts its effect on transcription, the next step is to perform promoter analysis using reporter assays. While the majority of regulatory sites have been identified within the first 5 kb of the promoter region, sites far upstream of the proximal promoter (i.e., 18–20 kb) have also been shown to exert important regulatory effects. *In silico* approaches using either software or Web-based shareware (i.e., MatInspector or TFSearch) may be used to identify putative DNA recognition sites for further analysis. The reporter gene most commonly used for these assays is luciferase, owing to the ease in adapting this system for rapid analysis and high-throughput screening. Current instrumentation also allows for simultaneous analyses of the enzyme activity generated from the *Renilla* reporter plasmid (available from Promega, Madison, WI). Cotransfection of the *Renilla* reporter plasmid and subsequent normalization of the luciferase/*Renilla* values will adjust for variations in plate-to-plate transfection efficiencies and nonspecific effects of the exogenous agents on gene transcription. These reporter plasmids are transfected into cultured cells using either the traditional calcium phosphate *(12)* or lipid based (i.e., Lipofectamine, Invitrogen) transfection protocols.

After verification that the reporter assay is appropriately responsive to the pharmacological or xenobiotic agent, the specific DNA recognition site(s) is (are) then identified following processive 5′ and 3′ deletion of the promoter fragment. This is classically demonstrated in the analyses of TCDD-responsiveness of the CYP1A1 promoter region *(13)*. The reporter constructs representative of deletion fragments may be generated either by subcloning the deletion fragments into the luciferase reporter vector following restriction digestions, amplification of specific segments using PCR, or using enzymes that progressively degrade double-stranded DNA, such as *Bal*31 *(14)*. Site-directed mutagenesis of the putative site within the context of the promoter fragment further strengthens the role of the putative site. Finally, analyses performed using constructs containing only the consensus site and its flanking regions indicate that the site is necessary and sufficient for mediating the response.

An example of these types of reporter analyses is shown in Fig. 2 in our recent characterization of pifithrin-α (PFTα) as a putative agonist of the AHR. In previous experiments, we found that PFTα was capable of inducing the mRNA levels of CYP1A1. To determine whether this event occurs via promoter activation of CYP1A1, we performed reporter assays using three constructs, that containing the 5′ flanking region of the human CYP1A1 (−1612 to +292), two copies of the consensus DRE, or two copies of the mutated

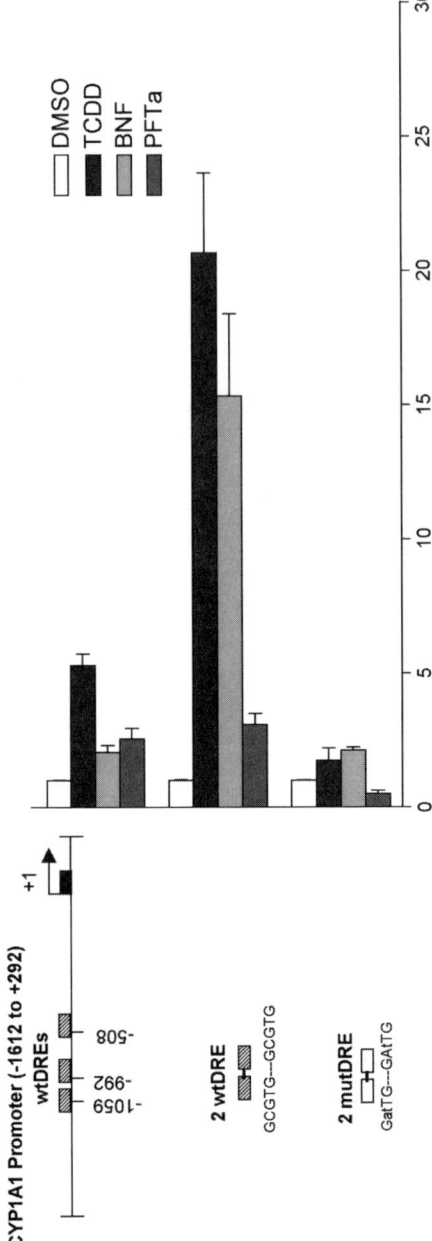

Fig. 2. Use of reporter assays to determine whether pharmacologica or /xenobiotic agents are capable of inducing CYP1A1 promoter activity via the DREs. HepG2 cells were transiently transfected with the indicated reporter constructs containing either the human CYP1A1 promoter, two copies of the wild-type DRE (GCGTG, 26), or two copies of the mutated DRE (GATTG). The human CYP1A1 reporter construct was that described previously (39) and contains three XREs at positions −1059, −992, and −508 (40). After the transfections, the cells were treated with either the vehicle control (0.1% DMSO), two previously characterized agonists of the AHR, TCDD (1 nM) and β-naphthoflavone (1 μM BNF), or the putative AHR agonist pifithrin-α (10 μM PFTα). After a 24-h incubation, the cells were harvested and luciferase and *Renilla* activities were determined. The values represent the normalized luciferase activities (luciferase/*Renilla*) and are expressed as fold change relative to the DMSO control.

dioxin-responsive element (DRE). As shown in Fig. 2, the 10-μM dose of PFTα is nearly as potent as the 1-μM dose of β-naphthoflavone in the induction of luciferase activity that is regulated by the CYP1A1 promoter. However, when the luciferase activities regulated by only two copies of the DRE were examined, the potency of PFTα was approx 20% that of BNF, indicating that sequences in addition to the DRE are required to elicit the actions of PFTα. Finally, using the mutated DRE, it can be seen that the effects of all three ligands require sequences that are recognized by the AHR–ARNT heterodimer.

4. DETERMINATION OF SPECIFIC PROTEIN–DNA INTERACTIONS IN VITRO

Once it has been determined that a discrete segment of the promoter region mediates the effect of interest, it must then be demonstrated that this sequence is capable of interacting with a specific protein. If the promoter and *in silico* analyses both support the idea that a previously identified transcription factor elicits the effect of interest, the subsequent experiments usually involve electromobility shift assays (EMSAs), using purified proteins and the appropriate antibodies that will recognize the transcription factor within the protein–DNA complex. However, if it is thought that the protein–DNA interaction may be novel, two classical methods may be employed: UV-crosslinking and Southwestern blot analysis. New advances in mass spectroscopy can also be coupled with these approaches to identify proteins definitively.

4.1. UV-Crosslinking

In this method, the thymine residues within the ^{32}P-labeled DNA probe are substituted with 5-bromo-2-deoxyuridine 5′-triphosphate by end-filling using the Klenow fragment *(15)*. UV-irradiation results in the formation of a covalent bond between the 5-bromo-2-deoxyuridine 5′-triphosphate residues and proteins that are in close contact with the DNA. However, the efficiency of the crosslinking is typically quite low, representing approx 10% of the protein–DNA complex. The UV-irradiation can be performed either on the protein–DNA mixture prior to sodium dodecyl sulfate-polyacrylamide gel electrophoresis (SDS-PAGE) or on the wet EMSA gel. In the latter case, the proteins are eluted from the EMSA gel and then subjected to SDS-PAGE. Using ^{14}C-labeled molecular mass markers, the molecular weight of the DNA-bound proteins may be estimated. It remains to be determined whether sufficient quantities of the protein can be recovered for protein identification using mass spectrophotometry analysis. UV-crosslinking has been used to determine that three discrete proteins interact in a TCDD-inducible manner with the TNGCGTG recognition site, representing the AHR, aryl hydrocarbon receptor nuclear translocator (ARNT), and an as yet unidentified protein (Fig. 3).

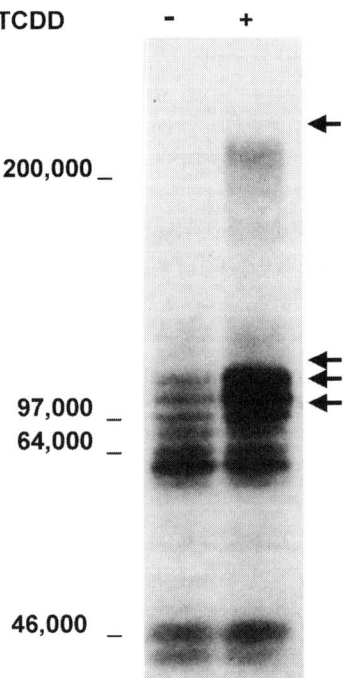

Fig. 3. Use of UV crosslinking to identify the molecular weights of proteins that interact with the DRE in response to TCDD treatment. Guinea pig hepatic cytosol (16 mg of protein/mL) was incubated with ^{32}P-labeled, BrdU-substituted (100,000 cpm, 0.5–1 ng) wild-type DRE as described previously *(15)*. The protein–DNA mixture was subjected to UV-irradiation for 30 min and subsequently analyzed by SDS-PAGE followed by autoradiography. The positions of the molecular weight markers are indicated on the left and the TCDD inducible bands are indicated by the *arrows* on the right. The upper band of approx 247,000 kDa is thought to be representative of two protein–DNA complexes *(15)*. (Reprinted with permission from ref. *15*. Copyright 1993, American Chemical Society.)

4.2. Southwestern Blot

Here, a cell-free preparation is subjected to SDS-PAGE and the proteins transferred to a nitrocellulose membrane *(16)*. Maximal results are obtained if high protein concentrations of the extracts can be used, that is, 30–150 µg of crude cell extract per lane using a 0.5–1-mm thick gel. The proteins are renatured using treatment with and withdrawal of protein denaturants such as urea. The membrane is then probed with radiolabeled DNA that contains the appropriate recognition site. Ideally, the radiolabeled probe will contain a single recognition site that is composed of the 6- to 10-base pair core and 10 base pairs of sequences that flank each side of the core. Again, this assay will only identify the molecular weight of the protein and will not be successful if protein dimerization is required for DNA recognition and binding. However, both the UV-crosslinking and Southwestern blot assays can facilitate identification of the protein of interest if the DNA containing the recognition site is then used to screen a cDNA expression library *(17)*. An alternate means of identifying the regulatory protein is to purify the protein from a matrix containing the immobilized DNA recognition site. Advances in mass spectrometry have made this a method of choice for the identification of novel proteins that interact with a known DNA sequences.

4.3. Yeast One-Hybrid Screening

Yeast one-hybrid screening is an alternative to proteomic techniques for cloning and identifying novel transcription factors given a known DNA binding sequence. This technique is an adaptation of the yeast two-hybrid screening technique *(18)*. Similar to the two-hybrid screen, the one-hybrid screen is based upon the discovery that the GAL4 transcription factor can be separated into an "activation domain" and a "DNA-binding domain." In fact, this domain structure is a property of most transcription factors and is the basis of the yeast one-hybrid screen. In this technique, the DNA-binding domain of the unknown transcription factor is directly cloned. A cDNA library is created that contains individual cDNA clones fused to the GAL4 activation domain. Among these GAL4-fusion cDNA clones is one encoding the DNA-binding domain of the unknown transcription factor. In the presence of the cognate DNA binding site, the desired fusion protein brings the GAL4 activation domain into proximity with a basal promoter, resulting in transcription of a selectable yeast marker and/or the color indicator gene, β-galactosidase. Because only the DNA-binding domain is cloned, this technique works equally well for transcriptional activators and repressors, as is schematically depicted for the repressor known as REST, shown in Fig. 4 *(19)*.

For the cloning of REST *(19)*, four copies of the multimerized DNA binding site, RE1, were inserted before the basal yeast *Gal1* promoter so that the RE1 site regulates expression of the *Gal1* promoter. This promoter was inserted before the yeast gene *HIS3* in a plasmid that contained a selectable marker for growth in media lacking uracil. The plasmid was linearized and introduced into the yeast W303 line using a standard lithium acetate method. Following selection in media lacking uracil, the resulting yeast transformant contains the desired promoter-marker gene integrated into its chromosomal DNA. A similar approach was used to introduce the same promoter driving expression of the bacterial *lacZ* gene. The resulting W303 yeast strain contained both the *HIS3* gene and the *lacZ* gene driven by the same RE1-containing promoter integrated

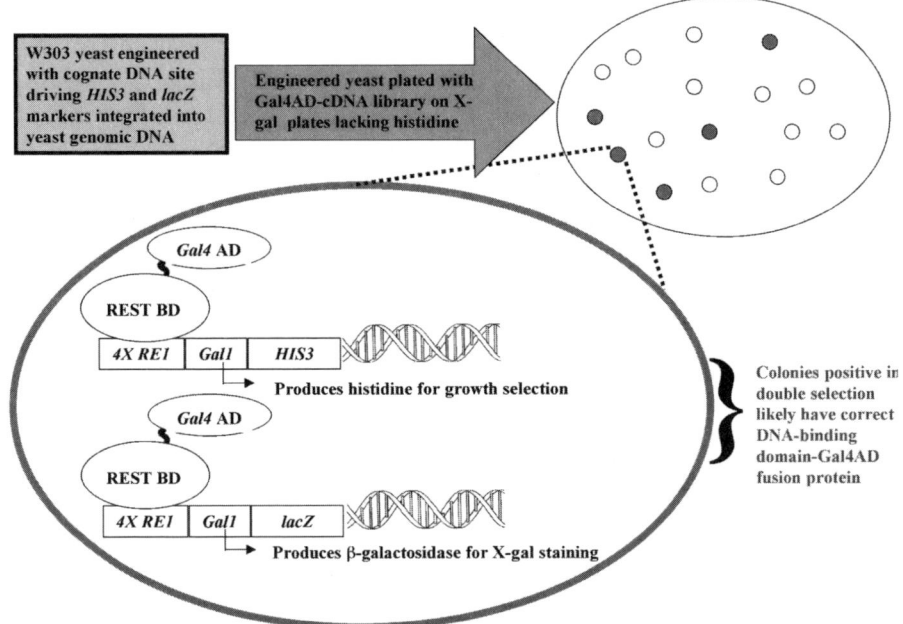

Fig. 4. A schematic depicting the yeast one-hybrid system.

into its chromosomal DNA. The *HIS3* marker allows yeast to grow in media lacking histidine, and the *lacZ* gene encodes β-galactosidase, which produces a blue color in the presence of the substrate 5-bromo-4-chloro-3-indoyl-β-D-galactosidase (X-gal).

This yeast strain was plated in the presence of a GAL4 activation domain-cDNA library from HeLa cells. In theory, the only yeast that survive plating in media lacking histidine are those that take up the "correct" GAL4-cDNA. However, yeast one-hybrid and two-hybrid screening are known for having large numbers of "false" positives. Thus, in cloning the REST transcription factor, 100 yeast clones grew in media lacking histidine, but only four were also positive in the colorimetric screen. To confirm that these colonies had the "correct" factor, they were screened against yeast containing a mutant-RE1–containing promoter. Three of the four passed this screen and were found to contain a cDNA encoding the same protein—the REST transcription factor.

The yeast one-hybrid approach is a powerful technique that allows for the direct cloning and identification of transcription factors. However, there are several disadvantages. As for Southwestern blotting, transcription factors that function as dimers or multimers cannot be identified. This approach is also labor intensive, as it requires the generation of several yeast transformants.

Finally, the resulting transcription factor candidate must be confirmed by other techniques such as supershift assays with antibodies developed to the cloned protein. Nevertheless, this approach is one of the most useful techniques in the "arsenal" of a molecular biologist studying gene regulation.

4.4. DNA Footprinting In Vitro

To identify the nucleotides involved in the protein–DNA interaction, two complementary approaches may be used, DNA footprinting and EMSAs. The advantage of the DNA footprinting analysis is that the length of DNA to be used can be relatively long (i.e., 500 base pairs) vs that used in the EMSAs (e.g., most commonly 25–50 nucleotides in length). An additional advantage is that the specific nucleotides required for the protein–DNA interaction may be directly identified.

Footprinting analysis uses a DNA fragment that is radiolabeled at one end and is allowed to equilibrate with the DNA binding proteins (typically present in a nuclear extract). The DNA fragment may be obtained following restriction digest, end-labeling, and removal of the radiolabel from one end using a second restriction digest. Alternatively, the DNA fragment may be obtained using PCR and ^{32}P-labeled primers. Two approaches are commonly used. The first is termed protection as the proteins that are bound to the DNA provide protection from either enzymatic (DNase I) or chemical cleavage. Of the footprinting techniques, DNase I is thought to be the least technically challenging. Systems for the use of DNase I are commercially available (e.g., from Promega, Madison, WI). In these assays, it is essential that the DNA probe be relatively free of contaminants. Toward this end, after the probe is labeled, it is purified using either diethylaminoethyl (DEAE) chromatography or glass powder (i.e., Geneclean®, Bio101). Alternatively, the probe may be gel purified. The amount of DNase I to be used should be diluted such that approx 50% of the labeled DNA probe is cleaved. The disadvantage of using DNase I is that the footprint observed may be much larger than that of the actual protein–DNA contacts. This is often attributable to steric hinderance of the DNase I. To circumvent this problem, hydroxyl radical footprinting may be used *(20)*. This method allows identification of the individual nucleotides that are in direct contact with the protein and does not display sequence dependency in its ability to cleave the DNA. The disadvantage to the hydroxyl radical approach is that it can be technically challenging owing to problems associated with the free radical formation.

Probably the most commonly used footprinting approach is the methylation interference assay, which is not as technically challenging as the hydroxyl radical footprinting, yet allows better resolution than that obtained using DNase I *(21)*. However, a limitation is that this assay only identifies the guanosines that are involved in the protein–DNA contacts. In this approach, the radiolabeled

DNA is first methylated using dimethyl sulfate, incubated with the DNA binding protein(s), and the protein–DNA complexes are resolved using EMSAs. After electrophoresis, the protein-bound and protein-free (that migrates at the bottom of the gel) DNA is excised and eluted. This is followed by incubation of the eluted DNA with piperidine that specifically cleaves at the methylated residues. The DNA ladder is then resolved following electrophoresis using a denaturing gel. We have obtained the best results when at least 10,000 cpm of that representing the bound DNA is analyzed. Problems frequently arise because of low purity of the eluted DNA and the low recoveries associated with most DNA purification schemes. One approach to avoiding these problems is through the use of biotin-labeled DNA, which will allow immobilization onto streptavidin beads and subsequent purification (22). A representation of the methylation interference assay used in the analysis of the interaction between the AHR/ARNT heterodimer and its GCGTG DNA recognition site is shown in Fig. 5.

4.5. EMSA

EMSAs may proceed directly from the promoter analysis, using oligonucleotides that correspond to the DNA sequences identified in mediating the observed event that contain putative consensus sites or following DNA footprinting, where the nucleotide–protein interactions have been characterized. Here, a double-stranded oligonucleotide is radiolabeled, often by end-labeling. Nuclear extracts from cells treated with the pharmacological or xenobiotic agent of interest are prepared and incubated with the radiolabeled probe. Prior to the addition of the probe, the nuclear extracts are incubated with nonspecific DNA, such as salmon sperm DNA or poly dI•dC. Optimization of this assay typically involves varying the concentrations of both the nuclear extracts and the nonspecific DNA. In addition, we have also optimized the time in which the cells are exposed to the pharmacological or xenobiotic agent. In our experiments, we have found that nuclear uptake of the AHR is maximum at 1 h when dioxin congeners are used, but that the time required for maximal nuclear uptake of the AHR may be ligand dependent (23).

Specificity of the protein–DNA interaction can be demonstrated using two approaches: (1) Antibodies to the putative proteins of interest and (2) competition of the protein/DNA complex, using unlabeled oligonucleotides as shown in Fig. 6 in the characterization of TCDD-induced DNA binding in human keratinocytes. Here, treatment of human keratinocytes with TCDD resulted in the formation of a single protein–DNA complex (lanes 1 and 2). Formation of this complex could be abolished following addition of the unlabeled wild-type, but not mutated, DRE (lanes 3 and 4). Further, incubation with antibodies that recognized either the AHR or ARNT proteins (lanes 5 and 6), but not

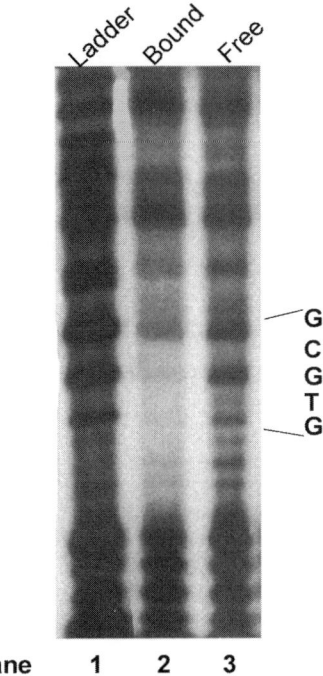

Fig. 5. Use of DNA methylation analysis to determine the nucleotide sequences involved in protein/DNA interactions. A 51-mer containing the consensus DRE *(26)* was amplified using a radiolabeled forward primer and an unlabeled reverse primer. After ethanol precipitation, the radiolabeled probe was methylated using dimethyl sulfate *(21)*. EMSAs were performed using 300,000 cpm of the radiolabeled probe as previously described except that the reactions were representative of a fivefold scale-up of the standard reactions *(26)*. The areas of the gel that contained either the AHR–ARNT complexes (Bound, *lane 2*) or the free probe (Free, *lane 3*) were excised and the DNA was eluted. Approximately 10,000 cpm of the eluted DNA was cleaved using piperidine, applied to a 12% sequencing gel, and the radiolabeled bands visualized following autoradiography. The ladder *(lane 1)* represents the methylated probe that was cleaved in the absence of protein binding.

the nonspecific IgG (lanes 7), indicated that both the AHR and ARNT proteins are contained within this complex.

Incubation of antibodies that recognize the DNA-bound proteins may either inhibit the ability of the protein to bind DNA or supershift the DNA-bound complex, depending on the site of antibody recognition. A supershift is defined as the formation of a complex that is higher than that of the original protein–DNA binding complex. Commercially available antibodies may be used to verify that the protein of interest is present within the observed protein–DNA

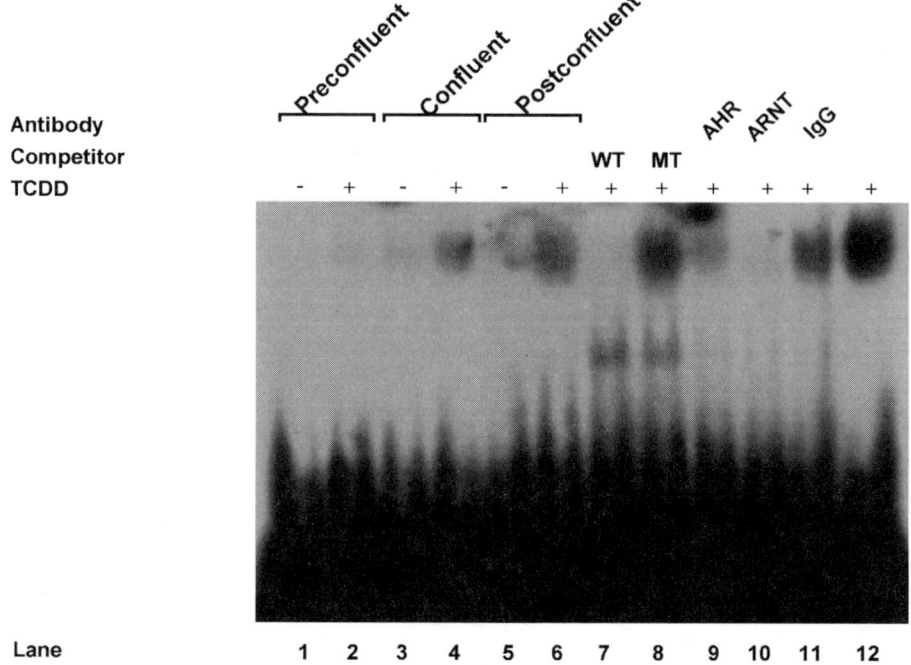

Fig. 6. Use of EMSA to identify specific protein–DNA interactions: Formation of the AHR/ARNT DNA binding complex is increased in differentiated keratinocytes. HaCaT cells that were proliferating (preconfluent, *lanes 1* and *2*), confluent (*lanes 3* and *4*), or differentiating (*lanes 5–11*) were treated with either DMSO (*lanes 1, 3, 5*) or 1 n*M* TCDD (*lanes 2, 4, 6–11*) 1 h prior to harvesting. Nuclear extracts were prepared and subjected to EMSA using 6 µg of the protein extract and a ^{32}P-labeled DRE as a probe as previously described *(41)*. The EMSAs were performed in the presence of a 50-fold molar excess of the wild-type DRE (GCGTG, *lane 7*), mutated DRE (GATTG, *lane 8*), or the following antibodies: AHR (*lane 9*), ARNT (*lane 10*), and nonspecific IgG (*lane 11*). *Lane 12* represents analysis of nuclear extracts isolated from HepG2 cells that were similarly treated with TCDD.

complex. Additional characterization of the protein–DNA complex may include the use of a battery of competitor oligonucleotides that contain varying nucleotide mutations, to define which nucleotides are essential for the protein–DNA interaction *(24)*. In these assays, competitive analyses are performed in which increasing concentrations of the unlabeled oligonucleotide is added and the amount of protein that remains bound to the DNA is quantitated.

An additional point to be considered is whether the parent compound or metabolite of the parent compound activates or interacts with the specific transcription factor. This question may be addressed using either purified transcription factors or those generated from an in vitro transcription/translation system (i.e., TNT reticulocyte lysates, Promega) *(25)* instead of the nuclear extracts.

4.6. Site Affinity Amplification Binding

Thus far, we have discussed approaches to be taken when the DNA sequences are known, but the proteins of interests that elicit the effect have not yet been determined. In the reverse scenario, where a putative DNA binding protein has been identified, but its DNA recognition site is unknown, the site affinity amplification binding assay (SAAB) may be used. Here, the protein of interest is incubated with a pool of oligonucleotides in which the central nucleotides represent all possible sequence combinations *(26,27)*. These oligonucleotides also contain enzyme restriction sites that allow subcloning of the selected oligonucleotides into the appropriate vector for either sequencing or analysis of reporter activity. In addition, they contain sequences that will allow for amplification using PCR. In this approach, the protein of interest is incubated with the DNA pool, the protein–DNA complexes separated from the free DNA following non-denaturing gel electrophoresis, and the bound DNA is isolated and amplified using PCR. This entire procedure is repeated approximately three to four times to obtain DNA sites that interact with the protein(s) with high specificity and affinity. The DNA recognition sites are then identified following subcloning and sequencing of the inserted DNA. Analysis of 20–25 distinct sequences by the chi square test will determine which nucleotides are essential for the protein–DNA interaction, and comprise the core consensus sequence.

5. DETERMINATION OF PROTEIN–DNA INTERACTIONS IN VIVO

While EMSAs indicate that a given protein has the capability of interacting with a given segment of DNA in vitro, additional analyses must be performed to determine whether these interactions occur within the context of the cell. Current approaches that may be used for the in vivo analysis of protein–DNA interactions have recently been described in an entire volume of Methods *(28)*. Two of the most commonly used approaches are the chromatin immunoprecipitation (ChIP) assays and in vivo footprinting.

5.1. Chromatin Immunoprecipitation

Currently, the method of choice in analyzing in vivo protein–DNA interactions is the chromatin immunoprecipitation assay (ChIP) *(29,30)*. This has proven to be a powerful approach owing to its high sensitivity and versatility. For example, it can be used to determine not only whether a specific protein interacts with a given DNA recognition site, but also whether this protein–DNA interaction involves the association of other proteins, whether chromatin modifications such as histone acetylation are involved, or whether protein–DNA interactions can promote phosphorylation of the C-terminus of RNA polymerase II, the initial step in transcriptional elongation *(28)*. An additional advantage to this method is that it can be used to analyze protein interactions with target genes that occur in cultured cell models as well as in vivo. For example, to determine whether family members of a given transcription factor may participate in compensatory activities in the absence of one particular member (i.e., null mouse models), the ChIP assay may be performed using tissues obtained from the null mouse model and antibodies that are specific to each family member *(29)*.

In this method, the cells or tissue *(29,30)* are isolated and the protein in close proximity to DNA are crosslinked using formaldehyde. Small fragments (i.e., 500 base pairs or fewer) of DNA are then generated following sonication. The DNA preparation is subjected to immunoprecipitation using a highly specific antibody that recognizes the protein of interest with high affinity. Obtaining the appropriate antibody for this step is often a critical component of the entire assay. The protein–DNA crosslinks are then reversed and the DNA purified and amplified using sequence-specific primers. Controls to be used include performing the assay using a nonspecific antibody, performing the amplification in the absence of antibody, or performing the immunoprecipitation using buffer instead of the DNA.

An example of the ChiP assay in analysis of CYP1A1 gene regulation is shown in Fig. 7. Using the ChiP assay and primers specific for the AHR/ARNT DNA recognition site on the CYP1A1 promoter (nucleotides –1098 to –779), recruitment of the AHR and ARNT can be observed after 30 min of TCDD treatment (Fig. 7, left side). Further analyses using primers specific for the TATA box demonstrate that recruitment of a number of factors including cyclin T1 and RNA polymerase II occurs after occupancy of the AHR/ARNT site (i.e., 1 h following TCDD treatment, Fig. 7, right side).

5.2. In Vivo DNA Footprinting

In vivo DNA footprinting was first reported in the analysis of the interaction of muscle-specific transcription factors with the muscle creatine kinase gene *(31)*. Here, the DNA is modified, most frequently using dimethyl sulfate owing to its cell permeable nature. DNA sequences that are occupied with transcription factors are protected from the methylation reaction. After purification, the DNA is cleaved using piperidine and denatured to separate the strands. To prepare the fragments for amplification, a genomic primer is annealed to one end and double-stranded DNA is generated following an extension reaction. The blunt ends on

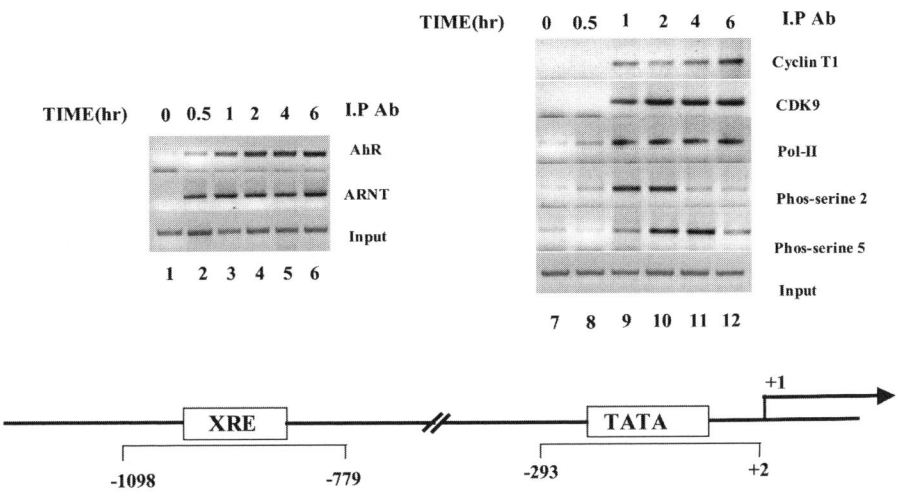

Fig. 7. Use of chromatin immunoprecipitation assays (ChIP) to characterize protein–DNA interactions that occur in cultured cells: activation of AHR by TCDD leads to sequential recruitment of AHR complex, RNA polymerase II, and positive transcription elongation factor (p-TEF) to the cyp1a1 promoter with differential phosphorylation of the C-terminal domain of RNA polymerase II. ChIP assays were performed to determine the time-dependent promoter occupancy following TCDD treatment of Hepa1c1c7 cells as previously described (42). Antibodies (Ab) used for the ChIP are indicated on the side of the panels. The associations of AHR complex with the cyp1a1 regulatory region was detected using antibodies against AHR and ARNT (lanes 1–6). The sequential recruitment of RNA polymerase II, p-TEF, and differential phosphorylations of the C-terminal domain of RNA polymerase II, phosphoserine 2, 5 of the C-terminal domain, cyclin T1, and CDK9 (lanes 7–12). The upstream regulatory and promoter regions are illustrated schematically in the **bottom panel**.

the other end of the DNA strand that were generated from the cleavage reaction then serve as the acceptor of a blunt-ended linker substrate in the subsequent ligation reaction. The DNA fragments are now bounded by the sequences contained within the first genomic primer and the linker substrate that contains a recognition site for a second primer in the PCR reaction. The PCR is performed using this second primer and a third primer that recognizes sequences that are internal to the first primer to ensure specificity of the PCR reaction. A modification of this approach is separation and identification of each allele prior to the ligation and PCR steps (32). Work with a repressor that inhibits the ability of TCDD to induce CYP1A1 gene transcription has illustrated an important point, that in some scenarios, in vitro assays may not appropriately mimic events that occur in vivo (33). In this study, it was discovered that in the mutant c31 cells, in which TCDD fails to induce CYP1A1 expression, an AHR-dependent interaction with its recognition site does not occur, as revealed by in vivo DNA footprinting. However, in vitro EMSAs contradicted these results, as the AHR obtained from nuclear extracts prepared from these cells was still capable of forming a DNA complex. To reconcile these differences, the authors suggested that a repressor protein interacts with the AHR recognition site in vivo, that this interaction is disrupted during the extraction procedure of the nuclear proteins, and hence, removal of the repressor protein allows for the in vitro formation of the AHR–DNA complex.

6. DETERMINATION OF A FUNCTIONAL ROLE FOR A SPECIFIC TRANSCRIPTION FACTOR

In the final verification that a specific transcription factor is required for regulating the gene of interest, experiments in which the transcription factor is overexpressed and/or in which expression of the transcription factor is inhibited are typically performed. The most commonly used approaches are described in the following subheadings.

6.1. Approaches To Be Used to Overexpress Proteins

6.1.1. Transient Transfections

The least time-consuming approach to overexpress a specific protein in cultured cells is that using transient transfections. During the last several years, significant improvements have been made in this area that have expanded the types of cultured cells that can effectively be transfected, increased the efficiencies of the transfections, and decreased the number of manipulations required. In many cases, the method of choice involves a lipid-mediated approach, such as LipofectAMINE (Invitrogen). To demonstrate that a particular transcription factor is required to mediate the pharmacogical or xenobiotic-induced event, the specific transcription factor can be transiently transfected into cells that do not normally express this transcription factor. For the steroid receptors and the AHR, the cells of choice have been CV-1 or COS cells that are derived from green monkey kidney. For example, we have used this approach to determine which amino acids contained within the basic region of ARNT that are bordered by amino acids 79 and 87 are essential for mediating its activities as a transcriptional activator (Fig. 8). As shown here, the glutamic acid residue is a critical amino acid, as its substitution to aspartic acid obliterates the ability of ARNT to activate gene transcription. A major problem with this approach is that the cellular milieu of the CV-1 or COS cells likely differs from that of the cell type of interest and the absence of unknown factors (i.e., coactivators or corepressors) may severely impact the ability of the particular transcription factor to partici-

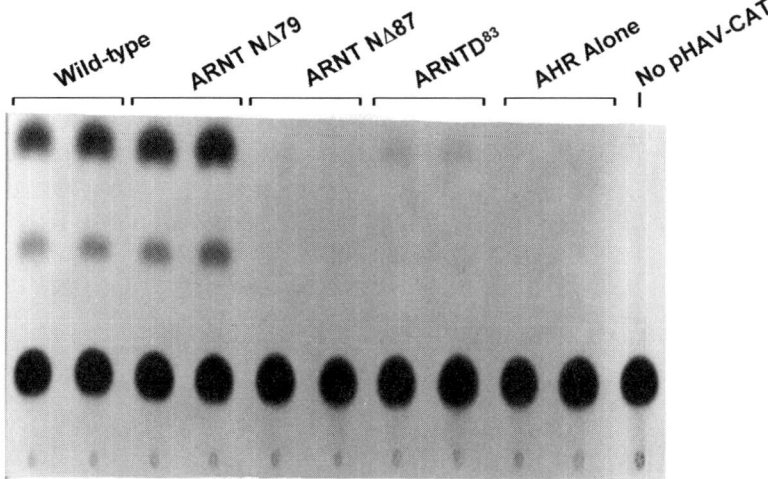

Fig. 8. Use of overexpression and chloramphenicol acetyl transferase (CAT) reporter assays to determine whether a specific transcription factor is essential for promoter activity. LA-II cells, a subclone of Hepa1c1c7 cells that lack functional expression of ARNT, were transiently transfected with plasmids encoding the indicated ARNT constructs (41) and the pHAV-CAT reporter construct containing the CAT reporter gene regulated by the upstream region of CYP1A1. The ARNT constructs analyzed consist of either the wild-type ARNT, those containing N-terminal deletions (NΔ79 and NΔ87), or single amino acid substitutions (i.e., glutamic acid residue 83 was substituted with aspartic acid). The cells were harvested and CAT activities were determined using thin-layer chromatography. (Reprinted with permission from ref. 41. Copyright 1996, American Society for Biochemistry and Molecular Biology.)

pate in gene regulation. For example, many of the cofactors that are recruited to DNA by the nuclear steroid receptors are expressed in a cell-type–specific manner (34). These cofactors, corepressors, and coactivators assist in the ability of these receptors to activate genes via their actions as either deacetylators or acetylators of the chromatin surrounding the DNA recognition sequence or promoter region. It is thought that the cell-type specific expression of these cofactors is essential in dictating whether the steroid receptor in a given cell can act as an activator or repressor of a particular target gene.

6.1.2. Generation of Stable Cell Lines

Disadvantages to using transient transfections in the overexpression of transcription factors are the relatively low transfection efficiencies (typically 10–30%), variations in cell-to-cell expression owing to variations in the ability

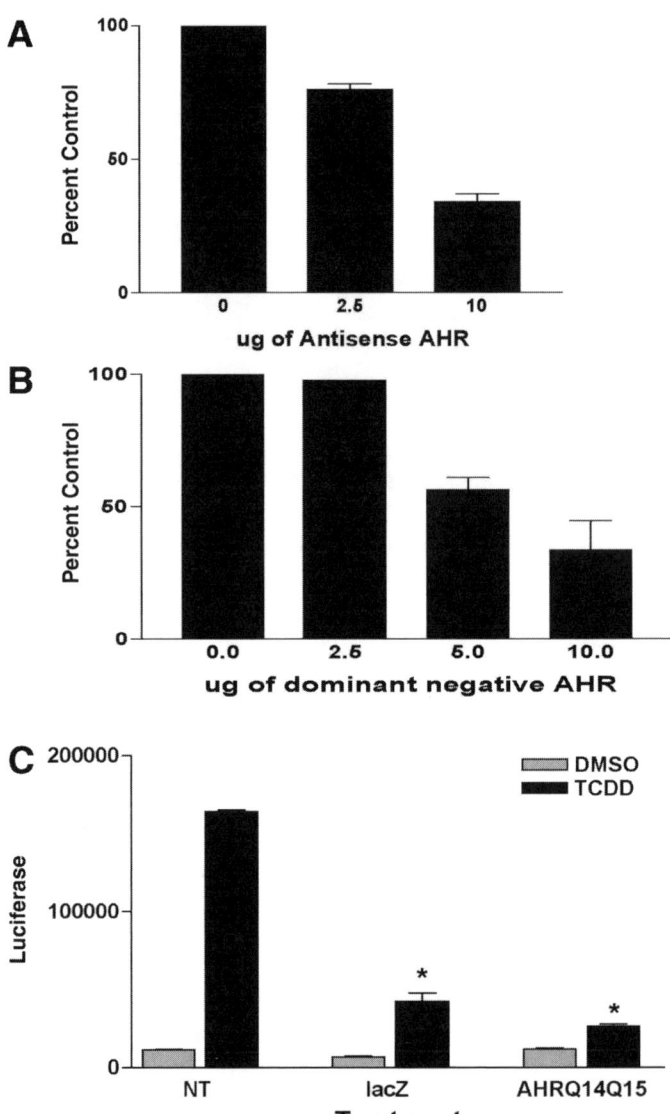

Fig. 9. Inhibition of AHR function by antisense and dominant-negative AHR cDNA. Proliferating HaCaT cells were cotransfected with the luciferase reporter vector that is regulated by two copies of the optimum DRE *(26)* and expression plasmids bearing either antisense (**A**) or dominant-negative AHR, AHR Q14Q15 *(41)* (**B**) using Tfx™-20 (Promega). Total DNA was normalized using the empty expression vector. Twenty-four hours following transfections, the cells were treated with either DMSO or 1 n*M* TCDD and incubated an additional 12 h. The cells were harvested, luciferase assays were performed, and the values normalized to that of the cotransfected β-galactosidase

Cytochrome P450 Gene Regulation

of cells to take up multiple copies of the expression plasmids, and the transient nature of the expression (up to approx 96 h). These problems may be circumvented by generating cell lines that stably express the transcription factor of interest. Here, the cells are first transiently transfected with the appropriate expression plasmid. To facilitate insertion of this plasmid into the chromosomal DNA of the cell, selective pressure is applied. The most commonly used approach is to use an expression plasmid that confers resistance to a given drug, such as resistance to neomycin or puromycin. Addition of either neomycin or puromycin to the cell culture media will result in the death of cells that do not harbor the resistant gene. The cells that have integrated the plasmid will survive and form colonies that are individually selected and expanded. In the final analyses, it is important to assay cell lines representative of several of these clones, as variations may occur owing to variations in the sites of integration. A major concern with this approach is that the manipulations required to generate the stable cell line may alter major characteristics of the cell of interest.

An additional problem is that overexpression of the transcription factor may interfere with cell growth, and thus stable transformants cannot be selected and expanded. In our experience, this has proven to be the case when working with the AHR. To circumvent this problem, a system that regulates the expression levels of the protein of interest may be used. The most commonly used approach is that regulated by tetracycline derivatives such as the Tet-On or Tet-Off systems (ClonTech).

6.1.3. Overexpression Using Viral Approaches

An alternative means of overexpressing the protein of interest is via viral-mediated approaches, using either adenoviruses, retroviruses, or lentiviruses. Here, homologous recombination is used to insert the cDNA into the genetic elements of the virus. Adenoviruses and lentiviruses can infect both dividing and nondividing cells whereas infection with retroviruses is permitted only in

---

Fig. 9. *(continued from opposite page)* reporter. The results are expressed as a percent of the TCDD-treated samples transfected with 10 µg of the empty expression vector. **(C)** Effect of the dominant-negative AHR when expressed by the adenovirus. The HepG2-p450luc cell line (HepG2 cells stably transfected with pLUC1A1 *(43)* were infected with 50 particles/cell of adenoviruses bearing either the dominant-negative AHR (AHR Q14Q15) or the *lacZ* gene (negative control) adenovirus when the cells were 60% confluent. After a 48-h incubation, the cells were treated with either 0.01% DMSO or 1 nM TCDD overnight and assayed for luciferase activity. NT represents untreated cells. The values denoted by the asterisks are statistically different from each other at the $p < 0.05$ level.

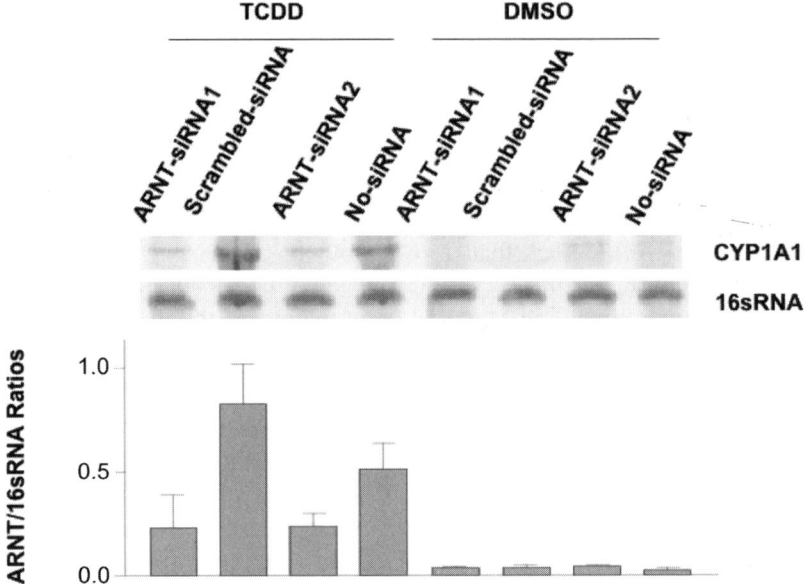

Fig. 10. Knockdown of ARNT decreases the ability of TCDD to induce CYP1A1 mRNA levels. The HepG2-p450luc cells were transfected with siRNA that targeted ARNT (Zheng et al., *manuscript in preparation*) using the Trans IT-TKO protocol (Mirus Corporation). After 24 h, the cells were treated with either 0.1% DMSO or 1 nM TCDD and incubated for an additional 20 h. The cells were harvested and mRNA levels of CYP1A1 and 16S determined using 2 µg of total RNA and RT-PCR. **(Top)** Detection of the RT-PCR products following staining of the acrylamide gels using SYBR® Green (Molecular Probes, Inc). **(Bottom)** The CYP1A1 and 16S bands were quantitated using densitometry. The values are representative of three independent experiments.

dividing cells. All of these viral approaches have been reported to result in infection rates of 70–100%. Given that viral infection is a receptor-mediated event, it is essential to first determine whether the cell type of interest is amendable to viral infection by performing a control experiment with either an adenovirus, retrovirus, or lentivirus that will allow determination of the infection rate. This is typically accomplished using viruses that encode either fluorescent proteins or lacZ. The ability to generate a virus that bears the protein of interest has been greatly facilitated by the commercial availability of a number of virus systems.

6.2. Approaches To Be Used for Inhibiting Protein Expression or Function

A number of approaches may be used to interfere with either the function of the transcription factor of interest or with its expression. Functional interference is typically achieved by overexpressing a dominant negative construct. For example, as shown in Fig. 9A, overexpression of plasmids containing either the antisense AHR or a dominant-negative construct (that is incapable of binding DNA) reduced that ability of the endogenous AHR to transactivate the DRE-regulated reporter gene by approx 50%. In an attempt to increase the effectiveness of inhibition, we turned to the use of adenoviruses. In this particular case, the control adenoviruses exerted a strong inhibitory effect on AHR-mediated transactivation such that the effect of the dominant-negative construct was minimal (Fig. 9C).

Currently, the method of choice for inhibiting gene expression is via siRNA. Here, administration of short (i.e., 21–25 nucleotides), double-stranded RNA to cultured cells has been shown to specifically inhibit gene expression by as much as 99% *(35)*. The advantages of this approach include the highly efficient knockdown capabilities and the relative ease of its use. While BLAST searches of the sequences to be targeted ensure that the probability of these RNA molecules interacting with other gene sequences is relatively low, the role of nonspecific interactions is not well defined. Disadvantages to the siRNA approach include the costliness of the synthesis of the double-stranded RNA molecules and the requirement for extensive screening owing to the unknown nature of the design specifications that will yield effective knockdown. Further, the effectiveness of the knockdown is often limited by the relatively low transfection efficiencies when introducing the molecules into the cells of interest. A number of technological advances have ameliorated these disadvantages. For example, a number of companies will perform both the design and synthesis of the double-stranded RNA molecule while guaranteeing at least a 70% knock-down rate. In addition, candidate RNA molecules can be inexpensively generated in vitro (as opposed to chemical synthesis) to screen for effective molecules. The optimum sequence can then be inserted into appropriate plasmids *(36)* or viruses *(37,38)* to allow for the stable expression of the desired siRNA in cultured cells.

An example of the use of siRNA in our laboratory is shown in Fig. 10. Here, double-stranded siRNA molecules directed toward ARNT were generated using in vitro synthesis. Two of the ten siRNA molecules were found to effectively inhibit both the expression of ARNT (data not shown) and the ability of TCDD to induce CYP1A1 mRNA levels.

REFERENCES

1. Frueh FW, Hayashibara KC, Brown PO, Whitlock JP Jr. Use of cDNA microarrays to analyze dioxin-induced changes in human liver gene expression. Toxicol Lett 2001;122:189–203.

2. Bushnell DA, Cramer P, Kornberg RD. Structural basis of transcription: α-amanitin-RNA polymerase II cocrystal at 2.8 Å resolution. Proc Natl Acad Sci USA 2002; 99:1218–1222.
3. Kimura H, Sugaya K, Cook PR. The transcription cycle of RNA polymerase II in living cells. J Cell Biol 2002;159:777–782.
4. Yamaguchi Y, Wada T, Handa H. Interplay between positive and negative elongation factors: drawing a new view of DRB. Genes Cells 1998;3:9–15.
5. Guo C, Savage L, Sarge KD, Park-Sarge O. Gonadotropins decrease estrogen receptor-β messenger ribonucleic acid stability in rat granulosa cells. Endocrinology 2001;142:2230–2237.
6. Dong L, Ma Q, Whitlock JP Jr. Down-regulation of major histocompatibility complex Q1 b gene expression by 2,3,7,8-tetrachlorodibenzo-p-dioxin. J Biol Chem 1997;272:29614–29619.
7. Ford LP, Wilusz J. An in vitro system using HeLa cytoplasmic extracts that reproduces regulated mRNA stability. In: Jacobson A, Peltz S, eds. Methods: A Companion to Methods in Enzymology. San Diego: Academic Press, 1999;17: 21–27.
8. Delany AM. Measuring transcription of metalloproteinase genes. In: Clark I, ed., Methods in Molecular Biology. Totowa, NJ: Human Press, 2000;151: 321–333.
9. Li L, Chaikof EL. Quantitative nuclear run-off transcription assay. BioTechniques 2002;33:1016–1017.
10. Elferink CJ, Reiners JJ Jr. Quantitative RT-PCR on CYP1A1 heterogeneous nuclear RNA: a surrogate for the in vitro transcription run-on assay. BioTechniques 1996;20:470–477.
11. Kwak M, Itoh K, Yamamoto M, Kensler TW. Enhanced expression of the transcription factor Nrf2 by cancer chemopreventive agents: role of antioxidant response element-like sequences in the nrf2 promoter. Mol Cell Biol 2002;22: 2883–2892.
12. Docherty K, Clark AR. Transcription of exogenous genes in mammalian cells. In: Hames BD and Higgins SJ, eds. Gene Transcription: A Practical Approach. Oxford: Oxford University Press, 1993:71–73.
13. Jones PB, Galeazzi DR, Fisher JM, Whitlock JP Jr. Control of cytochrome P-450 gene expression by dioxin. Science 1985;227:1499–1502.
14. Docherty K, Clark AR. Transcription of exogenous genes in mammalian cells. In: Hames BD, Higgins SJ, eds. Gene Transcription: A Practical Approach. Oxford: Oxford University Press, 1993;105–107.
15. Swanson H, Tullis K, Denison MS. Binding of transformed Ah receptor complex to a dioxin responsive transcriptional enhancer: evidence for two distinct heteromeric DNA-binding forms. Biochemistry 1993;32:12841–12849.
16. Liu B, Maul RS, Kaetzel DM Jr. Repression of platelet-derived growth factor A-chain gene transcription by an upstream silencer element. J Biol Chem 1996; 271:26281–26290.

17. Ma D, Xing Z, Liu B, et al. NM23-H1 and NM23-H2 repress transcriptional activities of nuclease-hypersensitive elements in the platelet-derived growth factor-A promoter. J Biol Chem 2002;277:1560–1567.
18. Fields S, Sternglanz R. The two-hyrid system: an assay for protein–protein interactions. Trends Genet 1994;10:286–292.
19. Chong JA, Tapia-Ramirez J, Kim S, et al. REST: a mammalian silencer protein that restricts sodium channel gene expression to neurons. Cell 1995;80:949–957.
20. Dixon WJ, Hayes JJ, Levin JR, Weidner MF, Dombroski BA, Tullius TD. Hydroxyl radical footprinting. Methods Enzymol 1991;208:380–413.
21. Struhl K. DNA-protein interactions. In: Ausubel FA, Brent R, Kingston RE, Moore DD, Seidman JG, Smith JA, Struhl K, eds. Current Protocols in Molecular Biology. New York: Greene Publishing and Wiley-Interscience, 1991:12.0.3–12.9.4.
22. Ragnhildstveit E, Fjose A, Becker PB, Quivy J-P. Solid phase technology improves coupled gel shift/footprinting analysis. Nucl Acids Res 1997;25:453–454.
23. Swanson HI, Whitelaw ML, Petrulis JR, Perdew GH. Use of [^{125}I]-4′-iodoflavone as a tool to characterize ligand-dependent differences in Ah receptor behavior. J Biochem Mol Toxicol 2002;16:298–310.
24. Yao EF, Denison MS. DNA sequence determinants for binding of transformed Ah receptor to a dioxin-responsive enhancer. Biochemistry 1992;31:5060–5067.
25. Dolwick KM, Swanson HI, Bradfield CA. In vitro analysis of Ah receptor domains involved in ligand-activated DNA recognition. Proc Natl Acad Sci USA 1993;90: 8566–570.
26. Swanson HI, Chan WK, Bradfield CA. DNA binding specificities and pairing rules of the Ah receptor, ARNT, and SIM proteins. J Biol Chem 1995;270:26292–26302.
27. Swanson HI, Yang J-H. Specificity of DNA binding of the c-Myc/Max and ARNT/ARNT dimers at the CACGTG recognition site. Nucl Acids Res 1999;27: 3205–3212.
28. Farnham PJ, ed. Methods, Vol. 26. San Diego: Academic Press, 2002.
29. Wells J, Farnham PJ. Characterizing transcription factor binding sites using formaldehyde cross-linking and immunoprecipitation. Methods 2002;26:48–56.
30. Boyd KE, Wells J, Gutman J, Bartley SM, Farnham PJ. c-Myc target gene specificity is determined by a post-DNA-binding mechanism. Proc Natl Acad Sci USA 1998;95:13887–13892.
31. Mueller PR, Wold B. In vivo footprinting of a muscle specific enhancer by ligation mediated PCR. Science 1989;246:780–786.
32. Heckman CA, Boxer LM. Allele-specific analysis of transcription factors binding to promoter regions. In: Farnham PJ, ed., Methods, Vol. 26. San Diego: Academic Press, 2002:19–26.
33. Watson AJ, Weir-Brown KI, Bannister RM, et al. Mechanism of action of a repressor of dioxin-dependent induction of Cyp1a1 gene transcription. Mol Cell Biol 1992;12:2115–2123.
34. Hermanson O., Glass CK, Rosenfeld MG. Nuclear receptor coregulators: multiple modes of modification. Trends Endocrinol Metab 2002;13:55–60.

35. McManus MT, Sharp PA. Gene silencing in mammals by small interfering RNAs. Nat Rev Genet 2002;3:737–747.
36. Czauderna F, Fechtner M, Aygun, H., et al. Functional studies of the PI(3)-kinase signaling pathway employing synthetic and expressed siRNA. Nucl Acids Res 2003;31:670–682.
37. Barton GM, Medzhitov R. Retroviral delivery of small interfering RNA into primary cells. Proc Natl Acad Sci USA 2002;99:14943–14945.
38. Tiscornia G, Singer O, Ikawa M, Verma IM. A general method for gene knockdown in mice by using lentiviral vector expressing small interfering RNA. Proc Natl Acad Sci USA 2003;100:1844–1848.
39. Postlind H, Vu, TP, Tukey RH, Quattrochi LC. Response of human CYP1-luciferase plasmids to 2,3,7,8-tetrachlorodibenzo-p-dioxin and polycyclic aromatic hydrocarbons. Toxicology 1993;118:255–262.
40. Hines RN, Mathis JN, Jacob CS. Identification of multiple regulatory elements on the cytochrome P4501A1 gene. Carcinogenesis 1988;9:1599–1605.
41. Swanson HI, Yang J. Mapping the protein/DNA contact sites of the Ah receptor and Ah receptor nuclear translocator. J Biol Chem 1996;271:31657–31665.
42. Tian Y, Ke S, Dension MS, Rabson AB, Gallo MA. Ah receptor and NF-κB interactions, a potential mechanism for dioxin toxicity. J Biol Chem 1999;274:510–515.
43. Heid SE, Walker MK, Swanson HI. Correlation of cardiotoxicity mediated by halogenated aromatic hydrocarbons to aryl hydrocarbon receptor activation. Toxicol Sci 2001;61:187–196.

3

Insulin and Growth Factor Signaling

Effects on Drug-Metabolizing Enzymes

Sang K. Kim, Kimberley J. Woodcroft, and Raymond F. Novak

Summary

Expression of drug-metabolizing enzymes may be altered in response to development, aging, gender, genetics, nutrition, pregnancy, disease states such as diabetes, long-term alcohol consumption, and inflammation, and by xenobiotics. Although the mechanisms by which xenobiotics regulate drug-metabolizing enzymes have been intensively studied, relatively little is known regarding the cellular mechanisms by which drug-metabolizing enzymes are regulated in response to endogenous factors such as hormones and growth factors. The first major section of the chapter defines the major insulin- and growth factor-mediated signaling pathways implicated in regulating drug-metabolizing enzyme expression, including those involving mitogen-activated protein and phosphatidyl inositol 3-kinases, small G proteins, and phosphatases. The second major section of the chapter presents a summary and evaluation of methods for determination of the role and function of signaling pathways that are involved in the regulation of drug-metabolizing enzyme gene and protein expression, including methods for determination of kinase activity and phosphorylation, the use of kinase inhibitors and dominant-negative protein kinase constructs, and the application of new RNA interference methods.

Key Words

Cytochrome P450; extracellular signal-regulated kinase; glutathione *S*-transferase; G proteins; green fluorescent protein; insulin; insulin receptor; jun N-terminal kinase; kinase assays; kinase inhibitors; mammalian target of rapamycin (mTOR); microsomal epoxide hydrolase; mitogen-activated protein kinase pathway; p38 mitogen-activated protein kinase; p70 ribosomal protein S6 kinase; p70 S6 kinase; phosphatase and tensin homologue deleted on chromosome ten; pleckstrin homology; primary culture; protein kinases; protein phosphatases; rat hepatocytes; receptor tyrosine kinase; small interfering RNA (siRNA); small temporal RNA; stress-activated protein kinases; sulfotransferase; UDP-glucuronosyltransferase.

From: *Methods in Pharmacology and Toxicology,
Drug Metabolism and Transport: Molecular Methods and Mechanisms*
Edited by: L. Lash © Humana Press Inc., Totowa, NJ

1. INTRODUCTION

The body is equipped with several mechanisms to ensure that xenobiotics do not accumulate. Polar molecules are often poorly absorbed into the body, but when absorbed they are readily eliminated via the kidneys. In contrast, nonpolar molecules are a special problem because of their affinity for membranes. Increasing the polarity of small, nonpolar molecules through metabolism generally promotes the excretion of the metabolites. Xenobiotic biotransformation is the principal mechanism for maintaining homeostasis during exposure of organisms to small foreign molecules and occurs predominantly in the liver, although it also occurs in nasal mucosa, intestine, kidneys, lungs, placenta, and skin.

The reactions catalyzed by xenobiotic-, or drug-metabolizing enzymes are generally divided into two groups, phase I and phase II. Phase I reactions introduce a functional group that increases hydrophilicity and are mediated by cytochrome P450 (CYP), flavin-containing monooxygenase, xanthine oxidase, prostaglandin H synthase, amine oxidase, alcohol dehydrogenase, aldehyde dehydrogenase, epoxide hydrolase, and esterase. Phase II reactions include glucuronidation, sulfation, methylation, glutathione conjugation, and amino acid conjugation. In general, these reactions, with the exception of methylation, result in a large increase in xenobiotic hydrophilicity.

It is generally recognized that the expression of drug-metabolizing enzymes may be altered in response to development, aging, gender, genetic factors, nutrition, pregnancy, and pathophysiological conditions such as diabetes, long-term alcohol consumption, inflammation, and protein-calorie malnutrition. The expression may also be altered by xenobiotics. Although the mechanisms by which xenobiotics regulate drug-metabolizing enzymes have been intensively studied, relatively less is known regarding the cellular mechanisms by which drug-metabolizing enzymes are regulated in response to endogenous factors such as hormones and growth factors. Recent findings, however, have revealed that hormones and growth factors play an important role in the regulation of drug-metabolizing enzyme expression. Furthermore, the cellular signaling pathways involved in hormone- and growth factor-mediated regulation of drug-metabolizing enzymes are currently being studied.

Pathophysiological conditions such as diabetes, fasting, obesity, and long-term alcohol consumption result in increased expression of several hepatic enzymes, including CYP1A1, 2B, 3A, 4A, 2E1, and bilirubin UDP-glucuronosyltransferase (UGT1A1), whereas decreased expression of CYP2C11, microsomal epoxide hydrolase (mEH) and sulfotransferases (SULTs), such as hydroxysteroid SULT-a (SULT2A1) and aryl SULT IV (SULT1A1), has been reported (Table 1) *(1–17)*. On the other hand, studies of the expression and activity of glutathione *S*-transferase (GST) during diabetes are inconclusive, with both increased and decreased GST expression being reported in vivo *(5,18–21)*. The reason for this discrepancy remains unknown. However, it may, in part, be associated with competing factors in vivo and with variations in oxidative stress, usually observed in diabetes. It has been reported that transcriptional activation of some GST genes may be associated with the change in the redox state in conjunction with oxidative stress *(22,23)*.

Because these pathophysiological states all result in altered hormone (insulin, glucagon, growth hormone) secretion, these hormones may be etiologic factors affecting the expression of hepatic drug-metabolizing enzymes. It has been reported that insulin or growth hormone administration to chemically induced or spontaneously diabetic rats restores drug-metabolizing enzyme activity and expression to control values (Table 1) *(5,6,9,24–29)*. Our laboratory and others have demonstrated that the activity and/or expression of hepatic drug-metabolizing enzymes such as CYP2B, CYP2E1, CYP2C11, CYP2A5, GST alpha class, GST pi class, UGT, and mEH are regulated by insulin and glucagon (Table 1) *(30–40)*. These results indicate that changes in drug-metabolizing enzyme mRNA or protein levels observed in pathophysiological conditions may be attributed to alterations in these hormone levels. Thus, it is of interest to identify which cellular signaling pathways are involved in regulating the expression of these genes in response to hormones.

In addition to altered expression of drug-metabolizing enzymes by pathophysiologic conditions, the pattern of drug-metabolizing enzyme expression is changed during development and aging and occurs in an organ-, sex-, and species-specific manner. Such observations also suggest that a cellular or organ context regulates the expression of drug-metabolizing enzymes. Growth factors, including epidermal growth factor (EGF) and hepatocyte growth factor (HGF), have a role in regulating drug-metabolizing enzyme gene expression. HGF results in decreased CYP2C11 expression in primary cultured rat hepatocytes *(41)* and decreased CYP1A1/2, 2A6, 2B6, and 2E1 activities in primary cultured human hepatocytes *(42)*. In primary cultured rat hepatocytes, addition of EGF suppresses constitutive and xenobiotic-inducible CYP expression including CYP2C11, CYP2C12, CYP1A1, CYP2B1/2 *(43–45)* and CYP2E1 (Woodcroft et al., *unpublished data*). EGF has also been reported to increase alpha and pi class GST expression *(46,47)*.

Our laboratory has demonstrated that the expression of CYP2E1 is suppressed by insulin (Fig. 1) and enhanced by glucagon in primary cultured rat hepatocytes *(35–37)*. In contrast, the expression of alpha-class GSTs (Fig. 2) and mEH is enhanced by insulin and decreased by glucagon *(33,40)*. Treatment of cells with glucagon also inhibits the expression of pi-class GST *(33)*. Phosphatidylinositol 3-kinase (PI3K) and p70 ribosomal protein S6 kinase (p70 S6 kinase) appear to play a central role in mediating the suppression of CYP2E1

Table 1
Effect of Diabetes, Insulin and Glucagon on Drug-Metabolizing Enzyme Expression and/or Activity

	Diabetes	Restored by insulin	Insulin	Glucagon
CYP2B	Increased (6)	Yes (6)	Decreased (34,35)	ND
CYP3A	Increased (7,12)	Yes (7,12)	Unchanged (35)	ND
CYP4A	Increased (7,12)	Yes (7,12)	Marginally increased (35)	ND
CYP2C11	Decreased (9,12)	Yes (12)	ND	Decreased (38)
CYP2E1	Increased (4,8,12,16)	Yes (12,24)	Decreased (34–37)	Increased (37)
mEH	Decreased (5)	Yes (5)	Increased (40)	Decreased (40)
UGT1A1	Increased (16)	Yes (16,29)	ND	Increased (30,31)
SULT2A1	Decreased (14)	Yes (14)	ND	ND
GSTs	Increase (18,20,21)/Decrease (5,19)	ND	Increased (32,33)	Decreased (32,33)
GST alpha	ND	ND	Increased (33)	Decreased (33)
GST pi	ND	ND	Unchanged (33)	Decreased (33)
GST mu	ND	ND	Unchanged (33)	Unchanged (33)

ND, Not determined.

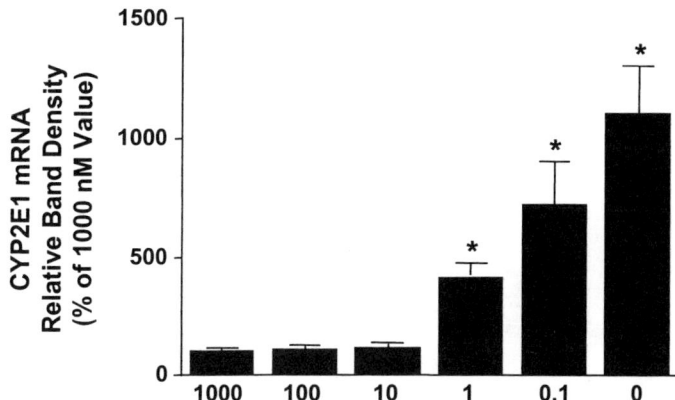

Fig. 1. Changes in CYP2E1 mRNA levels in primary cultured rat hepatocytes maintained in culture medium in the presence of various concentrations of insulin for 96 h. Values are shown as a percentage of the 1000 nM insulin value (100%). Columns and cross bars represent means ± SEM of Northern blot band densities of six to nine preparations of total RNA. Values were normalized for loading using 7S RNA. *Significantly different than 1000 nM insulin-treated cells, $p < 0.05$. (Reprinted from ref. *35*. Copyright 1997, with permission from Elsevier.)

expression *(48)* as well as enhancement of mEH *(40)* and alpha-class GSTs (Kim, Woodcroft and Novak, *unpublished data*). The regulation of CYP2E1 expression by insulin does not involve extracellular signal-regulated kinases (ERK1/2) or p38 mitogen activated protein kinase (p38 MAPK) *(48)*. This is in contrast to the findings for insulin-mediated expression of mEH, which appears to involve p38 MAPK *(40)*. Furthermore, our results implicate cAMP and protein kinase A (PKA) in mediating the effects of glucagon on CYP2E1, GSTs, and mEH expression *(33,37,40)*.

In this chapter, an overview of the signaling pathways implicated in regulating drug-metabolizing enzyme expression in response to insulin and growth factors is described along with the methods for identifying which signaling pathways and components are involved in mediating this regulation.

2. INSULIN- AND GROWTH FACTOR-MEDIATED SIGNALING PATHWAYS

The numerous and varied biological functions of insulin and growth factors are mediated by their corresponding cell surface receptors. The insulin receptor and growth factor receptors belong to the large family of receptor tyrosine kinase (RTK) cell surface receptors possessing intrinsic tyrosine kinase activity. After binding of their corresponding agonist, these receptors undergo

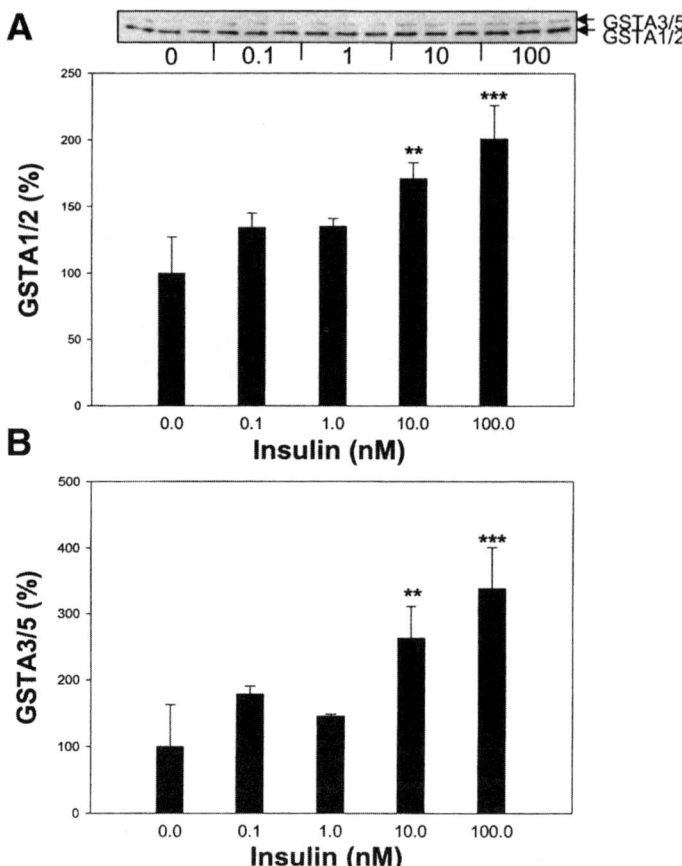

Fig. 2. Immunoblot analysis of GSTA1/2 (**A**) and GSTA3/5 (**B**) protein levels in primary cultured rat hepatocytes maintained in culture in the presence of various concentrations of insulin for 3 d. Values are shown as a percentage of the GST levels monitored in hepatocytes cultured in the absence of insulin (100%). Data are means ± SD of immunoblot band densities of three preparations of cell lysates. **,***Significantly different than levels monitored in hepatocytes cultured in the absence of insulin, $p < 0.01$ or $p < 0.001$, respectively. (Reprinted from ref. *33* with permission.)

autophosphorylation of tyrosine residues in the cytoplasmic domain and initiate a complex series of intracellular signaling cascades that ultimately result in diverse cellular responses.

Insulin and growth factors stimulate the recruitment of a family of lipid kinases known as class I PI3Ks to the plasma membrane. There, PI3Ks phosphorylate the glycerophospholipid phosphatidylinositol (PI) 4,5-bisphosphate at the D-3 position of the inositol ring, converting it to PI 3,4,5-triphosphate (PI[3,4,5]P$_3$). Recent evidence indicates that serine/threonine protein kinase Akt/PKB (protein kinase B), atypical protein kinase C (PKC), and p70 S6 kinase mediate many of the downstream events controlled by PI3K.

Insulin and growth factors also lead to activation of mitogen activated protein kinase (MAPK) signaling pathways. On recruitment and activation via phosphorylated RTKs, the small guanosine triphosphatase protein Ras activates Raf, which leads to a phosphorylation signaling cascade involving activation of the MAPKs. RTK signaling is regulated not only by a cascade of phosphorylation via protein kinases, but also by dephosphorylation via tyrosine and serine/threonine phosphatases and lipid phosphatases. A simplified scheme of insulin receptor signaling as discussed in this chapter is illustrated in Fig. 3.

2.1. Insulin Receptor

The insulin receptor is a transmembrane heterotetramer consisting of two α- (extracellular; 135 kDa) and two β- (transmembrane; 95 kDa) subunits linked by disulfide bonds *(49)*. During transport to the cell surface, a single high-molecular-weight proreceptor is proteolytically cleaved at a tetrabasic amino acid sequence (arginine-lysine-arginine-arginine) located at the junction of the α- and β-subunits, and oligosaccharide chains are added at specific sites of glycosylation. Interactions between the two α-subunits, and between the α and β subunit, are stabilized by disulfide bridges *(50,51)*.

Unoccupied α-subunits on the cell membrane surface inhibit the intrinsic tyrosine kinase activity of the β-subunit and may be viewed as a regulatory subunit of the catalytic intracellular subunit *(52)*. The β-subunit is composed of a short extracellular domain, a transmembrane domain, and a cytoplasmic domain that possesses intrinsic tyrosine kinase activity. The cytoplasmic domain contains the ATP binding site and autophosphorylation sites. Binding of insulin to the α-subunits of the receptor induces conformational changes leading to activation of the RTK activity, resulting in transphosphorylation of the β-subunits and endocytic internalization of the receptor via clathrin-coated vesicles *(51)*. Some of the tyrosine-phosphorylated residues of the β-subunits of the receptor present binding sites for the subsequent recruitment of signaling molecules. The insulin receptor uses a family of soluble adaptors or scaffolding molecules, such as insulin receptor substrates (IRSs 1–4) and Shc molecules, to initiate its signaling cascade through other effectors.

Whereas the IRSs lack intrinsic catalytic activity, they have pleckstrin homology (PH) and phosphotyrosine binding (PTB) domains, and multiple phosphorylation motifs. The PH domains are globular protein domains of about 100–120 amino acids found in more than 150 proteins to date. PH domains are primarily

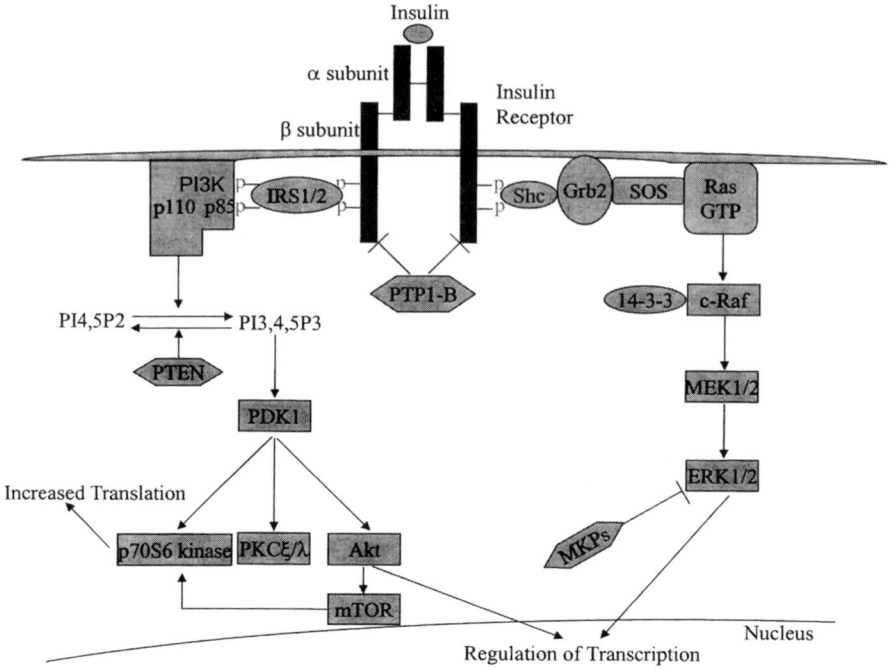

Fig. 3. Insulin-mediated signaling pathways.

lipid-binding modules, although they are also involved in mediating protein–protein interactions. The PTB domain of IRS binds to phosphorylated NPXP motifs in the insulin receptor and are subsequently phosphorylated on multiple tyrosine residues by the activated insulin receptor kinase. Following phosphorylation, IRS attracts and binds additional effector molecules to the vicinity of the receptor, thereby serving to increase the diversity of the signaling pathways initiated by the insulin receptor *(53,54)*. The primary effector that binds to IRSs in response to insulin receptor activation is the lipid kinase PI3K that produces PI(3,4,5)P_3 and subsequently activates Akt, PKC, and p70 S6 kinase (Fig. 3).

The adaptor protein Shc exists in p46, p52, and p66 isoforms and possesses Src homology-2 (SH2) and PTB domains and three tyrosine-phosphorylation sites. In response to extracellular signals, Shc is phosphorylated on tyrosine residues and binds the growth factor receptor binding protein 2 (Grb2), which is constitutively associated with the guanine nucleotide exchange factor Son of Sevenless (SOS) *(55)*. Recruitment of the Grb2–SOS complex to the vicinity of Shc induces exchange of GDP to GTP on the membrane-bound GTPase Ras, thereby activating Ras. Activated Ras binds Raf and activates the serine/threonine Raf/MAPK kinase (MKK)/MAPK signaling pathway (Fig. 3) *(56)*.

2.2. Growth Factor Receptor

The growth factor receptors are also members of a large family of cell surface receptors, including the EGF receptor; ErbB2, 3, and 4; and c-MET, which exhibit intrinsic protein tyrosine kinase activity. The EGF receptor is synthesized from a 1210-residue polypeptide precursor; after cleavage of the N-terminal sequence and glycosylation, the 1186-residue protein is inserted into the cell membrane *(57)*. The glycosylated extracellular domain of the EGF receptor contains conserved cysteine-rich clusters that comprise the ligand-binding domain. Within the intracellular domain, the juxtamembrane region is required for feedback attenuation by PKC, followed by the tyrosine kinase domain and C-terminal regulatory tail. The C-terminal tail contains the tyrosine autophosphorylation sites and motifs for internalization and degradation of the receptor. Binding of EGF to the receptor results in receptor dimerization and autophosphorylation. The resulting conformational change creates specific docking sites for recruitment and activation of additional signaling proteins that contain SH2 and PTB domains, including Shc and Grb2. In addition, the EGF receptor can be phosphorylated by other kinases, such as PKC and Src kinase, which regulate the distribution and kinase activity of the EGF receptor *(58,59)*. Following ligand binding and activation, EGF receptor dimers are recruited into clathrin-coated pits, which initiates a rapid endocytosis and degradation of the EGF receptor.

2.3. PI3K/Akt/p70 S6 Kinase/Atypical PKCs

There are four major classes of PI3Ks, designated class I–IV; class I is also subdivided into Ia and Ib subsets. Class IV PI3Ks are not known to possess lipid kinase activity, but are serine/threonine kinases. The different classes of PI3Ks catalyze phosphorylation of the 3′-OH position of phosphatidyl *myo*-inositol lipids, generating different 3′-phosphorylated lipid products that act as second messengers. Class Ia PI3Ks are primarily responsible for production of 3′-OH phosphoinositides in response to insulin and growth factors *(60)*. Class Ia enzymes are dimers composed of a 110-kDa catalytic subunit that is associated nonconvalently to an 85- or 55-kDa regulatory subunit (Fig. 3). The catalytic subunit in subclass Ia is subdivided into p110 α-, β-, and δ. The regulatory subunit maintains the catalytic subunit in a low-activity state in quiescent cells and mediates its activation through interactions between SH2 domains of the regulatory subunit and phosphotyrosine residues of activated growth factor receptors or adaptor proteins, such as the IRSs *(61)*. The single class Ib PI3K is the p110 γ catalytic subunit complexed with a p101 regulatory protein and mainly activated by heterotrimeric G protein-based signaling pathways. Direct binding of p110 to activated Ras plays an important role in the stimulation of PI3K in response to growth factor *(62)*, but the physiological significance of this interaction in insulin-mediated PI3K signaling is not entirely clear.

Following the recruitment of PI3K to the plasma membrane, the lipid kinase phosphorylates the 3′-OH position of the inositol ring to generate $PI(3,4,5)P_3$, $PI(3,4)P_2$, and $PI(3)P$. The preferred substrate of class I PI3Ks appears to be $PI(4,5)P_2$. These events occur within the first minute of insulin binding to its receptor and resulting lipid products then interact with a number of signaling proteins with PH domains, resulting in their membrane targeting and/or modulation of their enzyme activity.

The rapid increase in $PI(3,4,5)P_3$ concentration in response to insulin activates several protein kinases, such as phosphatidylinositide-dependent kinase 1 (PDK1), Akt, PKC isoforms, and p70 S6 kinase *(63–65)*. Among the $PI(3,4,5)P_3$-dependent kinases, Akt has received much attention. Akt/PKB was identified as a protein kinase with a high degree of homology to PKA and PKC, and is the cellular homologue of the viral oncoprotein v-Akt. Akt is a 57-kDa serine/threonine kinase with a PH domain and the three known isoforms of Akt (Akt1, 2, 3) are widely expressed *(66)*.

Akt exists in the cytoplasm of unstimulated cells in a low-activity conformation. The activation of Akt1 by insulin and growth factors is accompanied by its phosphorylation on threonine-308 in the kinase domain (T-loop) and serine-473 in the C-terminal regulatory domain (hydrophobic motif). Activation of Akt and phosphorylation of both these residues are abolished by pretreatment of cells with PI3K inhibitors such as wortmannin and LY294002 *(67)*. After activation of PI3K, association of $PI(3,4,5)P_3$ at the membrane brings Akt and PDK1 into proximity through their PH domains and facilitates phosphorylation of Akt at threonine-308 by PDK1 *(65)*. The mechanism mediating serine-473 phosphorylation remains to be clarified.

p70 S6 kinase catalyzes the phosphorylation of the S6 protein, a component of the 40S subunit of eukaryotic ribosomes, and thus plays a role in protein synthesis *(68,69)*. p70 S6 kinase participates in the translational control of mRNA transcripts that contain a polypyrimidine tract at their transcriptional start site. Although these transcripts represent only 100–200 genes, most of these transcripts encode components of the translational apparatus. The initial step in p70 S6 kinase activation appears to involve a phosphorylation-induced conformational change in the C-terminal domain, revealing additional phosphorylation sites. Subsequently, phosphorylation of the newly exposed sites (threonine 229, 389, and serine 371) occurs, which is dependent on both PI3K and the mammalian target of rapamycin (mTOR), based on wortmannin and rapamycin sensitivity, respectively.

Although expression of a constitutively membrane-anchored and active Akt variant induces the activation of p70 S6 kinase *(70)*, Akt does not appear to represent the immediate upstream effector of p70 S6 kinase. Conus et al. *(71)* suggested that p70 S6 kinase activation could be achieved independent of Akt. Dufner et al. *(72)* demonstrated that a constitutively active wortmannin-resistant form of Akt was sufficient to induce glycogen synthase kinase-3 and eIF4E-binding protein 1 phosphorylation, but not phosphorylation and activation of p70 S6 kinase. The data suggest that p70 S6 kinase activation by membrane-targeted forms of Akt may be an artifact of membrane localization and that Akt resides on a parallel PI3K-dependent signaling pathway to that described for p70 S6 kinase.

Recent findings indicate that atypical PKC isoforms (ζ, rat) and (λ, mouse) serve as downstream effectors for PI3K *(73)*. Increased activity of PKCζ/λ results from PDK1-dependent phosphorylation of the catalytic domain, via threonine-410 in rat PKCζ and threonine-411 in mouse PKCλ, followed by autophosphorylation of threonine-560 in rat PKCζ and threonine-563 in mouse PKCλ *(64,74)*. PI(3,4,5)P$_3$ may interact with the N-terminal lipid-binding domain of PKCζ to facilitate the interaction of threonine-410 with the catalytic site of PDK1 *(74)*. PI(3,4,5)P$_3$ also stimulates autophosphorylation of PKCζ and relieves the autoinhibition exerted by the N-terminal pseudosubstrate sequence on the C-terminal catalytic domain of PKCζ *(74,75)*. Insulin-stimulated glucose transport and protein synthesis are dependent on PI3K/PKCζ activity *(73,76)*. The latter is consistent with the observation that dominant-negative PKCζ antagonizes activation of p70 S6 kinase *(77)*. However, it is not known whether PKCζ can directly phosphorylate p70 S6 kinase or which residue(s) is/are involved.

2.4. Ras/Raf/MEK/ERK

Many RTKs, including the insulin and growth factor receptors, are known to activate intracellular protein serine/threonine kinases, termed MAPKs, that phosphorylate various cellular targets in a proline-directed manner, including transcription factors and other kinases. The MAPK family consists of subfamilies with multiple members (Fig. 4): these include the ERK1/2, the Jun N-terminal kinases/stress-activated protein kinases (JNKs/SAPKs), the p38 MAPKs and ERK5. Each MAPK is a member of a three-protein kinase cascade; a MAPK kinase kinase (MKKK) phosphorylates a MKK, which subsequently phosphorylates the MAPK. Of the various MAPKs, the ERK1/2 subfamily was the first to be characterized. The basic arrangement of the ERK signal cascade includes Ras, Raf (MKKK), MEK1/2 (MKK), and ERK1/2 (MAPK) (Fig. 4).

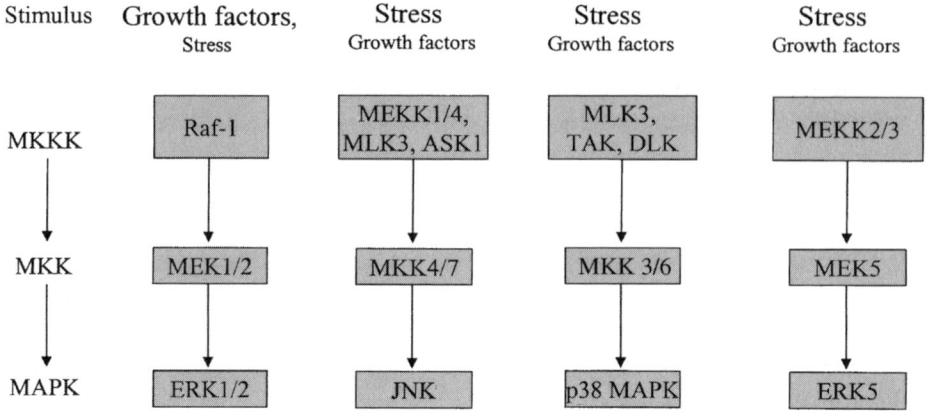

Fig. 4. MAPK signaling cascades. (Adapted from website of Cell Signaling Technology.)

Mammalian cells contain three different Ras genes that give rise to four Ras small GTPases—H-Ras, N-Ras, K_A-Ras and K_B-Ras—which are key regulators of signal transduction pathways controlling cell proliferation, differentiation, survival, and apoptosis *(78,79)*. In response to a great variety of extracellular stimuli, including hormones, growth factors, cell–extracellular matrix interactions, and oxidative stress, Ras proteins are activated through the GDP/GTP nucleotide exchange factor SOS, which induces the exchange of GDP for GTP, and thereby converts Ras to its active form. Ras cycles between the inactive GDP-bound and active GTP-bound states through the controlled activity of GTP nucleotide exchange factors and GTPase-activating proteins. After activation of insulin and growth factor receptors through agonist binding, the link between RTKs and Ras is provided by the GTP exchange factor SOS that exists in a complex with the adaptor protein Grb2 in the cytosol. Phosphorylated tyrosine residues in insulin and growth factor receptors are docking sites for Grb2. In addition, the interaction between Grb2/SOS and the receptors can be mediated by the adaptor protein Shc, which becomes tyrosine phosphorylated when recruited to the cytoplasmic domains of the activated receptors. This process brings SOS to the plasma membrane in close proximity to Ras, where it can promote GDP/GTP exchange. GTP-bound activated Ras recruits and activates three main classes of effector proteins, Raf kinases, PI3K, and RalGDS *(62)*.

Three genes encode for the Raf family of serine/threonine kinases found in mammalian cells: *A-Raf*, *B-Raf*, and *Raf-1* (*c-Raf*). The large majority of studies regarding the role of Raf in ERK activation have been performed with Raf-1. In resting cells, Raf-1 is located in the cytoplasm and is stabilized by a 14-3-3 scaffold protein dimer binding to phosphorylated serines 259 and 621, which are phosphorylated in resting cells *(80)*. The binding of Raf to Ras and translocation to the plasma membrane can displace 14-3-3 from phosphoserine 259, which makes it accessible to dephosphorylation and activation by protein phosphatase 2A (PP2A) *(81)*, although the role of dephosphorylation of serine-259 in Raf-1 activation was recently challenged *(82)*.

The activation of Raf-1 is required for the subsequent multistep events to occur at the plasma membrane following the relief from autoinhibition. Agonists such as insulin and growth factors stimulate the phosphorylation of several residues, including serine-338, tyrosine-341, tyrosine-491, and serine-494 *(83)*. Phosphorylation at serine-338 and tyrosine-341 is a critical step for Raf activation *(83)* and serine-338 phosphorylation appears to be a good qualitative indicator of Raf-1 activation.

MEK1 (MKK1) and MEK2 (MKK2) contain a proline-rich sequence necessary for the interaction of MEK with Raf-1 *(84)*. MEKs are phosphorylated by Raf-1 on two serine residues (serine-217 and -221), which are necessary for full activation. MEK1 and MEK2 activate ERK1 (p44 MAPK) and ERK2 (p42 MAPK) via phosphorylation of a threonine–glutamate–tyrosine motif in the activation loop. ERK is a proline-directed serine/threonine kinase at the end of this pathway with more than 50 identified substrates, including transcription factors, MAPK-activated protein kinase-2, and the p90 ribosomal S6 kinase *(85)*. ERK activation has traditionally been associated primarily with cell proliferation.

The stress-activated protein kinases (SAPKs) such as JNK, p38 MAPK, and ERK5 are slightly activated by insulin or growth factors but vigorously activated by stress signals (UV irradiation, heat or cold shock, osmotic stress, mechanical shear stress, oxidative stress), cytokines, and G protein–coupled receptor agonists *(86)*. The SAPKs are involved in the regulation of growth arrest, apoptosis, and proliferation. The SAPKs are activated through a similar kinase cascade as ERK, although some different mechanisms have been noted. MKK4/SEK1 and MKK7 phosphorylate and activate JNK, whereas p38 MAPK is activated by MKK3 and MKK6. At the level of the MKKK, many kinases activating either or both JNK and p38 MAPK have been identified by overexpression or dominant-negative experiments *(87)*.

2.5. Crosstalk Between PI3K and MAPKs

A number of studies have suggested that the MAPK and the PI3K pathways cross-talk on several levels *(88–96)*. But the interrelationship between MAPK and PI3K signaling pathways has been controversial. This may reflect differences associated with cell context and activators of the signaling cascades.

Studies of the relevance of PI3K signaling for the activation of ERK are inconclusive, with both increased and decreased ERK activation being reported.

Although ERK1/2 activation may occur independently of PI3K *(97–99)*, inhibitors of PI3K have been reported to inhibit insulin- and growth factor-induced increases in ERK1/2 activity in a number of cell types such as the rat skeletal muscle cell line L6, rat adipocytes, and hepatic stellate cells *(100–102)*. In contrast, Akt phosphorylates serine-259, located in the regulatory domain of Raf-1, resulting in the inactivation of Raf-1 *(103,104)*. Moelling et al. *(92)* showed that the PI3K/Akt pathway inhibited the Ras/Raf-1/MEK/ERK pathway at the level of Raf-1 and Akt. Thus, the PI3K-dependent signaling pathway can either stimulate or inhibit ERK activation and this likely depends on the cell context and the type of stimuli, as well as the concentration and period of treatment *(88,92)*.

JNK activity is elevated in obesity and an absence of JNK1 results in decreased adiposity, significantly improved insulin sensitivity and enhanced insulin receptor signaling capacity in two different models of mouse obesity *(105)*. Lee et al. *(96)* showed that insulin-stimulated JNK associated with IRS1 and phosphorylated IRS1 at serine-307 in mouse embryo fibroblasts and 3T3-L1 adipocytes, and that this interaction inhibited insulin signaling. These results suggest that prolonged activation of JNK inhibits IRS-associated PI3K activity and can be a crucial mediator of insulin resistance.

2.6. Phosphatases

The phosphorylation of tyrosine residues in proteins by kinases plays a key role in the regulation of cell signaling and gene expression. The level of tyrosine phosphorylation in receptors and their downstream substrates is dynamically and precisely regulated by two types of enzymes, protein tyrosine kinases, which catalyze the phosphorylation of tyrosine residues, and protein tyrosine phosphatases (PTPs), which dephosphorylate the phosphotyrosine residues *(106,107)*. Disregulated PTP activity may lead to aberrant tyrosine phosphorylation, which may contribute to disease, including cancer and diabetes *(108,109)*. PTPs can be divided into tyrosine-specific and dual-specific subfamilies, based on their substrate specificity. The dual-specificity subfamily recognizes phosphotyrosine, phosphothreonine and phosphoserine residues. Tyrosine-specific PTPs can be further classified as intracellular and receptor-like PTPs. Intracellular PTPs possess a single conserved catalytic domain, and the N- or C-terminus that appears to play a regulatory or targeting role. PTP-1B and SHP-2, an SH2-containing PTP-2, belong to this subfamily and are key regulators that control the intracellular phosphotyrosine level. Receptor-like PTPs, exemplified by CD45 and PTPα, contain one or two cytoplasmic catalytic domains, a single transmembrane region and an extracellular domain. The extracellular domains have structures found in cell-adhesion molecules, suggesting a role for this subfamily of PTPs in cell–cell and/or cell–extracellular matrix interactions. Dual-specificity PTPs include the MAPK phosphatases (MKPs) and cell cycle regulator Cdc25 phosphatases.

PTP-1B, the first mammalian PTP to be purified to homogeneity *(110)*, is widely expressed and localized predominantly to the endoplasmic reticulum through a cleavable proline-rich C-terminal segment *(111)*. Cleavage of the C-terminal 35 amino acids of PTP-1B appears to release this phosphatase from the endoplasmic reticulum and increase its specific activity *(112)*. PTP-1B deficiency in mice results in enhanced insulin sensitivity, as demonstrated by an increased insulin-stimulated phosphorylation of the insulin receptor in muscle and liver, an improved glucose clearance in glucose and insulin tolerance tests, and a significant reduction in fed glucose levels *(113)*. This study suggests that PTP-1B is a negative regulator of the insulin-stimulated signal transduction pathway by dephosphorylating the phosphotyrosine residues of the insulin receptor kinase *(114)*. The association between insulin receptor and PTP-1B has been demonstrated using the substrate trapping method, immunoprecipitation, and immunoblot analysis *(115,116)*. The mechanism(s) for regulation of PTP-1B activity is unclear. Recently, it has been reported that insulin-stimulated intracellular hydrogen peroxide production may reversibly oxidize PTP-1B, resulting in inhibition of PTP-1B and enhancement of the insulin signaling cascade *(117,118)*. Several groups have reported that phosphorylation of PTP-1B by the insulin receptor and other protein kinases affects PTP-1B enzyme activity *(119–121)*. In addition to the insulin receptor, PTP-1B has other targets such as EGF receptor and Src kinase *(122,123)*.

The SHP-2 phosphatase contains two tandem SH2 domains that mediate the binding of SHP-2 to phosphorylated tyrosine residues on other molecules. In the resting state, SHP-2 activity is repressed, but its mechanism of activation is unclear. SHP-2 plays a positive and/or negative role in transducing signals relayed from RTKs. For example, introduction of the catalytically inert SHP-2 markedly inhibited activation of ERK in response to EGF and insulin stimulation *(124,125)*. Chen et al. *(126)* also reported that overexpression of dominant-negative SHP-2 resulted in a modest impairment of insulin-stimulated glucose transporter 4 translocation, suggesting SHP-2 may play a minor role as a positive modulator of the metabolic effects of insulin. In contrast, Ouwens et al. *(127)* reported that expression of SHP-2 in cells resulted in a negative regulation of IRS-1 phosphorylation, PI3K activation, and stimulation of glycogen synthesis in response to insulin. Thus, it remains to be seen whether SHP-2 plays a major physiological role in insulin signaling.

The dual specificity MKPs are able to dephosphorylate both phosphotyrosine and phosphothreonine residues in the activation loop of MAPKs and inactivate them. In mammalian cells, at least 10 MKPs have been identified and individual MKPs display differential selectivity toward different MAPK family members and MKPs are localized to the nucleus or cytoplasm *(128–130)*.

In general, serine/threonine protein phosphatases can be classified into the phosphoprotein phosphatase *(PPP)* and Mg^{2+}-dependent protein phosphatase *(PPM)* gene families on the basis of similarity in the primary amino acid sequence between the different catalytic subunits *(131)*. The PPP family includes the most abundant protein phosphatases—PP1, PP2A, and PP2B (calcineurin)— as well as more recently cloned enzymes such as PP4 (also known as PPX), PP5, PP6, and PP7. Five PPC2 isoforms, together with the pyruvate dehydrogenase phosphatase, constitute the gene family *PPM*. The catalytic subunit of PP1 has four mammalian isoforms and this phosphatase is inhibited by the cell-permeable toxins okadaic acid and calyculin A and the membrane-impermeable agent microcystin *(132,133)*. PP2A is spontaneously active and inhibited by the inhibitors of PP1 whereas PP2B, a Ca^{2+}-dependent protein, is not inhibited by these inhibitors *(134)*. In response to insulin, PP1 is activated and catalyzes the insulin-mediated dephosphorylation of metabolic enzymes. The glycogen-associated form of PP1 dephosphorylates both glycogen synthase (resulting in enzyme activation) and glycogen phosphorylase (resulting in inactivation) to provide insulin-mediated coordination of glycogen metabolism *(135)*. PP2A contributes to the dephosphorylation and regulation of MAPKs *(81,136)*.

As discussed in Subheading 2.3., many different phosphorylated derivatives of PI play diverse roles in cellular signaling. The versatility of these molecules as cellular signals results from PH domain specificity in recognizing particular configurations of the inositol phosphate headgroup. Much attention has focused on $PI(3,4,5)P_3$ as an intracellular second messenger produced rapidly via the action of PI3K in response to many divergent cellular stimuli. Phosphatase and tensin homologue deleted on chromosome 10 (PTEN) was discovered in 1997 as a new tumor suppressor and serves as an unusual phosphatase whose primary target is $PI(3,4,5)P_3$. The 3-phosphorylated inositol lipids, $PI(3,4,5)P_3$ and $PI(3,4)P_2$, are the most efficient substrates for PTEN, which removes phosphate from the D-3 position of the inositol ring.

Evidence suggests that protein stability, localization, and transcription of the *PTEN* gene regulate the function of PTEN. The regulation of stability and localization appears to be achieved through the C-terminal tail of PTEN via phosphorylation of multiple serine and threonine residues. Recently, it has been shown that PI3K activation stimulates PTEN phosphorylation, suggesting that one of the kinases activated by PI3K is likely to be involved in PTEN phosphorylation *(137)*.

3. METHODS FOR DETERMINATION OF SIGNALING PATHWAYS INVOLVED IN THE REGULATION OF DRUG METABOLIZING ENZYME GENE AND PROTEIN EXPRESSION

3.1. Methods for Examination of Protein Kinase Activity and Phosphorylation

Phosphorylation plays an essential role in the regulation of most protein kinases. Phosphorylation of specific residues is a major determinant of protein kinase activity. For example, the activation of Akt by insulin or growth factors is accompanied by phosphorylation on threonine-308 in the kinase domain and serine-473 in the C-terminal regulatory domain. Activation of Akt and phosphorylation of both these residues are abolished by treatment with the PI3K inhibitors, wortmannin or LY294002, prior to stimulation with an agonist such as insulin.

3.1.1. Immunoblot Analysis

Since first reported by Ross et al. *(138)*, antibodies reactive with phospho-residues (e.g., phosphotyrosine, phosphoserine, and phosphothreonine) have become invaluable tools for isolating phosphorylated proteins and examining phosphorylation states. Phospho-specific antibodies for many protein kinases have been developed and these antibodies can be used for immunoblot analysis, immunoprecipitation, immunocytochemistry, and flow cytometry. In general, immunoblot analysis, coimmunoprecipitation, and kinase activity assays are the most frequently used methods for examination of protein kinase activation. Phospho-specific antibodies against a number of kinases and receptors are commercially available, and are used in standard immunoblotting procedures. If phospho-specific antibodies are not available, the kinase or receptor can be immunoprecipitated followed by immunoblotting with antiphosphotyrosine/serine/threonine antibodies.

Protein kinase activation usually occurs within a few minutes of agonist binding to a receptor (e.g., insulin and growth factors), suggesting that the phosphorylation state is dynamically regulated. Thus, inhibition of phosphatase activity is very important during preparation of cell lysates. Treatment of cells with phosphatase inhibitors may result in activation of kinases. Generally, cell lysis buffer contains phosphatase inhibitors such as sodium orthovanadate, sodium fluoride, ethylenebis(oxyethylenenitrilo)tetraacetic acid, and okadaic acid, to prevent dephosphorylation of protein kinases and other phosphoproteins. In immunoblot analysis, Laemmli sample buffer that contains sodium dodecyl sulfate and dithiothreitol can be used directly for making cell lysates.

3.1.2. Kinase Activity Assays

For protein kinase assays, phospho-specific antibodies to protein kinases have been used for selectively immunoprecipitating activated protein kinases from cell lysates. This method depends on the availability of a specific immunoprecipitating antibody that does not interfere with the kinase activity, but many of these are commercially available. Protein kinase activity can be assayed by incorporation of phosphate from ATP into a synthetic peptide substrate based on the sequences of the phosphorylation sites on the target substrate protein. Many protein kinases phosphorylate the short peptide substrate with kinetic parameters similar to those of the native target proteins. In some cases, however, protein kinases that recognize or require an aspect of 3-D structure for their target, in addition to the primary sequence, will phosphorylate synthetic peptides poorly or not at all. Kinases that fall into this class must be assayed using the native protein target as substrate, or at least an expressed domain of the substrate that contains the requisite recognition features. Most protein kinase assays using synthetic peptides use radioactive ATP, resulting in a radiolabeled phosphopeptide that can be quantified by scintillation counting. Recently, nonradioactive kinase assays employing phospho-specific antibodies to the substrate protein have been developed and allow detection and quantification of kinase activity following immunoprecipitation of an active kinase.

3.2. Chemical Inhibitors of Protein Kinases

A widely used approach for examining the role of a kinase or kinase family in a cell signaling pathway is the pharmacological inhibition of the kinase (Fig. 5). To elucidate the signaling function of individual protein kinases and phosphatases, inhibitors should be potent, highly specific, and cell-membrane permeable. Many inhibitors of protein kinases and phosphatases have been developed as therapy for diseases such as cancer, inflammation, and diabetes. The vast majority of protein kinase inhibitors have been designed to target the ATP-binding site of protein kinases *(139)*. Expectations for inhibitor specificity were initially poor because the number of protein kinases encoded in the human genome is estimated to be in excess of 500, and the significant number of other cellular enzymes that use ATP further complicates the issue. Nevertheless, several ATP-binding site-directed protein kinase inhibitors have been developed with a high degree of selectivity. Based on the numerous structures of complexes with ATP, it is clear that the ATP-binding cleft has regions that are not occupied by ATP and these regions show structural diversity among kinases *(140)*. In general, these inhibitors are added to cells prior to agonist addition. For longer periods of treatment (e.g., 24–48 h), the inhibitor may need to be replenished because the inhibitor half-life may be limited.

Insulin Regulation of Drug-Metabolizing Enzymes 63

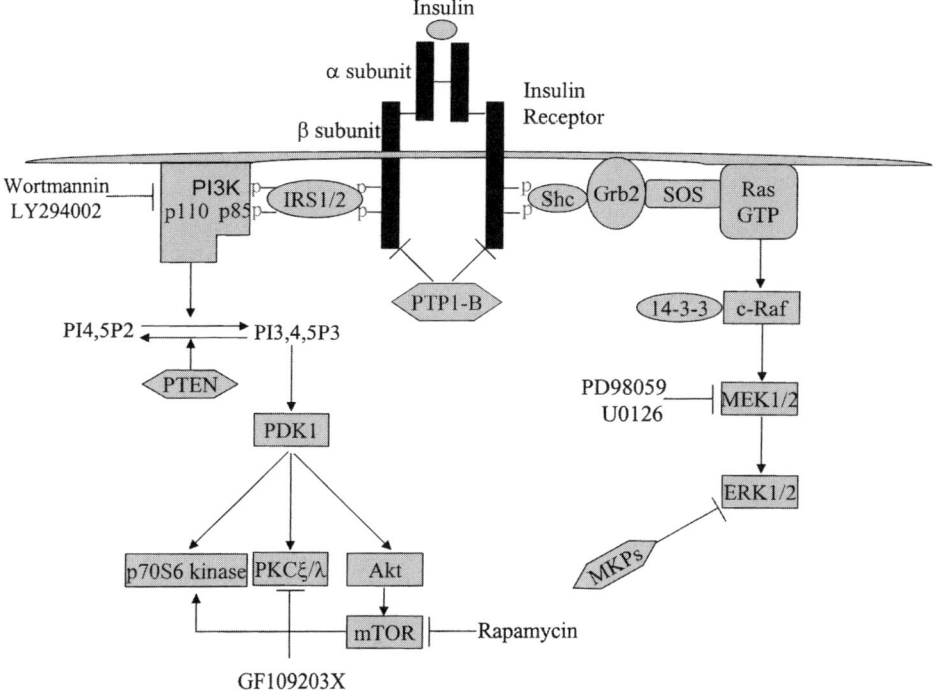

Fig. 5. Kinase inhibitors acting on insulin signaling pathways.

The inhibitors PD98059 and U0126 bind to the inactive form of MEK, preventing its activation by Raf-1 and other upstream activators *(141,142)*. These inhibitors do not compete with ATP and do not inhibit the phosphorylation of MEK, and thus are likely to have a distinct binding site on MEK. Quantitative evaluation of the steady-state kinetics of MEK inhibition by these compounds shows that U0126 has higher affinity than PD98059 *(142)*. In a comparison of multiple kinase inhibitors, the MEK1 and MEK2 inhibitors appeared to be the most specific kinase inhibitors tested *(143)*. But both of these inhibitors have recently been shown to inhibit activation of the ERK5 pathway through direct effects on MEK5 *(144)*. It is recommended that PD98059 or U0126 be added to cells at a concentration of 50–100 µM or 5–25 µM, respectively.

SB203580 and SB202190, a class of pyridinyl imidazoles, are relatively specific inhibitors of p38 MAPK α and β, but not p38 MAPK γ and δ, at a concentration of 10 µM *(145,146)*. However, these inhibitors were reported to inhibit the activation of PDK1 and its downstream effectors, including Akt and p70 S6 kinase *(147,148)*, although PDK1 activity remained unaffected by in vitro incubation with SB203580 or SB202190 *(143)*. We have found that in primary cultured rat hepatocytes, these p38 MAPK inhibitors failed to affect insulin-mediated Akt phosphorylation *(40)*. These compounds bind the ATP-binding cleft of the low-activity p38 MAPK, which binds ATP poorly *(149)*. As a consequence of binding the unphosphorylated form, these inhibitors appear to interfere with the activation of p38 MAPK. Generally, SB203580 and SB202190 completely inhibit p38 MAPK at a concentration of 10 μM.

SP600125, an anthrapyrazolone inhibitor of JNK1, JNK2 and JNK3, has been reported to inhibit JNKs through a reversible ATP-competition *(150)*. A number of studies have reported that the compound prevents the expression of several anti-inflammatory genes in cell-based assays and the activation of AP1 in synoviocytes *(150,151)*. The inhibitor is starting to be used more widely as a JNK inhibitor. However, Bain et al. *(152)* recently reported that SP600125 was a relatively weak inhibitor of JNK isoforms and also inhibited other protein kinases with similar or greater potency. Care must be used, therefore, when employing this inhibitor and in the interpretation of resulting data. For inhibition of JNKs, SP600126 has been used at a concentration of 10–25 μM.

SU6656 *(153)* and the related pyrazolopyrimidine, PP1 *(154)*, were developed as inhibitors of the Src family of enzymes. PP1 was originally described as a selective, ATP-competitive inhibitor of Src family kinases and has been widely used to investigate the contribution of Src kinases to a number of biological functions *(154)*. It is recommended that SU6656 be added to cells at a concentration of 1–5 μM.

Rapamycin, a potent immunosuppressant, rapidly inactivates p70 S6 kinase and prevents the activation of this kinase by all known agonists *(155,156)*. Rapamycin binds to the immunophilin FK506 binding protein 12, and the resultant complex interacts with the protein kinase mTOR/FKBP 12-rapamycin-associated protein, thereby inhibiting it. This leads to the dephosphorylation and inactivation of p70 S6 kinase *(157)*. Generally, rapamycin completely inhibits p70 S6 kinase at a concentration of 100 nM.

GF109203X (bisindolylmaleimide I; Gö6850) and Ro-31-8220 are bisindolylmaleimides that differ from each other in two functional groups and are analogues of staurosporine *(158,159)*. These inhibitors, which compete for the ATP binding site on PKC, have approx 100-fold selectivity for PKC over PKA *(160)*. They are both potent inhibitors of the α, β, and γ isoforms of PKC with IC_{50} values in the nanomolar range in vitro. However, micromolar concentrations of GF109203X are required to inhibit atypical PKCs *(161)*. These classes of compounds may also have the ability to selectivity inhibit PKC isoforms. Gö6976, another staurosporine-related compound, inhibits α- and β_1-PKCs when utilized at nanomolar concentrations, but fails to inhibit δ-, ϵ-, and ζ-PKC isoforms *(161)*. It is recommended that GF109203X be added to cells at a concentration of 1–10 μM.

Wortmannin and LY294002 are cell-permeable inhibitors of PI3K *(162,163)*. Wortmannin, an irreversible inhibitor, alkylates a lysine residue at the putative ATP binding site of p110α of PI3K and LY294002 is a pure competitive inhibitor of ATP. It is recommended that wortmannin or LY294002 be added to cells at a concentration of 100–500 nM or 10–20 µM, respectively. At higher concentrations, wortmannin inhibits a number of other kinases, including the class 2 PI3K *(164,165)*. If a longer incubation time is required, LY294002 is the inhibitor of choice rather than wortmannin, because of its higher stability in aqueous solution.

For longer treatment durations in highly metabolically competent cells, such as primary hepatocytes, the concentrations of protein kinase inhibitor recommended earlier may not be sufficient to inhibit each target protein kinase activity. Thus, higher concentrations of most of these inhibitors are often required to offset metabolism of the inhibitor, and care must therefore be exercised in the interpretation of these data.

In primary cultured rat hepatocytes, wortmannin and LY294002 effectively inhibit both basal and insulin-mediated Akt phosphorylation (Figs. 6 and 7). We have used these inhibitors to demonstrate that PI3K plays an obligatory role in the insulin-mediated induction of mEH protein (Fig. 8) and the insulin-mediated suppression of CYP2E1 mRNA expression *(37,48)*.

3.3. Dominant-Negative Protein Kinase Constructs

The activity of a protein kinase can be interfered with by expression of a dominant-negative mutant. The generation of dominant-negative mutants involves the design of an inactive form of the protein that can sequester interacting proteins. Some knowledge of the mechanism of regulation or function of the protein of interest is helpful when designing these molecules. In general, the activity of protein kinases requires the phosphorylation of specific residues for activation and the binding of ATP to a conserved protein motif for phosphorylation of effector proteins. Thus, the point mutation of the phosphorylation site or ATP-binding region can produce an inactivated kinase or kinase-dead mutant, respectively *(166,167)*. Overexpression of an inactive form of the kinase may act as a dominant-negative by sequestering interacting proteins or cofactors and thus inhibiting the activity of the endogenous wild-type kinase. Many protein kinases are inactive in resting cells and this basal inhibition is achieved by interaction with a regulatory protein or an inhibitory domain within the same polypeptide. Thus, in some cases, overexpression of a regulatory protein or an inhibitory domain can reduce or inhibit the ability of the pathway to stimulate the endogenous protein. Similarly, overexpression of a pseudosubstrate domain that can bind the enzyme but cannot be converted to product can often result in inhibition of signaling, as it will compete with the endogenous substrate *(168)*.

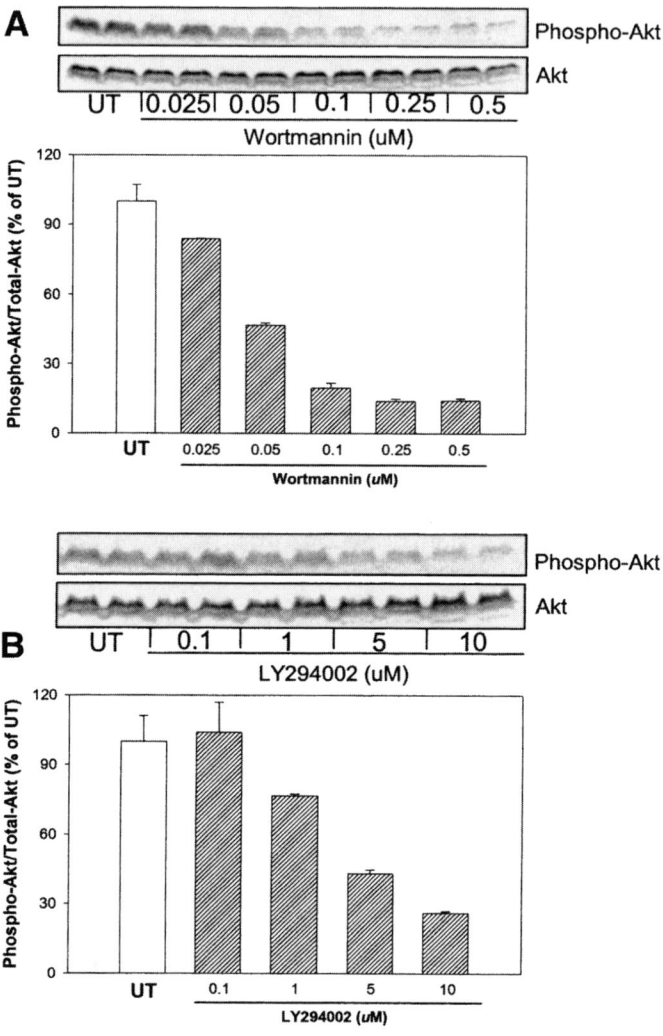

Fig. 6. The effects of the PI3K inhibitors, wortmannin (**A**) or LY294002 (**B**), on phosphorylation of Akt in rat hepatocytes cultured in the absence of insulin. Hepatocytes were treated with wortmannin or LY294002 for 4.5 h. Untreated (UT) hepatocytes were cultured in the absence of insulin and inhibitor. Phospho-Akt levels were normalized to total Akt levels. Values are shown as a percentage of the level of phospho-Akt/total-Akt in untreated hepatocytes (100% = 1245 arbitrary densitometry units of phospho-Akt and 1522 arbitrary densitometry units of Akt [A], 705 arbitrary densitometry units of phospho-Akt and 1471 arbitrary densitometry units of Akt [B]). Data are means ± SD of Western blot band densities of two preparations of cell lysates from a single hepatocyte preparation. (Reprinted from ref. *40* with permission.)

Insulin Regulation of Drug-Metabolizing Enzymes

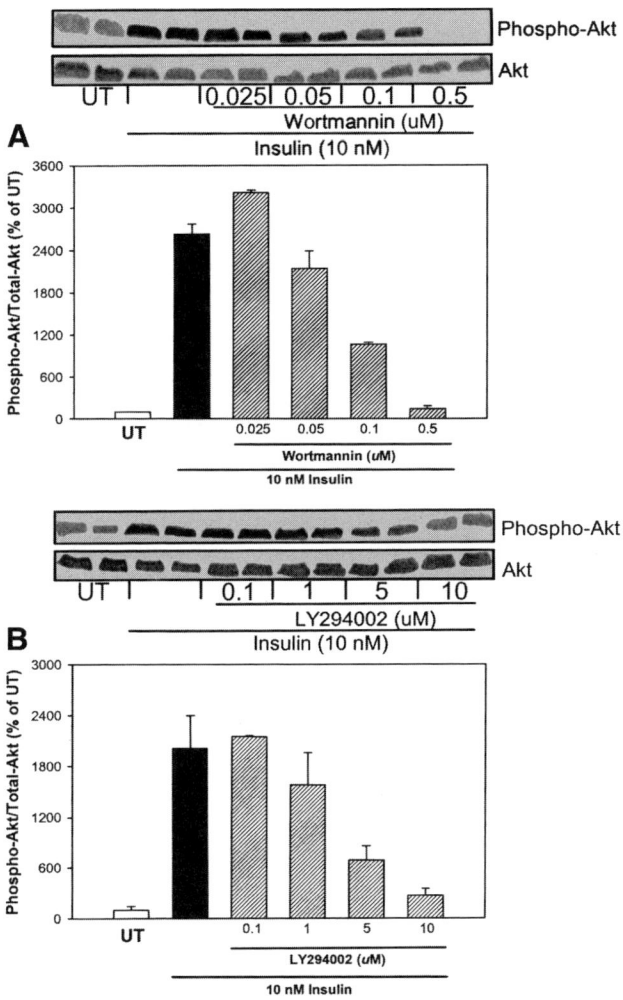

Fig. 7. The effects of the PI3K inhibitors, wortmannin (**A**) or LY294002 (**B**), on the insulin-mediated phosphorylation of Akt in primary cultured rat hepatocytes. Hepatocytes were treated with wortmannin or LY294002 for 1.5 h before addition of 10 nM insulin for 3 h. Untreated (UT) hepatocytes were cultured in the absence of insulin and inhibitor. Phospho-Akt levels were normalized to total Akt levels. Values are shown as a percentage of the level of phospho-Akt/total-Akt in untreated hepatocytes (100% = 84 arbitrary densitometry units of phospho-Akt and 776 arbitrary densitometry units of Akt [A], 36 arbitrary densitometry units of phospho-Akt and 473 arbitrary densitometry units of Akt [B]). Data are means ± SD of Western blot band densities of two preparations of cell lysates from a single hepatocyte preparation. (Reprinted from ref. *40* with permission.)

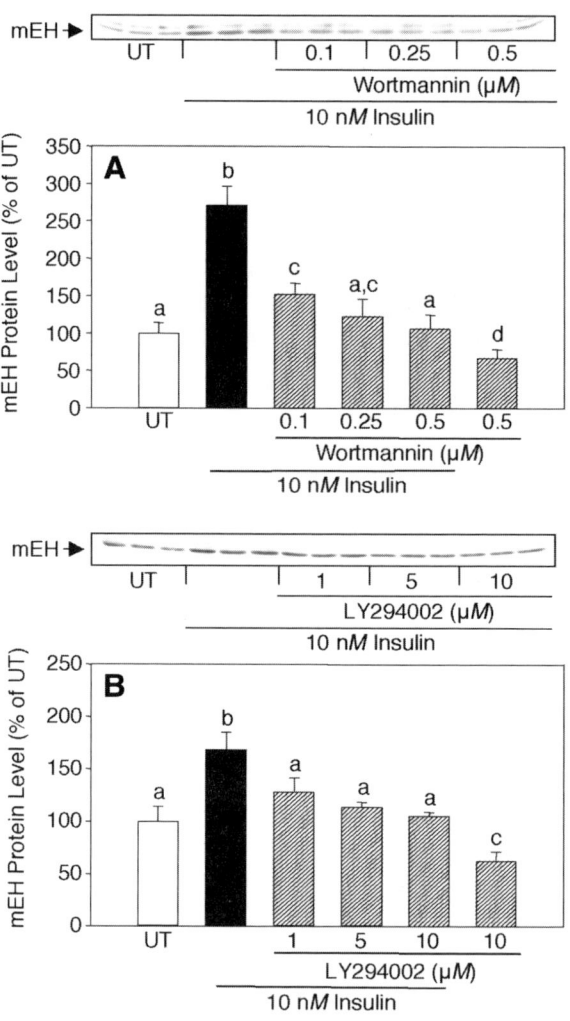

Fig. 8. Immunoblot analysis of the effects of the PI3K inhibitors, wortmannin (**A**) or LY294002 (**B**), on the insulin-mediated increase in mEH protein levels in primary cultured rat hepatocytes. (**A**) Hepatocytes were treated with wortmannin alone, or for 1.5 h prior to addition of 10 nM insulin for 24 h. (**B**) Hepatocytes were treated with LY294002 alone, or 1.5 h prior to addition of 10 nM insulin for 24 h. Untreated (UT) hepatocytes were cultured in the absence of insulin and inhibitors. Values are shown as a percentage of the level monitored in untreated hepatocytes (100% = 413 arbitrary densitometry units [A], 617 arbitrary densitometry units [B]). Data are means ± SD of Western blot band densities of three preparations of cell lysates from a single hepatocyte preparation. Values with different letters are significantly different from each other, $p < 0.05$. (Reprinted from Kim ref. *40* with permission.)

DNA constructs encoding inactive kinase mutants must be transported through the cell membrane and into the nucleus, to inhibit signaling pathways through their expression. There are several well-established techniques that allow transient transfection of recombinant DNA into cells in culture. These methods generally involve the permeabilization of cell membranes by chemical or electrical means, or the use of viral constructs that can recognize specific receptors on the cell surface, resulting in cellular uptake. A variety of viral systems, including adenoviruses and retroviruses, have become available for transporting recombinant DNA into cells *(169)*. The DNA can either be incorporated into the viral genome or be chemically linked to the exterior of the virion. After transfection of adenovirus into a mammalian cell, viral production may be monitored with green fluorescent protein (GFP), which is encoded by a gene incorporated into the viral backbone *(170)*. The most common methodologies have been reviewed in detail elsewhere *(170,171)*.

3.4. siRNA

In 1998, Fire and Mello described a new technology that was based on the silencing of specific genes by double-stranded RNA (dsRNA) and termed RNA interference (RNAi) *(172)*. RNAi consists of the presentation of a "triggering" dsRNA that is subsequently processed into 21–25 base-pair small interfering RNAs (siRNAs) through the action of the Dicer enzyme (RNase III endonuclease) *(173–175)*. siRNAs with 2-nucleotide 3'-end overhangs are then incorporated into a multisubunit RNA-induced silencing complex, which targets their complementary RNA transcript for enzymatic degradation *(176)*. The siRNA-induced degradation of mRNA is highly sequence-specific, to the extent that even a one- or two-nucleotide difference in the targeting recognition sequence hampers RNAi function.

In contrast to siRNAs, small temporal RNA (stRNA) molecules, which represent a large group of small transcripts called micro-RNAs, mediate gene suppression by inhibiting translation of target mRNA *(177,178)*. In common with siRNAs, Dicer is also involved in the processing of the 21- to 23-nucleotide stRNAs from approx 70-nucleotide stable hairpin precursors *(179)*. But stRNAs are stem-loops that are processed into an imperfect complementary dsRNA that inhibit protein translation of an imperfectly matched target sequence, which is almost invariably located at the 3'-untranslated region of the target mRNA *(180)*.

In mammalian somatic cells, dsRNAs longer than 30 nucleotides activate an antiviral defense mechanism that includes the production of interferon and activation of dsRNA-dependent protein kinase, resulting in inhibition of protein synthesis initiation and stimulation of apoptosis *(181,182)*. One mechanism for dealing with these nonspecific dsRNA responses is to create dsRNA triggers of fewer than 30 base pairs in length. Both siRNA and stRNA are long enough to induce sequence-specific suppression, but short enough to evade the host defense response. Although the use of siRNAs to silence genes in vertebrate cells was reported only a few years ago, the emerging literature indicates that most vertebrate genes can be studied with this technology.

Several laboratories demonstrated that synthesized dsRNAs induced sequence-specific gene silencing when transiently transfected into mammalian cells *(183,184)*. Factors that could ultimately limit the usefulness of siRNAs include a relatively short and transient period of activity. The longevity of silencing is dependent on abundance of mRNA and protein, stability of protein, the half-life of the silencing complex, and cell division rate. Generally the siRNA directs rapid reduction in mRNA levels that is readily observed in 18 h or less and siRNA-mediated RNAi lasts for 3–5 d for most cell lines *(185)*.

Recently a number of studies have reported the success of using RNA polymerase III promoters, such as U6 or H1, to direct in vivo synthesis of functional siRNAs *(186–191)*. These siRNAs have been expressed in two ways. In the first case, hairpin constructs are expressed from a single RNA polymerase III promoter. The resulting RNAs are predicted to form hairpins containing 19- to 29-nucleotide stems that match target sequences precisely, three- or nine-nucleotide loops and 3' overhangs of four or fewer uridines. It is believed that these hairpin RNAs are processed by Dicer to active siRNAs in vivo *(192)*. In the second case, coding and noncoding strands of a potential siRNA are driven from separate promoters and the expressed transcripts anneal in the cell nucleus. The hairpin siRNA strategy appears to inhibit gene expression more efficiently than the duplex siRNAs expressed from two separate plasmids *(192)*. The use of a plasmid-based RNA polymerase III promoter system to intracellularly produce siRNAs could allow for a longer period of expression as compared with exogenously added siRNAs.

An alternative approach to prolong siRNA-mediated inhibition of gene expression is the introduction of modified nucleotides into chemically synthesized RNA. Amarzguioui et al. *(193)* reported that siRNA generally tolerated mutations in the 5'-end, while the 3'-end exhibited low tolerance. An siRNA with two 2'-O-methyl RNA nucleotides at the 5'-end and four methylated monomers at the 3'-end was as active as its unmodified counterpart and led to a prolonged silencing effect in cell culture *(193)*.

The effectiveness of an siRNA is likely to be determined by the accessibility of its target sequence in the intended substrate. It has been suggested that the first 50–100 nucleotides of an mRNA sequence, downstream of the translation initiation sequence, should be used to target a gene and that 5'- or 3'-untranslated regions, as well as highly conserved domains (i.e., catalytic, ligand binding, etc.), should be avoided, as they are likely to contain regulatory protein binding sites *(190)*. However, successful gene inhibition has been reported for siRNAs targeting various sequences, including the 3′-untranslated region *(194)*. There are no reliable ways to predict or identify the "ideal" sequence for an siRNA. However, targeting different regions of a given mRNA might give different results *(185)*. Generally, siRNAs become susceptible to RNase H; therefore, the degree of the RNase H sensitivity of a given probe reflects the RNase H accessibility of the chosen sites. In practical terms, it might be just as easy to construct and test several siRNAs.

4. CONCLUSION

It is becoming increasingly clear that endogenous factors, including hormones and growth factors, play an important role in the regulation of drug-metabolizing enzyme expression in both physiological and pathophysiological conditions. Our laboratory has used phospho-specific antibodies and chemical inhibitors of protein kinases to define the signaling pathways involved in insulin- and glucagon-mediated regulation of several drug-metabolizing enzymes *(40,48)*. Small molecule chemical inhibitors of protein kinases used for this purpose in many studies, however, have been reported to have specificity problems, although many chemicals have been considered to be reasonably selective inhibitors for each target protein kinase. As with all pharmacological tools, interpretation of experiments with these protein kinase inhibitors requires caution. It is advisable to conduct experiments with at least two pharmacologically distinct inhibitors wherever possible. Dominant-negative kinase constructs allow for more kinase-specific inhibition. Recently, RNAi methods have opened new opportunities for investigators to study cell signaling pathways by leading to a highly specific mRNA degradation. Furthermore, retrovirus or adenovirus vectors have been developed for use in carrying dominant-negative kinase constructs or siRNA-expressing DNA templates into cells to mediate gene-specific silencing in cells or animals. Thus, RNAi using siRNAs to silence specific genes is a very promising method for determination of cell signaling pathways involved in protein expression in response to hormones and growth factors.

REFERENCES

1. Duvaldestin P, Mahu J-L, Berthelot P. Effect of fasting on substrate specificity of rat liver UDP-glucuronosyltransferase. Biochim Biophys Acta 1975;384:81–86.
2. Abernethy DR, Greenblatt DJ, Divoll M, Shader RI. Enhanced glucuronide conjugation of drugs in obesity: studies of lorazepam, oxazepam, and acetaminophen. J Lab Clin Med 1983;101:873–880.
3. Hong JY, Pan JM, Gonzalez FJ, Gelboin HV, Yang CS. The induction of a specific form of cytochrome P-450 (P-450j) by fasting. Biochem Biophys Res Commun 1987;142:1077–1083.

4. Bellward GD, Chang T, Rodrigues B, et al. Hepatic cytochrome P-450j induction in the spontaneously diabetic BB rat. Mol Pharmacol 1988;33:140–143.
5. Thomas H, Schladt L, Knehr M, Oesch F. Effect of diabetes and starvation on the activity of rat liver epoxide hydrolases, glutathione S-transferases and peroxisomal beta-oxidation. Biochem Pharmacol 1989;38:4291–4297.
6. Yamazoe Y, Murayama N, Shimada M, Yamauchi K, Kato R. Cytochrome P450 in livers of diabetic rats: regulation by growth hormone and insulin. Arch Biochem Biophys 1989;268:567–575.
7. Barnett CR, Gibson GG, Wolf CR, Flatt PR, Ioannides C. Induction of cytochrome P450III and P450IV family proteins in streptozotocin-induced diabetes. Biochem J 1990;268:765–769.
8. Song BJ, Veech RL, Saenger P. Cytochrome P450IIE1 is elevated in lymphocytes from poorly controlled insulin-dependent diabetics. J Clin Endocrinol Metab 1990; 71:1036–1040.
9. Donahue BS, Skottner-Lundin A, Morgan ET. Growth hormone-dependent and -independent regulation of cytochrome P-450 isozyme expression in streptozotocin-diabetic rats. Endocrinology 1991;128:2065–2076.
10. Chaudhary IP, Tuntaterdtum S, McNamara PJ, Robertson LW, Blouin RA. Effect of genetic obesity and phenobarbital treatment on the hepatic conjugation pathways. J Pharmacol Exp Ther 1993;265:1333–1338.
11. Ronis MJ, Huang J, Crouch J, et al. Cytochrome P450 CYP 2E1 induction during chronic alcohol exposure occurs by a two-step mechanism associated with blood alcohol concentrations in rats. J Pharmacol Exp Ther 1993;264:944–950.
12. Shimojo N, Ishizaki T, Imaoka S, Funae Y, Fujii S, Okuda K. Changes in amounts of cytochrome P450 isozymes and levels of catalytic activities in hepatic and renal microsomes of rats with streptozocin-induced diabetes. Biochem Pharmacol 1993; 46:621–627.
13. Van de Wiel JA, Fijneman PH, Teeuw KB, Van Ommen B, Noordhoek J, Bos RP. Influence of long-term ethanol treatment on rat liver biotransformation enzymes. Alcohol 1993;10:397–402.
14. Runge-Morris M, Vento C. Effects of streptozotocin-induced diabetes on rat liver sulfotransferase gene expression. Drug Metab Dispos 1995;23:455–459.
15. Visser TJ, van Haasteren GA, Linkels E, Kaptein E, van Toor H, de Greef WJ. Gender-specific changes in thyroid hormone-glucuronidating enzymes in rat liver during short-term fasting and long-term food restriction. Eur J Endocrinol 1996; 135:489–497.
16. Braun L, Coffey MJ, Puskas F, et al. Molecular basis of bilirubin UDP-glucuronosyltransferase induction in spontaneously diabetic rats, acetone-treated rats and starved rats. Biochem J 1998;336:587–592.
17. Kardon T, Coffey MJ, Banhegyi G, et al. Transcriptional induction of bilirubin UDP-glucuronosyltransrase by ethanol in rat liver. Alcohol 2000;21:251–257.
18. Agius C, Gidari AS. Effect of streptozotocin on the glutathione S-transferases of mouse liver cytosol. Biochem Pharmacol 1985;34:811–819.

19. Grant MH, Duthie SJ. Conjugation reactions in hepatocytes isolated from streptozotocin-induced diabetic rats. Biochem Pharmacol 1987;36:3647–3655.
20. Mukherjee B, Mukherjee JR, Chatterjee M. Lipid peroxidation, glutathione levels and changes in glutathione-related enzyme activities in streptozotocin-induced diabetic rats. Immunol Cell Biol 1994;72:109–114.
21. Raza H, Ahmed I, Lakhani MS, Sharma AK, Pallot D, Montague W. Effect of bitter melon (Momordica charantia) fruit juice on the hepatic cytochrome P450-dependent monooxygenases and glutathione S-transferases in streptozotocin-induced diabetic rats. Biochem Pharmacol 1996;52:1639–1642.
22. Wasserman WW, Fahl WE. Functional antioxidant responsive elements. Proc Natl Acad Sci USA 1997;94:5361–5366.
23. Kang KW, Cho MK, Lee CH, Kim SG. Activation of phosphatidylinositol 3-kinase and Akt by tert-butylhydroquinone is responsible for antioxidant response element-mediated rGSTA2 induction in H4IIE cells. Mol Pharmacol 2001;59:1147–1156.
24. Dong ZG, Hong JY, Ma QA, et al. Mechanism of induction of cytochrome P-450ac (P-450j) in chemically induced and spontaneously diabetic rats. Arch Biochem Biophys 1988;263:29–35.
25. Favreau LV, Schenkman JB. Composition changes in hepatic microsomal cytochrome P-450 during onset of streptozotocin-induced diabetes and during insulin treatment. Diabetes 1988;37:577–584.
26. Yamazoe Y, Murayama N, Shimada M, Imaoka S, Funae Y, Kato R. Suppression of hepatic levels of an ethanol-inducible P-450DM/j by growth hormone: relationship between the increased level of P-450DM/j and depletion of growth hormone in diabetes. Mol Pharmacol 1989;36:716–722.
27. Donahue BS, Morgan ET. Effects of vanadate on hepatic cytochrome P-450 expression in streptozotocin-diabetic rats. Drug Metab Dispos 1990;18:519–526.
28. Thummel KE, Schenkman JB. Effects of testosterone and growth hormone treatment on hepatic microsomal P450 expression in the diabetic rat. Mol Pharmacol 1990;37:119–129.
29. Tunon MJ, Gonzalez P, Garcia-Pardo LA, Gonzalez J. Hepatic transport of bilirubin in rats with streptozotocin-induced diabetes. J Hepatol 1991;13:71–77.
30. Constantopoulos A, Matsaniotis N. Augmentation of uridine diphosphate glucuronyltransferase activity in rat liver by adenosine 3′,5′-monophosphate. Gastroenterology 1978;75:486–491.
31. Ricci GL, Fevery J. Treatment of rats with glucagon, vasointestinal peptide or secretin has a different effect on bilirubin and p-nitrophenol UDP-glucuronyltransferase. Biochem Pharmacol 1988;37:3526–3528.
32. Carrillo MC, Monti JA, Favre C, Carnovale CE. Acute regulation of hepatic glutathione S-transferase by insulin and glucagon. Toxicol Lett 1995;76:105–111.
33. Kim SK, Woodcroft KJ, Novak RF. Insulin and glucagon regulation of glutathione S-transferase expression in primary cultured rat hepatocytes. J Pharmacol Exp Ther 2003;305:353–361.

34. De Waziers I, Garlatti M, Bouguet J, Beaune PH, Barouki R. Insulin down-regulates cytochrome P450 2B and 2E expression at the post-transcriptional level in the rat hepatoma cell line. Mol Pharmacol 1995;47:474–479.
35. Woodcroft KJ, Novak RF. Insulin effects on CYP2E1, 2B, 3A, and 4A expression in primary cultured rat hepatocytes. Chem Biol Interact 1997;107:75–91.
36. Woodcroft KJ, Novak RF. Insulin differentially affects xenobiotic-enhanced, cytochrome P-450 (CYP)2E1, CYP2B, CYP3A, and CYP4A expression in primary cultured rat hepatocytes. J Pharmacol Exp Ther 1999;289:1121–1127.
37. Woodcroft KJ, Novak RF. The role of phosphatidylinositol 3-kinase, Src kinase, and protein kinase A signaling pathways in insulin and glucagon regulation of CYP2E1 expression. Biochem Biophys Res Commun 1999;266:304–307.
38. Iber H, Li-Masters T, Chen Q, Yu S, Morgan ET. Regulation of hepatic cytochrome P450 2C11 via cAMP: implications for down-regulation in diabetes, fasting, and inflammation. J Pharmacol Exp Ther 2001;297:174–180.
39. Viitala P, Posti K, Lindfors A, Pelkonen O, Raunio H. cAMP mediated upregulation of CYP2A5 in mouse hepatocytes. Biochem Biophys Res Commun 2001;280: 761–767.
40. Kim SK, Woodcroft KJ, Kim SG, Novak RF. Insulin and glucagon signaling in regulation of microsomal epoxide hydrolase expression in primary cultured rat hepatocytes. Drug Metab Dispos 2003;31:1260–1268.
41. Iber H, Morgan ET. Regulation of hepatic cytochrome P450 2C11 by transforming growth factor-beta, hepatocyte growth factor, and interleukin-11. Drug Metab Dispos 1998;26:1042–1044.
42. Donato MT, Gomez-Lechon MJ, Jover R, Nakamura T, Castell JV. Human hepatocyte growth factor down-regulates the expression of cytochrome P450 isozymes in human hepatocytes in primary culture. J Pharmacol Exp Ther 1998;284:760–767.
43. Ching KZ, Tenney KA, Chen J, Morgan ET. Suppression of constitutive cytochrome P450 gene expression by epidermal growth factor receptor ligands in cultured rat hepatocytes. Drug Metab Dispos 1996;24:542–546.
44. De Smet K, Loyer P, Gilot D, Vercruysse A, Rogiers V, Guguen-Guillouzo C. Effects of epidermal growth factor on CYP inducibility by xenobiotics, DNA replication, and caspase activations in collagen I gel sandwich cultures of rat hepatocytes. Biochem Pharmacol 2001;61:1293–1303.
45. Garcia MC, Thangavel C, Shapiro BH. Epidermal growth factor regulation of female-dependent CYP2A1 and CYP2C12 in primary rat hepatocyte culture. Drug Metab Dispos 2001;29:111–120.
46. Matsumoto M, Imagawa M, Aoki Y. Epidermal growth factor regulation of glutathione S-transferase gene expression in the rat is mediated by class Pi glutathione S-transferase enhancer I. Biochem J 2000;349:225–230.
47. Desmots F, Rissel M, Gilot D, et al. Pro-inflammatory cytokines tumor necrosis factor α and interleukin-6 and survival factor epidermal growth factor positively regulate the murine GSTA4 enzyme in hepatocytes. J Biol Chem 2002;277: 17892–17900.

48. Woodcroft KJ, Hafner MS, Novak RF. Insulin signaling in the transcriptional and posttranscriptional regulation of CYP2E1 expression. Hepatology 2002;35: 263–273.
49. Perz M, Torlinska T. Insulin receptor—structural and functional characteristics. Med Sci Monit 2001;7:169–177.
50. Sparrow LG, McKern NM, Gorman JJ, et al. The disulfide bonds in the C-terminal domains of the human insulin receptor ectodomain. J Biol Chem 1997;272: 29460–29467.
51. Cheatham B, Kahn CR. Cysteine 647 in the insulin receptor is required for normal covalent interaction between α- and β-subunits and signal transduction. J Biol Chem 1992;267:7108–7115.
52. Kahn CR. Banting Lecture. Insulin action, diabetogenes, and the cause of type II diabetes. Diabetes 1994;43:1066–1084.
53. White MF, Kahn CR. The insulin signaling system. J Biol Chem 1994;269:1–4.
54. White MF. IRS proteins and the common path to diabetes. Am J Physiol 2002; 283:E413–E422.
55. Kao AW, Waters SB, Okada S, Pessin JE. Insulin stimulates the phosphorylation of the 66- and 52-kilodalton Shc isoforms by distinct pathways. Endocrinology 1997; 138:2474–2480.
56. Sasaoka T, Kobayashi M. The functional significance of Shc in insulin signaling as a substrate of the insulin receptor. Endocr J 2000;47:373–381.
57. Jorissen RN, Walker F, Pouliot N, Garrett TP, Ward CW, Burgess AW. Epidermal growth factor receptor: mechanisms of activation and signalling. Exp Cell Res 2003;284:31–53.
58. Whiteley B, Glaser L. Epidermal growth factor (EGF) promotes phosphorylation at threonine-654 of the EGF receptor: possible role of protein kinase C in homologous regulation of the EGF receptor. J Cell Biol 1986;103:1355–1362.
59. Tice DA, Biscardi JS, Nickles AL, Parsons SJ. Mechanism of biological synergy between cellular Src and epidermal growth factor receptor. Proc Natl Acad Sci USA 1999;96:1415–1420.
60. Fruman DA, Meyers RE, Cantley LC. Phosphoinositide kinases. Annu Rev Biochem 1998;67:481–507.
61. Cantley LC. The phosphoinositide 3-kinase pathway. Science 2002;296:1655–1657.
62. Shields JM, Pruitt K, McFall A, Shaub A, Der CJ. Understanding Ras: 'it ain't over 'til it's over'. Trends Cell Biol 2000;10:147–154.
63. Alessi DR, Deak M, Casamayor A, et al. 3-Phosphoinositide-dependent protein kinase-1 (PDK1): structural and functional homology with the Drosophila DSTPK61 kinase. Curr Biol 1997;7:776–789.
64. Le Good JA, Ziegler WH, Parekh DB, Alessi DR, Cohen P, Parker PJ. Protein kinase C isotypes controlled by phosphoinositide 3-kinase through the protein kinase PDK1. Science 1998;281:2042–2045.
65. Vanhaesebroeck B, Alessi DR. The PI3K-PDK1 connection: more than just a road to PKB. Biochem J 2000;346:561–576.

66. Chan TO, Rittenhouse SE, Tsichlis PN. AKT/PKB and other D3 phosphoinositide-regulated kinases: kinase activation by phosphoinositide-dependent phosphorylation. Annu Rev Biochem 1999;68:965–1014.
67. Alessi DR, Andjelkovic M, Caudwell B, et al. Mechanism of activation of protein kinase B by insulin and IGF-1. EMBO J 1996;15:6541–6551.
68. Jefferies HB, Fumagalli S, Dennis PB, Reinhard C, Pearson RB, Thomas G. Rapamycin suppresses 5'TOP mRNA translation through inhibition of p70s6k. EMBO J 1997;16:3693–3704.
69. Kawasome H, Papst P, Webb S, et al. Targeted disruption of p70(s6k) defines its role in protein synthesis and rapamycin sensitivity. Proc Natl Acad Sci USA 1998; 95:5033–5038.
70. Kohn AD, Takeuchi F, Roth RA. Akt, a pleckstrin homology domain containing kinase, is activated primarily by phosphorylation. J Biol Chem 1996;271: 21920–21926.
71. Conus NM, Hemmings BA, Pearson RB. Differential regulation by calcium reveals distinct signaling requirements for the activation of Akt and p70S6k. J Biol Chem 1998;273:4776–4782.
72. Dufner A, Andjelkovic M, Burgering BM, Hemmings BA, Thomas G. Protein kinase B localization and activation differentially affect S6 kinase 1 activity and eukaryotic translation initiation factor 4E-binding protein 1 phosphorylation. Mol Cell Biol 1999;19:4525–4534.
73. Farese RV. Insulin-sensitive phospholipid signaling systems and glucose transport. Update II. Exp Biol Med (Maywood) 2001;226:283–295.
74. Standaert ML, Bandyopadhyay G, Perez L, et al. Insulin activates protein kinases C-zeta and C-lambda by an autophosphorylation-dependent mechanism and stimulates their translocation to GLUT4 vesicles and other membrane fractions in rat adipocytes. J Biol Chem 1999;274:25308–25316.
75. Standaert ML, Bandyopadhyay G, Kanoh Y, Sajan MP, Farese RV. Insulin and PIP3 activate PKC-zeta by mechanisms that are both dependent and independent of phosphorylation of activation loop (T410) and autophosphorylation (T560) sites. Biochemistry 2001;40:249–255.
76. Mendez R, Kollmorgen G, White MF, Rhoads RE. Requirement of protein kinase C zeta for stimulation of protein synthesis by insulin. Mol Cell Biol 1997;17: 5184–5192.
77. Romanelli A, Martin KA, Toker A, Blenis J. p70 S6 kinase is regulated by protein kinase Czeta and participates in a phosphoinositide 3-kinase-regulated signalling complex. Mol Cell Biol 1999;19:2921–2928.
78. Khosravi-Far R, Campbell S, Rossman KL, Der CJ. Increasing complexity of Ras signal transduction: involvement of Rho family proteins. Adv Cancer Res 1998;72: 57–107.
79. Chong H, Vikis HG, Guan KL. Mechanisms of regulating the Raf kinase family. Cell Signal 2003;15:463–469.
80. Tzivion G, Luo Z, Avruch J. A dimeric 14-3-3 protein is an essential cofactor for Raf kinase activity. Nature 1998;394:88–92.

81. Kubicek M, Pacher M, Abraham D, Podar K, Eulitz M, Baccarini M. Dephosphorylation of Ser-259 regulates Raf-1 membrane association. J Biol Chem 2002; 277:7913–7919.
82. Light Y, Paterson H, Marais R. 14-3-3 antagonizes Ras-mediated Raf-1 recruitment to the plasma membrane to maintain signaling fidelity. Mol Cell Biol 2002;22:4984–4996.
83. Mason CS, Springer CJ, Cooper RG, Superti-Furga G, Marshall CJ, Marais R. Serine and tyrosine phosphorylations cooperate in Raf-1, but not B-Raf activation. EMBO J 1999;18:2137–2148.
84. Catling AD, Schaeffer HJ, Reuter CW, Reddy GR, Weber MJ. A proline-rich sequence unique to MEK1 and MEK2 is required for raf binding and regulates MEK function. Mol Cell Biol 1995;15:5214–5225.
85. Lewis TS, Shapiro PS, Ahn NG. Signal transduction through MAP kinase cascades. Adv Cancer Res 1998;74:49–139.
86. Kyriakis JM, Avruch J. Mammalian mitogen-activated protein kinase signal transduction pathways activated by stress and inflammation. Physiol Rev 2001;81: 807–869.
87. Hagemann C, Blank JL. The ups and downs of MEK kinase interactions. Cell Signal 2001;13:863–875.
88. Duckworth BC, Cantley LC. Conditional inhibition of the mitogen-activated protein kinase cascade by wortmannin. Dependence on signal strength. J Biol Chem 1997;272:27665–27670.
89. Bisotto S, Fixman ED. Src-family tyrosine kinases, phosphoinositide 3-kinase and Gab1 regulate extracellular signal-regulated kinase 1 activation induced by the type A endothelin-1 G-protein-coupled receptor. Biochem J 2001;360:77–85.
90. Yu CF, Roshan B, Liu ZX, Cantley LG. ERK regulates the hepatocyte growth factor-mediated interaction of Gab1 and the phosphatidylinositol 3-kinase. J Biol Chem 2001;276:32552–3558.
91. Yu CF, Liu ZX, Cantley LG. ERK negatively regulates the epidermal growth factor-mediated interaction of Gab1 and the phosphatidylinositol 3-kinase. J Biol Chem 2002;277:19382–19388.
92. Moelling K, Schad K, Bosse M, Zimmermann S, Schweneker M. Regulation of Raf-Akt Cross-talk. J Biol Chem 2002;277:31099–31106.
93. Park HS, Kim MS, Huh SH, et al. Akt (protein kinase B) negatively regulates SEK1 by means of protein phosphorylation. J Biol Chem 2002;277:2573–2578.
94. Fujishiro M, Gotoh Y, Katagiri H, et al. Three mitogen-activated protein kinases inhibit insulin signaling by different mechanisms in 3T3-L1 adipocytes. Mol Endocrinol 2003;17:487–497.
95. Kim JW, Lee JE, Kim MJ, Cho EG, Cho SG, Choi EJ. Glycogen synthase kinase 3 beta is a natural activator of mitogen-activated protein kinase/extracellular signal-regulated kinase kinase kinase 1 (MEKK1). J Biol Chem 2003;278:13995–14001.
96. Lee YH, Giraud J, Davis RJ, White MF. c-Jun N-terminal kinase (JNK) mediates feedback inhibition of the insulin signaling cascade. J Biol Chem 2003;278: 2896–2902.

97. Yamamoto-Honda R, Tobe K, Kaburagi Y, et al. Upstream mechanisms of glycogen synthase activation by insulin and insulin-like growth factor-I. Glycogen synthase activation is antagonized by wortmannin or LY294002 but not by rapamycin or by inhibiting p21ras. J Biol Chem 1995;270:2729–2734.
98. Nakamura K, Zhou CJ, Parente J, Chew CS. Parietal cell MAP kinases: multiple activation pathways. Am J Physiol 1996;271:G640–G649.
99. Scheid MP, Duronio V. Phosphatidylinositol 3-OH kinase activity is not required for activation of mitogen-activated protein kinase by cytokines. J Biol Chem 1996; 271:18134–18139.
100. Cross DA, Alessi DR, Vandenheede JR, McDowell HE, Hundal HS, Cohen P. The inhibition of glycogen synthase kinase-3 by insulin or insulin-like growth factor 1 in the rat skeletal muscle cell line L6 is blocked by wortmannin, but not by rapamycin: evidence that wortmannin blocks activation of the mitogen-activated protein kinase pathway in L6 cells between Ras and Raf. Biochem J 1994;303:21–26.
101. Standaert ML, Bandyopadhyay G, Farese RV. Studies with wortmannin suggest a role for phosphatidylinositol 3-kinase in the activation of glycogen synthase and mitogen-activated protein kinase by insulin in rat adipocytes: comparison of insulin and protein kinase C modulators. Biochem Biophys Res Commun 1995; 209:1082–1088.
102. Marra F, Pinzani M, DeFranco R, Laffi G, Gentilini P. Involvement of phosphatidylinositol 3-kinase in the activation of extracellular signal-regulated kinase by PDGF in hepatic stellate cells. FEBS Lett 1995;376:141–145.
103. Zimmermann S, Moelling K. Phosphorylation and regulation of Raf by Akt (protein kinase B). Science 1999;286:1741–1744.
104. Rommel C, Clarke BA, Zimmermann S, et al. Differentiation stage-specific inhibition of the Raf-MEK-ERK pathway by Akt. Science 1999;286:1738–1741.
105. Hirosumi J, Tuncman G, Chang L, et al. A central role for JNK in obesity and insulin resistance. Nature 2002;420:333–336.
106. Zhang ZY, Zhou B, Xie L. Modulation of protein kinase signaling by protein phosphatases and inhibitors. Pharmacol Ther 2002;93:307–317.
107. Asante-Appiah E, Kennedy BP. Protein tyrosine phosphatases: the quest for negative regulators of insulin action. Am J Physiol 2003;284:E663–E670.
108. Wu C, Sun M, Liu L, Zhou GW. The function of the protein tyrosine phosphatase SHP-1 in cancer. Gene 2003;306:1–12.
109. Elchebly M, Cheng A, Tremblay ML. Modulation of insulin signaling by protein tyrosine phosphatases. J Mol Med 2000;78:473–482.
110. Tonks NK, Diltz CD, Fischer EH. Characterization of the major protein-tyrosine-phosphatases of human placenta. J Biol Chem 1988;263:6731–6737.
111. Charbonneau H, Tonks NK, Kumar S, et al. Human placenta protein-tyrosine-phosphatase: amino acid sequence and relationship to a family of receptor-like proteins. Proc Natl Acad Sci USA 1989;86:5252–5256.
112. Frangioni JV, Oda A, Smith M, Salzman EW, Neel BG. Calpain-catalyzed cleavage and subcellular relocation of protein phosphotyrosine phosphatase 1B (PTP-1B) in human platelets. EMBO J 1993;12:4843–4856.

113. Elchebly M, Payette P, Michaliszyn E, et al. Increased insulin sensitivity and obesity resistance in mice lacking the protein tyrosine phosphatase-1B gene. Science 1999;283:1544–1548.
114. Salmeen A, Andersen JN, Myers MP, Tonks NK, Barford D. Molecular basis for the dephosphorylation of the activation segment of the insulin receptor by protein tyrosine phosphatase 1B. Mol Cell 2000;6:1401–1412.
115. Seely BL, Staubs PA, Reichart DR, et al. Protein tyrosine phosphatase 1B interacts with the activated insulin receptor. Diabetes 1996;45:1379–1385.
116. Bandyopadhyay D, Kusari A, Kenner KA, et al. Protein-tyrosine phosphatase 1B complexes with the insulin receptor in vivo and is tyrosine-phosphorylated in the presence of insulin. J Biol Chem 1997;272:1639–1645.
117. Mahadev K, Zilbering A, Zhu L, Goldstein BJ. Insulin-stimulated hydrogen peroxide reversibly inhibits protein-tyrosine phosphatase 1b in vivo and enhances the early insulin action cascade. J Biol Chem 2001;276:21938–21942.
118. Wu X, Hoffstedt J, Deeb W, et al. Depot-specific variation in protein-tyrosine phosphatase activities in human omental and subcutaneous adipose tissue: a potential contribution to differential insulin sensitivity. J Clin Endocrinol Metab 2001; 86:5973–5980.
119. Dadke S, Kusari A, Kusari J. Phosphorylation and activation of protein tyrosine phosphatase (PTP) 1B by insulin receptor. Mol Cell Biochem 2001;221:147–154.
120. Ravichandran LV, Chen H, Li Y, Quon MJ. Phosphorylation of PTP1B at Ser(50) by Akt impairs its ability to dephosphorylate the insulin receptor. Mol Endocrinol 2001;15:1768–1780.
121. Tao J, Malbon CC, Wang HY. Insulin stimulates tyrosine phosphorylation and inactivation of protein-tyrosine phosphatase 1B in vivo. J Biol Chem 2001;276: 29520–29525.
122. Liu F, Chernoff J. Protein tyrosine phosphatase 1B interacts with and is tyrosine phosphorylated by the epidermal growth factor receptor. Biochem J 1997;327: 139–145.
123. Bjorge JD, Pang A, Fujita DJ. Identification of protein-tyrosine phosphatase 1B as the major tyrosine phosphatase activity capable of dephosphorylating and activating c-Src in several human breast cancer cell lines. J Biol Chem 2000;275:41439–41446.
124. Milarski KL, Saltiel AR. Expression of catalytically inactive Syp phosphatase in 3T3 cells blocks stimulation of mitogen-activated protein kinase by insulin. J Biol Chem 1994;269:21239–21243.
125. Bennett AM, Hausdorff SF, O'Reilly AM, Freeman RM, Neel BG. Multiple requirements for SHPTP2 in epidermal growth factor-mediated cell cycle progression. Mol Cell Biol 1996;16:1189–1202.
126. Chen H, Wertheimer SJ, Lin CH, et al. Protein-tyrosine phosphatases PTP1B and syp are modulators of insulin-stimulated translocation of GLUT4 in transfected rat adipose cells. J Biol Chem 1997;272:8026–8031.
127. Ouwens DM, van der Zon GC, Maassen JA. Modulation of insulin-stimulated glycogen synthesis by Src homology phosphatase 2. Mol Cell Endocrinol 2001; 175:131–140.

128. Nichols A, Camps M, Gillieron C, et al. Substrate recognition domains within extracellular signal-regulated kinase mediate binding and catalytic activation of mitogen-activated protein kinase phosphatase-3. J Biol Chem 2000;275: 24613–24621.
129. Masuda K, Shima H, Watanabe M, Kikuchi K. MKP-7, a novel mitogen-activated protein kinase phosphatase, functions as a shuttle protein. J Biol Chem 2001;276: 39002–39011.
130. Camps M, Nichols A, Arkinstall S. Dual specificity phosphatases: a gene family for control of MAP kinase function. FASEB J 2000;14:6–16.
131. Sim AT, Baldwin ML, Rostas JA, Holst J, Ludowyke RI. The role of serine/threonine protein phosphatases in exocytosis. Biochem J 2003;373:641–659.
132. Cohen P. The structure and regulation of protein phosphatases. Annu Rev Biochem 1989;58:453–508.
133. Winder DG, Sweatt JD. Roles of serine/threonine phosphatases in hippocampal synaptic plasticity. Nat Rev Neurosci 2001;2:461–474.
134. Klumpp S, Krieglstein J. Serine/threonine protein phosphatases in apoptosis. Curr Opin Pharmacol 2002;2:458–462.
135. Brady MJ, Saltiel AR. The role of protein phosphatase-1 in insulin action. Recent Prog Horm Res 2001;56:157–173.
136. Keyse SM. Protein phosphatases and the regulation of mitogen-activated protein kinase signalling. Curr Opin Cell Biol 2000;12:186–192.
137. Birle D, Bottini N, Williams S, Huynh H, deBelle I, Adamson E, Mustelin T. Negative feedback regulation of the tumor suppressor PTEN by phosphoinositide-induced serine phosphorylation. J Immunol 2002;169:286–291.
138. Ross AH, Baltimore D, Eisen HN. Phosphotyrosine-containing proteins isolated by affinity chromatography with antibodies to a synthetic hapten. Nature 1981; 294:654–656.
139. Fabbro D, Parkinson D, Matter A. Protein tyrosine kinase inhibitors: new treatment modalities? Curr Opin Pharmacol 2002;2:374–381.
140. Toledo LM, Lydon NB, Elbaum D. The structure-based design of ATP-site directed protein kinase inhibitors. Curr Med Chem 1999;6:775–805.
141. Alessi DR, Cuenda A, Cohen P, Dudley DT, Saltiel AR. PD 098059 is a specific inhibitor of the activation of mitogen-activated protein kinase kinase in vitro and in vivo. J Biol Chem 1995;270:27489–27494.
142. Favata MF, Horiuchi KY, Manos EJ, et al. Identification of a novel inhibitor of mitogen-activated protein kinase kinase. J Biol Chem 1998;273:18623–18632.
143. Davies SP, Reddy H, Caivano M, Cohen P. Specificity and mechanism of action of some commonly used protein kinase inhibitors. Biochem J 2000;351:95–105.
144. Karihaloo A, O'Rourke DA, Nickel C, Spokes K, Cantley LG. Differential MAPK pathways utilized for HGF- and EGF-dependent renal epithelial morphogenesis. J Biol Chem 2001;276:9166–9173.
145. Cuenda A, Rouse J, Doza YN, et al. SB 203580 is a specific inhibitor of a MAP kinase homologue which is stimulated by cellular stresses and interleukin-1. FEBS Lett 1995;364:229–233.

146. Eyers PA, Craxton M, Morrice N, Cohen P, Goedert M. Conversion of SB 203580-insensitive MAP kinase family members to drug-sensitive forms by a single amino-acid substitution. Chem Biol 1998;5:321–328.
147. Lali FV, Hunt AE, Turner SJ, Foxwell BM. The pyridinyl imidazole inhibitor SB203580 blocks phosphoinositide-dependent protein kinase activity, protein kinase B phosphorylation, and retinoblastoma hyperphosphorylation in interleukin-2-stimulated T cells independently of p38 mitogen-activated protein kinase. J Biol Chem 2000;275:7395–7402.
148. Wang L, Gout I, Proud CG. Cross-talk between the ERK and p70 S6 kinase (S6K) signaling pathways. MEK-dependent activation of S6K2 in cardiomyocytes. J Biol Chem 2001;276:32670–32677.
149. Frantz B, Klatt T, Pang M, et al. The activation state of p38 mitogen-activated protein kinase determines the efficiency of ATP competition for pyridinylimidazole inhibitor binding. Biochemistry 1998;37:13846–13853.
150. Bennett BL, Sasaki DT, Murray BW, et al. SP600125, an anthrapyrazolone inhibitor of Jun N-terminal kinase. Proc Natl Acad Sci USA 2001;98: 13681–13686.
151. Han Z, Boyle DL, Chang L, et al. c-Jun N-terminal kinase is required for metalloproteinase expression and joint destruction in inflammatory arthritis. J Clin Invest 2001;108:73–81.
152. Bain J, McLauchlan H, Elliott M, Cohen P. The specificities of protein kinase inhibitors: an update. Biochem J 2003;371:199–204.
153. Blake RA, Broome MA, Liu X, et al. SU6656, a selective src family kinase inhibitor, used to probe growth factor signaling. Mol Cell Biol 2000;20:9018–9027.
154. Hanke JH, Gardner JP, Dow RL, et al. Discovery of a novel, potent, and Src family-selective tyrosine kinase inhibitor. Study of Lck- and FynT-dependent T cell activation. J Biol Chem 1996;271:695–701.
155. Price DJ, Grove JR, Calvo V, Avruch J, Bierer BE. Rapamycin-induced inhibition of the 70-kilodalton S6 protein kinase. Science 1992;257:973–977.
156. Kuo CJ, Chung J, Fiorentino DF, Flanagan WM, Blenis J, Crabtree GR. Rapamycin selectively inhibits interleukin-2 activation of p70 S6 kinase. Nature 1992;358:70–73.
157. Hidalgo M, Rowinsky EK. The rapamycin-sensitive signal transduction pathway as a target for cancer therapy. Oncogene 2000;19:6680–6686.
158. Toullec D, Pianetti P, Coste H, et al. The bisindolylmaleimide GF 109203X is a potent and selective inhibitor of protein kinase C. J Biol Chem 1991;266: 15771–15781.
159. Davis PD, Hill CH, Keech E, et al. Potent selective inhibitors of protein kinase C. FEBS Lett 1989;259:61–63.
160. Gordge PC, Ryves WJ. Inhibitors of protein kinase C. Cell Signal 1994;6: 871–882.
161. Martiny-Baron G, Kazanietz MG, Mischak H, et al. Selective inhibition of protein kinase C isozymes by the indolocarbazole Go 6976. J Biol Chem 1993;268: 9194–9197.

162. Vlahos CJ, Matter WF, Hui KY, Brown RF. A specific inhibitor of phosphatidylinositol 3-kinase, 2-(4-morpholinyl)-8-phenyl-4*H*-1-benzopyran-4-one (LY294002). J Biol Chem 1994;269:5241–5248.
163. Stein RC. Prospects for phosphoinositide 3-kinase inhibition as a cancer treatment. Endocr Relat Cancer 2001;8:237–248.
164. Brunn GJ, Williams J, Sabers C, Wiederrecht G, Lawrence JC Jr, Abraham RT. Direct inhibition of the signaling functions of the mammalian target of rapamycin by the phosphoinositide 3-kinase inhibitors, wortmannin and LY294002. EMBO J 1996;15:5256–5267.
165. Izzard RA, Jackson SP, Smith GC. Competitive and noncompetitive inhibition of the DNA-dependent protein kinase. Cancer Res 1999;59:2581–2586.
166. Wang D, Sul HS. Insulin stimulation of the fatty acid synthase promoter is mediated by the phosphatidylinositol 3-kinase pathway. Involvement of protein kinase B/Akt. J Biol Chem 1998;273:25420–25426.
167. Kitamura T, Ogawa W, Sakaue H, et al. Requirement for activation of the serine-threonine kinase Akt (protein kinase B) in insulin stimulation of protein synthesis but not of glucose transport. Mol Cell Biol 1998;18:3708–3717.
168. House C, Kemp BE. Protein kinase C contains a pseudosubstrate prototope in its regulatory domain. Science 1987;238:1726–1728.
169. Yeh P, Perricaudet M. Advances in adenoviral vectors: from genetic engineering to their biology. FASEB J 1997;11:615–623.
170. He TC, Zhou S, da Costa LT, Yu J, Kinzler KW, Vogelstein B. A simplified system for generating recombinant adenoviruses. Proc Natl Acad Sci USA 1998;95:2509–2514.
171. Becker TC, Noel RJ, Coats WS, et al. Use of recombinant adenovirus for metabolic engineering of mammalian cells. Methods Cell Biol 1994;43:161–189.
172. Fire A, Xu S, Montgomery MK, Kostas SA, Driver SE, Mello CC. Potent and specific genetic interference by double-stranded RNA in *Caenorhabditis elegans*. Nature 1998;391:806–811.
173. Hamilton AJ, Baulcombe DC. A species of small antisense RNA in posttranscriptional gene silencing in plants. Science 1999;286:950–952.
174. Zamore PD, Tuschl T, Sharp PA, Bartel DP. RNAi: double-stranded RNA directs the ATP-dependent cleavage of mRNA at 21 to 23 nucleotide intervals. Cell 2000;101:25–33.
175. Elbashir SM, Lendeckel W, Tuschl T. RNA interference is mediated by 21- and 22-nucleotide RNAs. Genes Dev 2001;15:188–200.
176. McManus MT, Sharp PA. Gene silencing in mammals by small interfering RNAs. Nat Rev Genet 2002;3:737–747.
177. Reinhart BJ, Slack FJ, Basson M, et al. The 21-nucleotide let-7 RNA regulates developmental timing in *Caenorhabditis elegans*. Nature 2000;403:901–906.
178. Pasquinelli AE, Reinhart BJ, Slack F, et al. Conservation of the sequence and temporal expression of let-7 heterochronic regulatory RNA. Nature 2000;408:86–89.

179. Grishok A, Pasquinelli AE, Conte D, et al. Genes and mechanisms related to RNA interference regulate expression of the small temporal RNAs that control *C. elegans* developmental timing. Cell 2001;106:23–34.
180. Dykxhoorn DM, Novina CD, Sharp PA. Killing the messenger: short RNAs that silence gene expression. Nat Rev Mol Cell Biol 2003;4:457–467.
181. Baglioni C, Nilsen TW. Mechanisms of antiviral action of interferon. Interferon. 1983;5:23–42.
182. Williams BR. Role of the double-stranded RNA-activated protein kinase (PKR) in cell regulation. Biochem Soc Trans 1997;25:509–513.
183. Caplen NJ, Parrish S, Imani F, Fire A, Morgan RA. Specific inhibition of gene expression by small double-stranded RNAs in invertebrate and vertebrate systems. Proc Natl Acad Sci USA 2001;98:9742–9747.
184. Elbashir SM, Harborth J, Lendeckel W, Yalcin A, Weber K, Tuschl T. Duplexes of 21-nucleotide RNAs mediate RNA interference in cultured mammalian cells. Nature 2001;411:494–498.
185. McManus MT, Haines BB, Dillon CP, et al. Small interfering RNA-mediated gene silencing in T lymphocytes. J Immunol 2002;169:5754–5760.
186. Brummelkamp TR, Bernards R, Agami R. A system for stable expression of short interfering RNAs in mammalian cells. Science 2002;296:550–553.
187. Lee NS, Dohjima T, Bauer G, et al. Expression of small interfering RNAs targeted against HIV-1 rev transcripts in human cells. Nat Biotechnol 2002;20:500–555.
188. Miyagishi M, Taira K. U6 promoter-driven siRNAs with four uridine 3′ overhangs efficiently suppress targeted gene expression in mammalian cells. Nat Biotechnol 2002;20:497–500.
189. Paul CP, Good PD, Winer I, Engelke DR. Effective expression of small interfering RNA in human cells. Nat Biotechnol 2002;20:505–508.
190. Sui G, Soohoo C, Affar el B, et al. A DNA vector-based RNAi technology to suppress gene expression in mammalian cells. Proc Natl Acad Sci USA 2002;99:5515–5520.
191. Yu JY, DeRuiter SL, Turner DL. RNA interference by expression of short-interfering RNAs and hairpin RNAs in mammalian cells. Proc Natl Acad Sci USA 2002;99:6047–6052.
192. Paddison PJ, Caudy AA, Hannon GJ. Stable suppression of gene expression by RNAi in mammalian cells. Proc Natl Acad Sci USA 2002;99:1443–1448.
193. Amarzguioui M, Holen T, Babaie E, Prydz H. Tolerance for mutations and chemical modifications in a siRNA. Nucl Acids Res 2003;31:589–595.
194. McManus MT, Petersen CP, Haines BB, Chen J, Sharp PA. Gene silencing using micro-RNA designed hairpins. RNA 2002;8:842–850.

4

Catalytic Function and Expression of Glutathione Transferase Zeta

Philip G. Board, M. W. Anders, and Anneke C. Blackburn

Summary

The zeta class of glutathione S-transferases (GSTZ) is one of the most recently discovered soluble GST classes and has proved to be of considerable interest because of its contribution to the catabolism of phenylalanine and tyrosine and its role in α-halo acid metabolism. GSTZ was originally discovered as a result of a bioinformatic approach to gene discovery in the mid-1990s. This approach and others have also led to the discovery of several polymorphic forms of GSTZ. This chapter summarizes methods and approaches that have been used to express recombinant GSTZ, determine its crystal structure, measure its activity and characterize its kinetic properties, and study the function and importance of GSTZ in the metabolism of dichloroacetate (DCA), which is of great toxicological and public health interest. DCA is a multisite toxicant and carcinogen that is a byproduct of water chlorination and is a breakdown product of the industrial chemical and environmental contaminant trichloroethylene.

Key Words

Bioinformatics; BLAST programs; dichloroacetic acid; expressed sequence tag; fumarylacetoacetate hydrolase; gene knockout; glutathione S-transferase-zeta; glyoxylic acid; α-halo acids; leukotrienes; maleylacetoacetate isomerase; polymorphisms; single nucleotide polymorphisms.

1. THE GLUTATHIONE TRANSFERASES

Proteins known as glutathione transferases have a diverse range of structures and functions and belong to at least three gene families. These enzymes can be broadly divided into the membrane-bound and soluble superfamilies. The membrane-bound glutathione transferases, known collectively as the MAPEG (membrane-associated proteins involved in eicosanoid and glutathione

From: *Methods in Pharmacology and Toxicology,*
Drug Metabolism and Transport: Molecular Methods and Mechanisms
Edited by: L. Lash © Humana Press Inc., Totowa, NJ

metabolism) family, include enzymes such as microsomal glutathione transferase, prostaglandin E synthase and leukotriene C_4 synthase *(1)*.

The soluble glutathione transferases (GSTs) are an independent superfamily of multifunctional proteins that share tertiary structural homology *(2)*. The super family can be further subdivided into a number of classes where the members share closer primary sequence similarities. The classes of soluble GSTs have been named after letters in the Greek alphabet, and in mammals the alpha, mu, omega, pi, sigma, theta, and zeta classes have been clearly identified *(3)*. Other classes termed lambda, phi, tau, delta, and epsilon have been defined in plants and insects *(4,5)*. There are variable numbers of genes within each class in humans, ranging from five in the mu class to one in the zeta and pi classes. The multiple members of each class appear to have resulted from gene duplication events, because the genes encoding all the members of each class have been located in clusters on distinct chromosomes: alpha, 6p12 *(6)*; mu, 1p13.3 *(7)*; omega, 10q24.3 *(8)*; pi, 11q13 *(9)*; sigma, 4q21-22 *(10)*; theta, 22q11.1 *(11)*; zeta 14q24.3 *(12)*. To complicate the picture further, a group of proteins known collectively as CLIC proteins (ChLoride Intracellular Channel) that are at times either soluble or membrane-bound have recently been shown to be members of the soluble glutathione transferase structural family *(13)*. So far the CLIC proteins have not revealed any substantial glutathione-dependent enzymatic activity. A soluble GST has also been isolated from mitochondria and termed kappa *(14)*. However the sequence of GST kappa has little similarity with any of the other soluble GSTs and phylogenetic analysis suggests strongly that kappa is not related to the other soluble GSTs *(15)*. From the evidence currently available, it seems likely that GST kappa is a representative of a third group of proteins that catalyze glutathione-transferase reactions. The resolution of this question will probably require the solution of the crystal structure.

1.1. Glutathione-Transferase Functions

Members of the various classes within the soluble GST superfamily exhibit a broad range of catalytic activities and functions. The first GSTs studied were known for their ability to conjugate glutathione to a range of xenobiotic electrophiles and to physically bind and sequester a range of hydrophobic compounds of endogenous and xenobiotic origins *(16,17)*. Consequently the GSTs have become known for their major contributions to the metabolism of xenobiotics that include therapeutic drugs as well as carcinogens and other toxins. More recently a number of GSTs have been identified that catalyze glutathione-dependent reactions with a range of endogenous compounds. Notably, the alpha class isoenzyme GSTA4-4 catalyzes the conjugation of 4-hydroxynonenal, a cytotoxic α,β-unsaturated aldehyde that is generated during lipid peroxidation *(18,19)*. Additionally, GSTA3-3 plays a significant role in the isomerization of

Δ⁵-androstene-3, 17-dione *(20)*, and the sigma class GST is known as prostaglandin D-synthase because of its role in the isomerization of prostaglandin H_2 to prostaglandin D_2 *(21)*. The zeta class isoenzyme GSTZ1-1 appears to have dual activities with endogenous and exogenous substrates. GST zeta plays a significant role in the catabolism of tyrosine *(22)* and is also important for the biotransformation of α-halo acids *(23)* (*see* Fig. 7).

Some soluble GSTs appear to have nonenzymatic functions. The sigma class GSTs function as lens crystallins in squid and related species *(24)*. Recent studies have indicated a role for some GSTs in cell signaling pathways. GSTP1-1 regulates the activity of Jun N-terminal kinase *(25)* and a mu-class GST regulates apoptosis stimulating kinase (ASK1) *(26)*. In addition, GSTO1-1 modulates the activity of ryanodine receptor Ca^{2+} ion channels *(13)*. The protein CLIC 1 is clearly a member of the GST structural family and forms ion channels *(27)*. In our unpublished studies, neither CLIC1 nor CLIC2 have demonstrated any GST-like catalytic activity.

2. GLUTATHIONE TRANSFERASE ZETA (GSTZ)

The zeta class is one of the most recently discovered soluble GST classes and has proved to be of considerable interest because of its contribution to the catabolism of phenylalanine and tyrosine and its role in α-halo acid metabolism.

2.1. The Discovery of GSTZ by Bioinformatic Analysis

The zeta-class GST was originally discovered as a result of a bioinformatic approach to gene discovery *(15)*. It had become evident that most known members of the GST superfamily had been discovered and characterized by their ability to conjugate the xenobiotic substrate 1-chloro-2,4-dinitrobenzene and their simple purification by affinity chromatography on immobilized glutathione. In the mid-1990s we considered that there may be additional members of the glutathione transferase family that were active with novel endogenous and exogenous substrates and may not bind to glutathione agarose. To test this hypothesis we used the BLAST program *(28)* to search the human expressed sequence tag (EST) database for sequences that were similar to GST-like sequences that had been detected in nonmammalian species. These studies revealed two new classes of GSTs that we termed zeta and omega *(15,29)*. The EST database currently contains more than five million entries, so transcripts of most human genes are represented. Application of this strategy can be readily applied to identify all the members of gene families that are of interest *(30)*.

Several studies have shown that the zeta-class GSTs occur in a range of species from plants and fungi to mammals *(4,15,22)*. The extensive conservation of this enzyme over an evolutionary range that was far beyond that of other

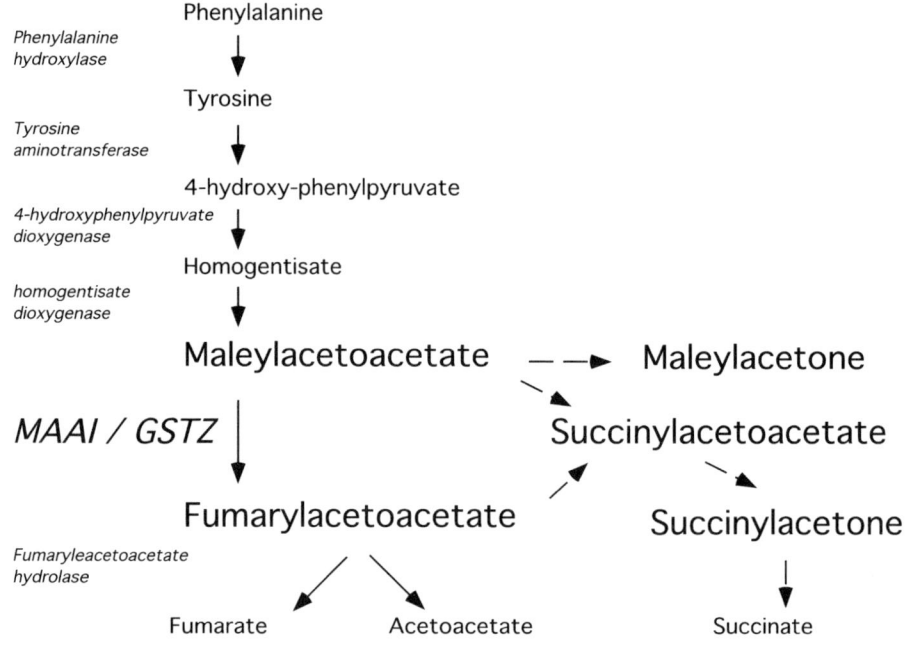

Fig. 1. The catabolic pathway for phenylalanine and tyrosine.

GSTs strongly suggested that it catalyzed an important, if not essential reaction. The studies of Fernández-Cañón and Peñalva *(22)* demonstrated that GSTZ and maleylacetoacetate isomerase (MAAI) are identical. As MAAI catalyses the penultimate step in the tyrosine catabolism pathway (Fig. 1), it seems likely that the maintenance of this role has been an important factor in the conservation of the zeta-class GSTs.

2.2. Detection of Polymorphism by Bioinformatic Analysis

Polymorphisms in genes can give rise to significant functional variations. In the case of drug and xenobiotic metabolizing enzymes, polymorphisms can translate into differences in drug response and toxicity as well as susceptibility to environmental carcinogens. Our initial comparison of several cDNA sequences extracted from the EST database suggested the presence of polymorphisms in the human *GSTZ* gene *(15)*. To explore the extent of this polymorphism, we developed a new bioinformatic approach to the detection of genetic polymorphisms *(31,32)*. This approach relies on the fact that the EST database has been compiled from cDNA sequences that are derived from a large number of cDNA libraries. As each library usually represents the genome of a different individual, screening the EST database is equivalent to sequencing genes of interest in a small multiracial sample.

```
Query         298  tggaatcaccattcaccagtcactggccatcattgagtatctagaggagacgcgtcccac 357
gi30641554    839  ............................................................ 780
gi31031019    357  ............................................................ 416
gi31278259    367  ............................................................ 426
gi30460826    372  ............................................................ 431
gi19895559    303  ............................................................ 362
gi22342438    298  ...............................................t............ 357
gi30641556    401  ............................................................ 460
gi22371232    768  ............................................................ 709
gi19817864    300  ............................................................ 359
gi19813966    304  ............................................................ 363
gi24035243    313  ...............................................t............ 372
gi21769805    326  ............................................................ 385
gi15019490    290  ...........c................................................ 349
gi13964804    112  ............................................................ 171
gi21796105    304  ............................................................ 363
gi24041445    313  ...............................................t............ 372
gi23547560    731  .........................................................  707
gi16535033    305  ............................................................ 364
gi14502716    289  ............................................................ 348
gi21786506    300  ............................................................ 359
gi30048337    733  .........................................................  708
gi12420195    132  ............................................................ 191
gi24472255    722  ...............................................t............ 707
gi10141565    282  ............................................................ 341
gi22683496    357  ............................................................ 416
```

Fig. 2. Typical output from a BLAST search of the EST database in the "flat query-anchored with identities" format. Polymorphic sites can be rapidly identified by eye.

To facilitate the screening process, we again used the BLAST alignment program and the "Flat query-anchored with identities" output format at the National Center for Biological Information (NCBI) website (www.ncbi.nlm.nih.gov/). The typical output from this approach is illustrated in Fig. 2, and shows part of the alignment of the human GSTZ cDNA sequence with a series of ESTs. The C-to-T transition that occurs in some of the ESTs is readily detectable. This base substitution encodes a threonine-82 to methionine substitution that has an allele frequency of about 0.16 in Europeans. Thus far, we have identified several polymorphisms in human GSTZ by this simple procedure *(33,34)*. Because the different substitutions occur in different combinations, we have defined several common haplotypes (Table 1).

The single nucleotide polymorphism (SNP) SNP finder program (Table 2) is an additional means of searching the EST database and permits the user to confirm variations in the original sequence trace. In addition to these direct-searching strategies, there are several databases of compiled SNPs that can be searched (Table 2). Theoretically, analysis of the SNP databases and strategies for the alignment of EST sequences provide a rapid means of identifying genetic polymorphisms in genes of pharmacological interest. In practice, although the approach successfully identifies real polymorphisms, it is now evident that no single program or method identifies all the variants in the EST database and a large number of false positives have to be eliminated by

Table 1
GSTZ Haplotypes in a Normal European Population (*n* = 128)

Haplotype	Residue position			Frequency
	32	42	82	
Z1A	Lys	Arg	Thr	.086
Z1B	Lys	Gly	Thr	.285
Z1C	Glu	Gly	Thr	.473
Z1D	Glu	Gly	Met	.156

Data derived from Blackburn et al. *(34)*.

Table 2
Sequence Database Analysis Programs and SNP Databases

Program/database	Web address
BLAST	http://www.ncbi.nlm.nih.gov/
SNP Finder	http://lpg.nci.nih.gov/GAI
SNPper	http://snpper.chip.org/
db SNP	http://www.ncbi.nlm.nih.gov/SNP/
TSC	http://snp.cshl.org/
CGAP	http://lpg.nci.nih.gov
HGVbase	http://hgvbase.cgb.ki.se/
refseq	http://www.ncbi.nlm.nih.gov/RefSeq/
UUGC Gene SNPs	http://www.genome.utah.edu/genesnps

genotyping in large population samples. In a recent study of the omega-class GST genes, we confirmed only 2 polymorphic sites out of 28 possibilities identified by database analysis *(8)*. This approach has other limitations: genes that show limited expression in particular tissues or are expressed only under specific conditions are likely to be poorly represented in the EST database and variants are less likely to be included. In addition, SNPs within large cDNAs may not be well represented in the databases, as the majority of ESTs are derived from the 5'- and 3'-ends. Finally, this bioinformatic approach does not identify SNPs in noncoding regions and SNPs in promoter regions may be important sources of individual variation.

3. EXPRESSION AND CHARACTERIZATION OF RECOMBINANT GSTZ

Expression of recombinant GSTs in *E. coli* has facilitated their structural and functional analysis *(35)*. Recombinant GSTs from the alpha, mu, and pi classes can be readily purified from *E. coli* extracts by affinity chromatography on glutathione agarose *(35–37)*. In contrast, the zeta-class GSTs do not bind to immobilized glutathione and another approach is required to effect the purification of the recombinant enzymes.

The addition of a poly-His tag at the N-terminal and purification by immobilized metal-ion affinity chromatography (IMAC) proved to be a useful strategy for the preparation of the zeta-, theta- and omega-class GSTs *(15,29,38)*. Constructs for the expression of these isoenzymes have been made in the pQE vectors available from QIAGEN.

3.1. Expression of GSTZ in E. coli

To express and purify GSTZ1-1, cultures of M15 [pREP4] containing the appropriate pQEZ1 plasmid were grown in Luria broth supplemented with 100 mg/mL of ampicillin and 25 mg/mL of kanamycin (kanamycin is unstable in solution and should be prepared fresh) at 37°C until the culture reached an OD_{600} of 0.5. Isopropylthio-β-D-thiogalactocide was added to a final concentration of 0.1 mM and the culture was allowed to grow for a minimum of 3 h. The bacteria were collected by centrifugation and resuspended at a dilution of 25 mL/500 mL of culture in buffer A (50 mM sodium phosphate, 300 mM NaCl, pH 7.5) containing 1 mg/mL of lysozyme. After standing on ice for 1 h, the bacteria were ultrasonicated and centrifuged at 10,000g for 15 min at 4°C. The bacterial pellet was discarded and the supernatant mixed gently with Ni-agarose beads (~1 mL/500 mL of culture) at 4°C for 1 h. Immobilized nickel agarose is readily prepared by the methods described originally by Porath and Olin *(39)*. The Ni-agarose was collected by gentle centrifugation, washed extensively with buffer A, and then packed under gravity into a small column. The column was equilibrated with buffer A containing 10% glycerol, and the proteins were subsequently eluted in two steps with 50 and 500 mM imidazole in buffer A containing 10% glycerol. Highly purified GSTZ eluted with 500 mM imidazole, was dialyzed overnight in 5 mM N-(2-hydroxyethyl)piperazine-N'-(2-ethanesulfonic acid) (HEPES), pH 7.0, 1 mM dithiothreitol, and 10% glycerol, and was stored frozen at –20°C.

Recombinant GSTZ1 expressed in *E. coli* is enzymatically active and has been used to study the function of the various polymorphic isoforms of the human enzyme. These studies revealed significant functional differences. In particular, the GSTZ1a–1a isoform, which has an arginine at position 42, has a range of

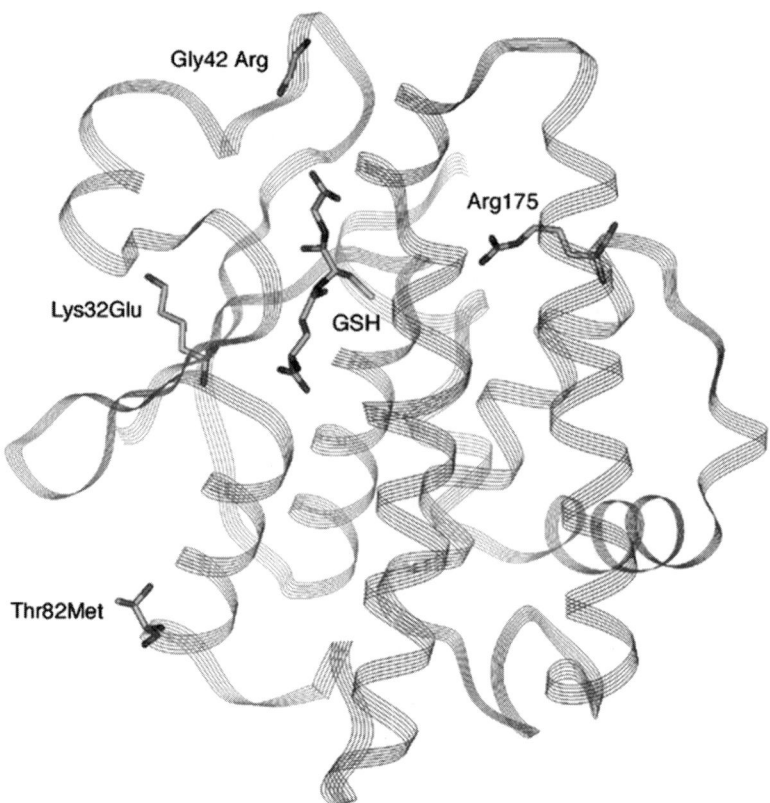

Fig. 3. A ribbon representation of a human GSTZ subunit. The position of glutathione and the side chains of the polymorphic residues are indicated. Arg-175 is in a position to form a salt bridge with the substrate carboxylate *(42)*.

distinct properties including enantiomeric selectivity with 2-chloropropionates, resistance to inactivation by dichloroacetic acid (DCA), and low isomerase activity with maleylacetone (Table 3) *(33,34,40,41)*.

3.2. Determination of the Crystal Structure of GSTZ1-1

We also used recombinant enzyme to determine the crystal structure of human GSTZ1A (Fig. 3) *(42)* and similar studies have determined the structure of the zeta-class GST from *Arabidopsis thaliana (43)*. Figure 3 also shows the position of the polymorphic residues listed in Table 1. The crystal structure of the human enzyme shows that it adopts the canonical GST fold with a number of functional differences. The glutathione-binding site is at the base of a deep crevice (about 25 Å in depth), which explains the difficulty in purifying zeta-class GSTs by affinity chromatography on immobilized glutathione. The struc-

Table 3
Specific Activities and Inactivation Half-Lives of Naturally Occurring GSTZ Variants

Enzyme	BNPP[a] (μmol/min/mg)	CFA[b] (μmol/min/mg)	(R)-2-Chloropropionate[c] (μmol/min/mg)	(S)-2-Chloropropionate[b] (μmol/min/mg)	MA[b] (μmol/min/mg)	DCA inactivation[c] half-life (min)
GSTZ1a-1a	2.3 ± 0.15	1.35 ± 0.05	1.11 ± 0.04	0.07 ± .002	318 ± 91	23 ± 1
GSTZ1b-1b	1.5 ± 0.03	1.34 ± 0.03	0.28 ± 0.009	0.21 ± .004	1010 ± 217	9.6 ± 0.3
GSTZ1c-1c	1.6 ± 0.04	1.29 ± 0.05	0.29 ± 0.009	0.22 ± .005	1856 ± 716	10.1 ± 0.5
GSTZ1d-1d	1.2 ± 0.08	1.27 ± 0.025	0.26 ± 0.002	0.25 ± .004	464 ± 215	9.5 ± 0.3

[a]Data from ref. 47.
[b]Data from ref. 34.
[c]Data from ref. 40.

ture also provides insight into the molecular bases for the different reactions catalyzed by the zeta-class GSTs (*see* Section 4).

3.3. Generation of Antiserum to GSTZ1-1

Recombinant GSTs expressed in *E. coli* can also be used to generate antiserum. Recombinant antigens are free from contamination with other mammalian proteins and are more likely to be highly specific. We have used antibodies raised in rabbits against recombinant human GSTZ1-1 to study the distribution of GSTZ in rat tissues *(44)* and to study the inactivation of GSTZ by some substrates *(40,45)*. We have also used antiserum to human GSTZ1-1 to evaluate GSTZ expression in GSTZ knockout mice *(45a)*.

4. THE CATALYTIC ACTIVITIES OF GSTZ

Our initial investigations of the zeta-class GST revealed that apart from some minor glutathione peroxidase activity with cumene hydroperoxide, human GSTZ1-1 was largely devoid of activity with known substrates for other GSTs *(15)*. Subsequent studies revealed that GSTZ has activities with novel endogenous and exogenous substrates. Fernández-Cañon and colleagues revealed that GSTZ was identical with maleylacetoactetate isomerase and we have confirmed that GSTZ has MAAI activity *(22,33)*. We have also discovered that GSTZ1-1 catalyzes the biotransformation of α-halo acids, a reaction of considerable toxicological importance *(23,46)*. Although the zeta-class GSTs have these two distinct activities, there is a vast difference in the efficiency of the two reactions. In comparative studies, we showed that the k_{cat}/K_M is around 1000-fold greater for the MA isomerase reaction than for the reaction with α-halo acid substrates *(41,47)*.

4.1. Maleylacetoacetate Isomerase Activity

The glutathione-dependent isomerization of maleylacetoacetate by GSTZ/MAAI is an important step in the catabolism of phenylalanine and tyrosine to fumarate and acetoacetate (Fig. 1). With the notable exception of GSTZ/MAAI, deficiencies of each of the enzymes in this pathway have been shown to cause diseases of varying severity in humans. The most severe of these disorders, hereditary tyrosinemia type 1 (HT-1), is caused by a deficiency of fumarylacetoacetate hydrolase (FAH), the last step in the pathway (Fig. 1). Patients with HT-1 suffer from liver failure and renal tubule defects and frequently develop liver cancer at an early age *(48,49)*. The deleterious symptoms that accompany FAH deficiency are thought to result from the accumulation of FAA and MAA as well as their derivatives succinylacetoacetate (SAA) and succinylacetone (SA) *(50–52)*. It has previously been considered that MAA, FAA, and SA would accumulate and cause a tyrosinemia-like syndrome in cases of GSTZ/MAAI deficiency. The absence of any proven cases of GSTZ/MAAI deficiency and the early death of a suspected case, suggested that this deficiency may have a very severe, if not lethal phenotype *(53)* (*see* Subheading 6).

4.1.1. Determination of GSTZ/MAAI Activity

The isomerization of MAA to FAA is a difficult reaction to measure because of the instability of MAA. Maleylacetone (MA) is more stable and can be synthesized by published procedures *(54)*. Several laboratories have reported methods for measuring the isomerization of MA to fumarylacetone (FA) *(55,56)*. In our laboratory, we developed a relatively rapid procedure for the separation and quantification of FA by reverse-phase HPLC *(47)*. The reaction mixture contained 0.01 *M* sodium phosphate (pH 7.6), 500 µ*M* glutathione, 500 µ*M* MA, and 0.1–1.0 µg/mL of enzyme in a final volume of 500 µL. The reaction mixture was incubated at 25°C and was stopped after 30 s by addition of 100 µL of ice-cold stop solution (a 1:1 mixture of 1 *M* HCl and 5 µ*M* salicylic acid as an internal standard). The samples were chilled to 4°C and the quantity of FA produced was determined by HPLC. MA, FA, and SA were separated on a Waters muBondapak C18 column (3.9 × 300 mm) eluted at a flow rate of 1.5 mL/min. The mobile phase consisted of 40% acetonitrile, 1% triethylamine, 59% MilliQ water; the pH of the mixture was brought to 3.1–3.2 with phosphoric acid, and the mixture was sparged with helium. The absorbance of the eluate was monitored at 312 nm; under these conditions, MA eluted at 2.4 min, FA at 3.4 min, and the internal standard salicylic acid at 4 min (Fig. 4). FA formation was quantified by reference to a standard curve prepared with pure FA. The concentration of MA used in these studies was determined by conversion of a sample of MA to FA in the presence of glutathione and hGSTZ1c-1c.

4.2. α-Halo Acids as Substrates for GSTZ

Previous studies showed that glyoxylate is the major metabolite of DCA and that the oxygenation of DCA to glyoxylic acid is catalyzed by cytosolic enzymes that require glutathione *(57,58)*. The discovery that the reaction is catalyzed by GSTZ has allowed a rapid expansion of our understanding of the metabolism of DCA and other α-halo acids *(23)*. Studies by Tong and colleagues *(46)* revealed that GSTZ catalyzes the oxygenation of bromochloro-, bromofluoro-, chlorofluoro-, dibromo-, and dichloroacetic acid, but not difluoroacetic acid, to glyoxylic acid. GSTZ also catalyzes the biotransformation of *(R,S)*-2-bromopropionic acid, *(R)*-, *(S)*-, and *(R,S)*-2-chloropropionic acid and *(R,S)*-2-iodopropionic acid, but not *(R,S)*-2-fluoropropionic acid, to *S*-(α-methylcarboxymethyl)glutathione. The same study also established that 2,2-dichloropropionic acid is converted to pyruvate. However, no reaction was detected with 3,3-dichloropropionic acid, indicating that β-halo acids are not substrates. Similarly, no reaction was detected with fluoroacetamide or

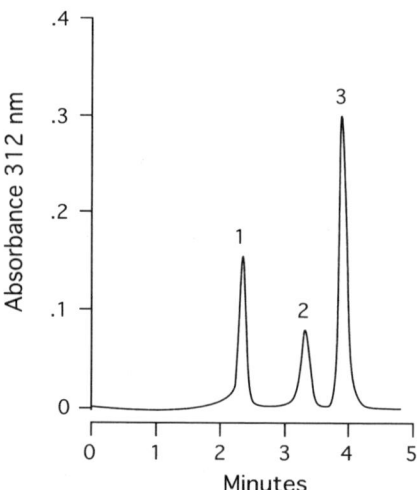

Fig. 4. HPLC separation of maleylacetone isomerase reaction products. Peak 1, maleylacetone; peak 2, fumarylacetone; peak 3, salicylic acid (internal standard).

ethyl fluoroacetate, indicating the importance of the carboxylate on the α carbon. The crystal structure and mutagenic studies have clarified this requirement (*see* Subheading 5).

The role of GSTZ1-1 in the metabolism of α-halo acids has been of great interest. Several studies have shown that DCA causes multiorgan toxicities (reviewed in ref. *59*) and is carcinogenic in rats and mice *(60,61)*. Humans are exposed to DCA, as it is a contaminant of chlorinated drinking water *(62,63)* and as a breakdown product of the sedative chloral hydrate and the industrial solvent trichloroethylene *(64)*. Despite its apparent carcinogenicity in mice and rats, DCA is used for the clinical management of congenital lactic acidosis *(65)*. Whereas GSTZ1-1 catalyzes the biotransformation of DCA to glyoxylate, DCA is also a mechanism-based inactivator of GSTZ1-1 *(23,40,45,66)*. In addition, we have shown that there is genetically determined heterogeneity in the susceptibility of GSTZ1-1 to inactivation by DCA *(40)* (Table 3). This could lead to significant individual variation in the pharmacokinetics of DCA in humans. Thus, many previous studies of the toxicology of DCA could have been confounded by the variable inactivation of the enzyme that is of prime importance in its metabolism.

4.2.1. Determination of GSTZ Activity With α-Halo Acid Substrates

In the presence of glutathione, GSTZ catalyzes the biotransformation of α-halo acids such as dichloroacetic acid and chlorofluoroacetic acid to glyoxylate. The reaction can be measured by the determination of glyoxylate formation *(23)*, but

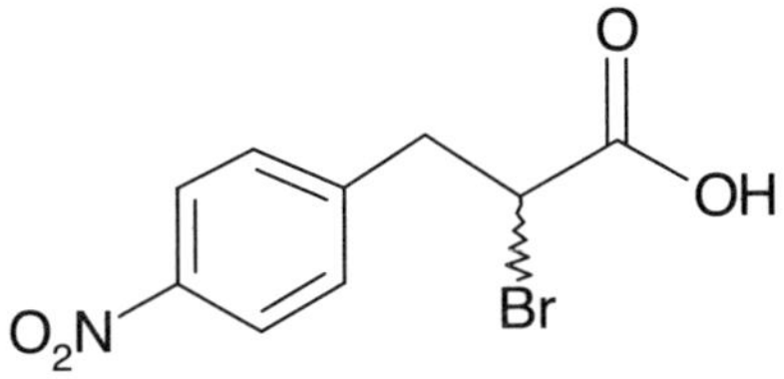

Fig. 5. Structure of (±)-2-bromo-3-(4-nitrophenyl)propionic acid (BNPP).

the assay is cumbersome and time consuming. 2-Halopropionic acids are also good substrates for GSTZ, but the measurement of the reaction product, S-(α methylcarboxymethyl)-glutathione, is also cumbersome *(46)*. To facilitate the further study of GSTZ and the characterization of its reaction with α-halo acids, we have developed a direct-reading spectrophotometric assay with a novel α-halo acid substrate, ±-2-bromo-3-(4-nitrophenyl)propionic acid (BNPP) (Fig. 5) *(47)*. The reaction mixture contained 0.1 M sodium phosphate, pH 7.4, 1 mM glutathione, and 0.75 mM BNPP and was incubated at 37°C. The absorbance of the reaction mixture was recorded at 310 nm and a molar absorptivity of 420 for the reaction product, 2-glutathion-S-yl-3-(4-nitrophenyl) propionic acid (GS-NPP), was used to calculate the reaction rate. Because of the high absorbance of BNPP at 310 nm, it is necessary to use a dual-beam spectrophotometer with a blank reaction without enzyme in the reference cuvette. While this assay allows kinetic analysis of purified enzymes, the low increase in absorbance of the reaction product relative to the high absorbance of the substrate limits its sensitivity and precludes its use with unpurified enzymes. We found that GST1a-1a has a higher specific activity with BNPP than the other naturally occurring polymorphic variants (Table 3) *(47)*. This variant shows high enantiomeric selectivity with *(R)*-2-chloropropionate compared with *(S)*-2-chloropropionate *(34)*, and it is possible that the elevated activity of hGSTZ1a-1a with BNPP may reflect similar enantiomeric selectivity.

5. ACTIVE-SITE RESIDUES AND THE REACTION MECHANISM

A knowledge of 3D structure and the capacity to express recombinant enzyme allows the formulation and testing of hypotheses concerning residues involved in substrate binding and catalysis. We used site-directed mutagenesis to construct specific mutations that probe the active site and the reaction mechanism *(47)*. Previous studies implicated tyrosine, serine, arginine, and cysteine residues in the catalytic mechanism of a range of GSTs. Typically, a hydrogen bond from the active-site tyrosine or serine residue lowers the pK_a of the glutathione thiol group and stabilizes the cysteinyl thiol as a thiolate ion *(67)*. The zeta-class GSTs have a characteristic sequence motif (SSCX (W/H) RVIAL) in

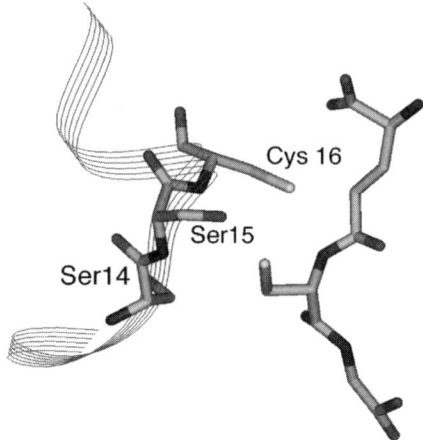

Fig. 6. The position of Ser-14, Ser-15, and Cys-16 side chains relative to glutathione in the human GSTZ structure *(42)*.

the N-terminal region that is strongly conserved. Based on their position in the 3D structure and alignment with other GST sequences, it is possible to argue that either of the first three residues (SSC) within the GST zeta motif could be of primary importance in the catalytic mechanism (Fig. 6) *(47)*. Mutation of these residues to alanine indicated that only the first serine (Ser-14) is essential for activity in the MAAI reaction or in the halide-displacement reaction. Although Ser-14 aligns with the active-site serine residues in the mammalian theta-class and the insect delta-class GSTs, the crystal structure of GSTZ1-1 indicates that the hydroxyl of Ser-14 is to distant (4.7 Å) and pointing in the wrong direction to form a hydrogen bond with the thiol of glutathione (Fig. 6) *(42)*. On structural grounds, Ser-15 (3.95 Å) and Cys-16 (2.8 Å) are possibly better positioned to play a role in catalysis, but this was not supported by their mutation to alanine, as both mutant enzymes retained activity *(47)*. An involvement of Ser-14 would require a significant conformational change to reposition the serine hydroxyl and the glutathione thiol. There is a precedent for such a change in the pi-class GST. Protonation of glutathione causes a loss of direct interaction between the catalytic tyrosine and glutathione and the thiol sulfur points in a different direction than that seen in other glutathione complexes *(68)*. If a similar mechanism occurs in GSTZ, it is possible that the glutathione in the GSTZ structure is protonated. The structure of GSTZ1-1 also suggests that Gln-111 and the helix dipole of α helix 1 could play a role in the activation of glutathione, but these possibilities are yet to be tested *(42)*.

5.1. The Role of Cys-16

Although Cys-16 is not essential for activity, mutation of this residue to alanine results in a striking increase in the K_M for glutathione, suggesting that it plays a significant role in binding glutathione rather than in catalysis *(47)*. In addition, this residue appears to be the primary target for modification during the mechanism-based inactivation of GSTZ by DCA *(69)*.

5.2. Orientation of Substrates for Catalysis

The crystal structure of GSTZ contained a sulfate ion coordinated by the side chain of Arg-175, and this suggested a role for this residue in the productive binding and orientation of the carboxyl groups of substrates such as MA and DCA. When DCA is modeled into the crystal structure of GSTZ1-1, it fits best in the active site if it is oriented such that the carboxylate moiety forms a salt bridge with Arg-175 *(42)*. This optimally orients DCA for attack by glutathione on the α-carbon and the displacement of one of the chlorides. Mutagenesis of Arg-175 to alanine or lysine confirmed the importance of the amide of Arg-175 in orienting substrates in the active site. The R175A mutation caused a diminished k_{cat} and elevated K_M for MA compared with GSTZ1c-1c and the R175K mutant *(47)*. The crystal structure also indicates that β-halo acids such as 3,3-dichloropropionic acid are not substrates because the binding site cannot orient the β-carbon for attack by glutathione.

5.3. Inactivation of GSTZ by α-Halo Acids

It was originally noted that the plasma half-life of DCA in humans is prolonged after repeated exposure to DCA and that the capacity of hepatic cytosol to convert DCA to glyoxylate is diminished in rats given DCA *(58,70)*. These phenomena were explained by the observation that GSTZ is inactivated by DCA and other fluorine-lacking α-halo acids *(45)*. The inability of fluorine-lacking α-halo acids to inactivate GSTZ explains the higher specific activity of GSTZ with fluorine-containing substrates such as chlorofluoroacetic acid *(46)*.

Tzeng and colleagues demonstrated that the inactivation of GSTZ by DCA was the result of a covalent modification of the enzyme by a reactive intermediate *(40)*. In the proposed reaction with DCA, GSTZ catalyzes the displacement of one chloride by glutathione via an S_N2 reaction to yield *S*-(α-chlorocarboxymethyl)glutathione. In a second step, the remaining chloride is lost to yield a carbonium/sulfonium intermediate. This intermediate is then either hydrolyzed to yield glyoxylate and glutathione or it reacts with a nucleophilic residue in the enzyme to form a covalently linked inactive enzyme–substrate complex (Fig. 7). Experiments with [^{35}S]glutathione and

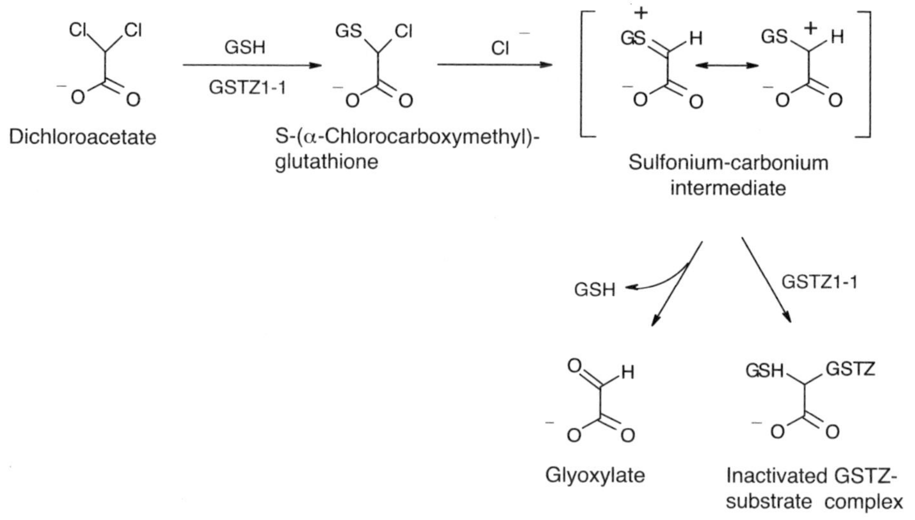

Fig. 7. The GSTZ1-1-catalyzed oxygenation of dichloroacetic acid.

[^{14}C]DCA demonstrated the covalent addition of both substrates to the inactivated enzyme-substrate complex *(40)*. By mass-spectral analysis and site-directed mutagenesis, we showed that Cys-16 is the nucleophilic target of the *S*-(α-carboxymethyl)glutathione intermediate formed during the reaction *(69)*. This is consistent with its position in the active site in close proximity to the bound glutathione (Fig. 6). Although Cys-16 itself is not essential for activity, the inclusion of the bulky adduct within the active-site pocket prevents the normal turnover of substrate.

6. DEFICIENCY OF GSTZ/MAAI

As noted earlier, with the exception of GSTZ/MAAI, deficiencies of all the enzymes in the tyrosine catabolism pathway cause disease in humans. The absence of rare cases of MAAI deficiency and the severity of HT-1 resulting from fumarylacetoacetate-hydrolase deficiency (the subsequent step in the tyrosine catabolic pathway) suggested that MAAI deficiency may have a very severe or lethal phenotype. The effects of GSTZ/MAAI deficiency have been studied by knocking out the gene and by inactivating the enzyme by treatment with DCA.

6.1. GSTZ/MAAI Gene Knockouts

The *GSTZ/MAAI* gene was first knocked out in *Aspergillus nidulans* and the deficient variant failed to grow on phenylalanine-supplemented media *(22)*. Fernández-Cañón and colleagues recently inactivated the *GSTZ/MAAI* gene in 129Sv4 mice *(71)* and in our own laboratory we have knocked out the gene in

BALB/c mice *(45a)*. Both strains of mice survive and breed successfully but are severely affected by increased dietary phenylalanine or tyrosine. By 6 mo of age, the BALB/c null mice show multifocal hepatitis and a high incidence of pleomorphic mitochondria, which are features consistent with the chronic accumulation of a toxic metabolite. It was proposed that the lack of a severe phenotype in the 129Sv4 mice was attributable to nonenzymatic isomerization of MAA in the presence of glutathione *(71)*. Similarly, we found no evidence for the enzymatic redundancy of GSTZ/MAAI in BALB/c *Gstz* $^{-/-}$ mice. In other unpublished studies, we found no evidence for even low-level MAAI activity in a range of purified recombinant GSTs, including GSTA1-1, GSTA2-2, GSTA4-4, GSTM1-1, GSTM2-2, GSTM3-3, GSTP1-1, GSTT2-2, GSTO1-1, and GSTK. This is unusual, because many GSTs have some degree of overlap in their substrate specificities. Thus, based on the phenotype of the mice, it appears that GSTZ/MAAI deficiency in humans may be a benign disorder that does not become clinically apparent. However, long-term exposure of deficient individuals to a high-protein diet rich in tyrosine and phenylalanine may potentially cause liver and kidney damage. Additional studies are underway in our laboratory to determine the effects of GSTZ/MAAI deficiency in BALB/c mice over the long term.

6.2. Inactivation of GSTZ

Because GSTZ is irreversibly inactivated by DCA, transient deficiency of GSTZ can be created by repeated treatment with DCA. This technique has been used to determine the turnover of GSTZ in rat liver ($t_{1/2}$ = 3.3 d) and to study the metabolic changes that result from GSTZ/MAAI deficiency and decreased flux through the tyrosine degradation pathway *(45,72)*. Mass-spectral analysis of urine from rats given 1.2 mmol of DCA/kg/d for 5 d showed the presence of MAA and its decarboxylated product maleylacetone (MA). The reduced analogue of MA, succinylacetone (SA), was not detected *(72)*.

DCA is a carcinogen in mice and in rats, but at this stage it is not clear if DCA itself is carcinogenic or if the carcinogenicity results from the accumulation of MAA and MA that occurs when DCA inhibits GSTZ. Both MAA and MA are cytotoxic electrophiles and could react with a range of intracellular macromolecules *(72)*. The apparent carcinogenicity is important, considering the potential exposure of humans to DCA in chlorinated drinking water and from the metabolism of trichloroethylene and chloral hydrate. In addition, DCA is used clinically for the treatment of lactic acidosis by virtue of its capacity to activate the pyruvate dehydrogenase complex *(65)*. The inhibition of GSTZ by DCA has a distinct effect on the pharmacokinetics of DCA. This effect was considered in recent studies but earlier studies may need to be reinterpreted *(73–75)*.

Genetic polymorphism may also play a role in the pharmacokinetics of DCA in humans. We previously showed that there are significant differences in the susceptibility of some GSTZ1-1 isoforms to inactivation by DCA. Because of its resistance to inactivation (Table 3), individuals with the GSTZ1a-1a isoform would be expected to maintain their GSTZ activity and have a higher clearance of DCA after multiple exposures. A difference in clearance may translate to a difference in efficacy that could be considered when determining dose rates for DCA therapy. Adverse effects from DCA therapy have been noted in a patient with a mitochondrial disorder but it is unknown if this was related to her GSTZ genotype *(76)*. In Europeans, the *GSTZ1a* allele is the least frequent, suggesting that homozygotes will be rare. Further studies of other ethnic groups are warranted to determine if there are large differences in the frequency of the different alleles or the existence of additional alleles.

REFERENCES

1. Jakobsson PJ, Morgenstern R, Mancini J, Ford-Hutchinson A, Persson B. Common structural features of MAPEG—a widespread superfamily of membrane associated proteins with highly divergent functions in eicosanoid and glutathione metabolism. Protein Sci 1999;8:689–692.
2. Sheehan D, Meade G, Foley VM, Dowd, CA. Structure, function and evolution of glutathione transferases: implications for classification of non-mammalian members of an ancient enzyme superfamily. Biochem J 2001;360:1–16.
3. Mannervik B, Awasthi YC, Board PG, et al. Nomenclature for human glutathione transferases. Biochem J 1992;282:305–306.
4. Wagner U, Edwards R, Dixon DP, Mauch F. Probing the diversity of the *Arabidopsis* glutathione *S*-transferase gene family. Plant Mol Biol 2002;49:515–532.
5. Sawicki R, Singh SP, Mondal AK, Benes H, Zimniak P. Cloning, expression and biochemical characterization of one epsilon-class (GST-3) and ten delta-class (GST-1) glutathione *S*-transferases from *Drosophila melanogaster*, and identification of additional nine members of the epsilon class. Biochem J 2003;370:661–669.
6. Board PG, Webb GC. Isolation of a cDNA clone and localization of human glutathione *S*-transferase 2 genes to chromosome band 6p12. Proc Natl Acad Sci USA 1987;84:2377–2381.
7. Ross VL, Board PG, Webb GC. Chromosomal mapping of the human Mu class glutathione *S*-transferases to 1p13. Genomics 1993;18:87–91.
8. Whitbread AK, Tetlow N, Eyre HJ, Sutherland GR, Board PG. Characterization of the human omega class glutathione transferase genes and associated polymorphisms. Pharmacogenetics 2003;13:131–144.
9. Board PG, Webb GC, Coggan M. Isolation of a cDNA clone and localization of the human glutathione S-transferase 3 genes to chromosome bands 11q13 and 12q13-14. Ann Hum Genet 1989;53:205–213.
10. Kanaoka Y, Fujimori K, Kikuno R, Sakaguchi Y, Urade Y, Hayaishi O. Structure and chromosomal localization of human and mouse genes for hematopoietic

prostaglandin D synthase. Conservation of the ancestral genomic structure of sigma-class glutathione S-transferase. Eur J Biochem 2000;267:3315–3322.
11. Tan KL, Webb GC, Baker RT, Board PG. Molecular cloning of a cDNA and chromosomal localization of a human theta-class glutathione S-transferase gene (GSTT2) to chromosome 22. Genomics 1995;25:381–387.
12. Blackburn AC, Woollatt E, Sutherland GR, Board PG. Characterization and chromosome location of the gene GSTZ1 encoding the human zeta class glutathione transferase and maleylacetoacetate isomerase. Cytogenet Cell Genet 1998;83: 109–114.
13. Dulhunty A, Gage P, Curtis S, Chelvanayagam G, Board P. The glutathione transferase structural family includes a nuclear chloride channel and a ryanodine receptor calcium release channel modulator. J Biol Chem 2001;276:3319–3323.
14. Pemble SE, Wardle AF, Taylor JB. Glutathione S-transferase class kappa: characterization by the cloning of rat mitochondrial GST and identification of a human homologue. Biochem J 1996;319:749–754.
15. Board PG, Baker RT, Chelvanayagam G, Jermiin LS. Zeta, a novel class of glutathione transferases in a range of species from plants to humans. Biochem J 1997; 328:929–935.
16. Litwack G, Ketterer B, Arias IM. Ligandin: a hepatic protein which binds steroids, bilirubin, carcinogens and a number of exogenous organic anions. Nature 1971; 234:466–467.
17. Mannervik B, Danielson UH. Glutathione transferases—structure and catalytic activity. CRC Crit Rev Biochem 1988;23:283–337.
18. Board PG. Identification of cDNAs encoding two human alpha class glutathione transferases (GSTA3 and GSTA4) and the heterologous expression of GSTA4-4. Biochem J 1998;330:827–831.
19. Hubatsch I, Ridderstrom M, Mannervik B. Human glutathione transferase A4-4: an alpha class enzyme with high catalytic efficiency in the conjugation of 4-hydroxynonenal and other genotoxic products of lipid peroxidation. Biochem J 1998;330: 175–179.
20. Johansson AS, Mannervik B. Human glutathione transferase A3-3, a highly efficient catalyst of double-bond isomerization in the biosynthetic pathway of steroid hormones. J Biol Chem 2001;276: 33061–33065.
21. Kanaoka Y, Ago H, Inagaki E, et al. Cloning and crystal structure of hematopoietic prostaglandin D synthase. Cell 1997;90:1085–1095.
22. Fernández-Cñóon JM, Penalva MA. Characterization of a fungal maleylacetoacetate isomerase gene and identification of its human homologue. J Biol Chem 1998;273:329–337.
23. Tong Z, Board PG, Anders MW. Glutathione transferase zeta catalyses the oxygenation of the carcinogen dichloroacetic acid to glyoxylic acid. Biochem J 1998; 331:371–374.
24. Tomarev SI, Zinovieva RD, Piatigorsky J. Characterization of squid crystallin genes. Comparison with mammalian glutathione S-transferase genes. J Biol Chem 1992;267:8604–8612.

25. Adler V, Yin Z, Fuchs SY, et al. Regulation of JNK signaling by GSTp. EMBO J 1999;18:1321–1334.
26. Cho SG, Lee YH, Park HS, et al. Glutathione S-transferase mu modulates the stress-activated signals by suppressing apoptosis signal-regulating kinase 1. J Biol Chem 2001;276:12749–12755.
27. Harrop SJ, DeMaere MZ, Fairlie WD, et al. Crystal structure of a soluble form of the intracellular chloride ion channel CLIC1 (NCC27) at 1.4-A resolution. J Biol Chem 2001;276:44993–5000.
28. Altschul SF, Madden TL, Schaffer AA, et al. Gapped BLAST and PSI-BLAST: a new generation of protein database search programs. Nucl Acids Res 1997;25:3389–3402.
29. Board PG, Coggan M, Chelvanayagam G, et al. Identification, characterization and crystal structure of the omega class glutathione transferases. J Biol Chem 2000;275:24798–24806.
30. Board P, Tetlow N, Blackburn A, Chelvanayagam G. Database analysis and gene discovery in pharmacogenetics. Clin Chem Lab Med 2000;38:863–867.
31. Board P, Blackburn A, Jermiin LS, Chelvanayagam G. Polymorphism of phase II enzymes: identification of new enzymes and polymorphic variants by database analysis. Toxicol Lett 1998;102–103:149–154.
32. Tetlow N, Liu D, Board P. Polymorphism of human alpha class glutathione transferases. Pharmacogenetics 2001;11:609–617.
33. Blackburn AC, Tzeng HF, Anders MW, Board PG. Discovery of a functional polymorphism in human glutathione transferase zeta by expressed sequence tag database analysis. Pharmacogenetics 2000;10:49–57.
34. Blackburn AC, Coggan M, Tzeng HF, et al. GSTZ1d: a new allele of glutathione transferase zeta and maleylacetoacetate isomerase. Pharmacogenetics 2001;11:671–678.
35. Board PG, Pierce K. Expression of human glutathione S-transferase 2 in *Escherichia coli*. Immunological comparison with the basic glutathione S-transferases isoenzymes from human liver. Biochem J 1987;248:937–941.
36. Ross VL, Board PG. Molecular cloning and heterologous expression of an alternatively spliced human Mu class glutathione S-transferase transcript. Biochem J 1993;294 (Pt 2):373–380.
37. Baker RT, Smith SA, Marano R, McKee J, Board PG. Protein expression using cotranslational fusion and cleavage of ubiquitin. Mutagenesis of the glutathione-binding site of human Pi class glutathione S-transferase. J Biol Chem 1994;269: 25381–25386.
38. Tan KL, Chelvanayagam G, Parker MW, Board PG. Mutagenesis of the active site of the human theta-class glutathione transferase GSTT2-2: catalysis with different substrates involves different residues. Biochem J 1996;319:315–321.
39. Porath J, Olin B. Immobilized metal ion affinity adsorption and immobilized metal ion affinity chromatography of biomaterials. Serum protein affinities for gel-immobilized iron and nickel ions. Biochemistry 1983;22:1621–1630.
40. Tzeng HF, Blackburn AC, Board PG, Anders MW. Polymorphism- and species-dependent inactivation of glutathione transferase zeta by dichloroacetate. Chem Res Toxicol 2000;13:231–236.

41. Lantum HB, Board PG, Anders MW. Kinetics of the biotransformation of maleylacetone and chlorofluoroacetic acid by polymorphic variants of human glutathione transferase zeta (hGSTZ1-1). Chem Res Toxicol 2002;15:957–963.
42. Polekhina G, Board PG, Blackburn AC, Parker MW. Crystal structure of maleylacetoacetate isomerase/glutathione transferase zeta reveals the molecular basis for its remarkable catalytic promiscuity. Biochemistry 2001;40:1567–1576.
43. Thom R, Dixon DP, Edwards R, Cole, DJ, Lapthorn AJ. The structure of a zeta class glutathione S-transferase from *Arabidopsis thaliana*: characterisation of a GST with novel active-site architecture and a putative role in tyrosine catabolism. J Mol Biol 2001;308:949–962.
44. Lantum HB, Baggs RB, Krenitsky DM, Board PG, Anders MW. Immunohistochemical localization and activity of glutathione transferase zeta (GSTZ1-1) in rat tissues. Drug Metab Dispos 2002;30:616–625.
45. Anderson WB, Board PG, Gargano B, Anders MW. Inactivation of glutathione transferase zeta by dichloroacetic acid and other fluorine-lacking alpha-haloalkanoic acids. Chem Res Toxicol 1999;12:1144–1149.
45a. Lim CE, Matthaei KL, Blackburn AC, et al., Mice deficient in glutathione transferase zeta/maleylacetoacetate isomerase exhibit a range of pathological changes and elevated expression of alpha, mu, and pi class glutathione transferases. Am J Pathol 2004;165:679–693.
46. Tong Z, Board PG, Anders MW. Glutathione transferase zeta-catalyzed biotransformation of dichloroacetic acid and other alpha-haloacids. Chem Res Toxicol 1998;11:1332–1338.
47. Board PG, Taylor MC, Coggan M, Parker MW, Lantum HB, Anders MW. Clarification of the role of key active site residues of glutathione transferase zeta/ maleylacetoacetate isomerase by a new spectrophotometric technique. Biochem J 2003;374:731–737.
48. Russo P, O'Regan S. Visceral pathology of hereditary tyrosinemia type I. Am J Hum Genet 1990;47:317–324.
49. Mitchell GA, Grompe M, Lambert M, Tanquay RM. Hypertyrosiemia. In: Scriver CR, Beaudet AL, Sly WS, Valle D, eds. The Metabolic Basis of Inherited Disease, Vol. 2. New York: McGraw-Hill, 2001, pp. 1777–1805.
50. Lindblad B, Steen G. Identification of 4,6-dioxoheptanoic acid (succinylacetone), 3,5-dioxooctanedioic acid (succinylacetoacetate) and 4-oxo-6-hydroxyheptanoic acid in the urine from patients with hereditary tyrosinemia. Biomed Mass Spectrom 1982;9:419–424.
51. Lindblad B, Lindstedt S, Steen G. On the enzymic defects in hereditary tyrosinemia. Proc Natl Acad Sci USA 1977;74:4641–4645.
52. Sassa S, Kappas A. Hereditary tyrosinemia and the heme biosynthetic pathway. Profound inhibition of delta-aminolevulinic acid dehydratase activity by succinylacetone. J Clin Invest 1983;71:625–634.
53. Berger R, Michals K, Galbraeth J, Matalon R. Tyrosinemia type 1b caused by maleylacetoacetate isomerase deficiency: a new enzyme defect. Pediatr Res 1988; 23:328A.

54. Fowler J, Seltzer S. Synthesis of model compounds for maleylacetoacetic acid. J Org Chem 1970;35:3529–3532.
55. Seltzer S. Purification and properties of maleylacetone cis-trans isomerase from vibrio 01. J Biol Chem 1973;248:215–222.
56. Anandarajah K, Kiefer PM Jr, Donohoe BS, Copley SD. Recruitment of a double bond isomerase to serve as a reductive dehalogenase during biodegradation of pentachlorophenol. Biochemistry 2000;39:5303–5311.
57. Lipscomb JC, Mahle DA, Brashear WT, Barton HA. Dichloroacetic acid: metabolism in cytosol. Drug Metab Dispos 1995;23:1202–1205.
58. James MO, Cornett R, Yan Z, Henderson GN, Stacpoole PW. Glutathione-dependent conversion to glyoxylate, a major pathway of dichloroacetate biotransformation in hepatic cytosol from humans and rats, is reduced in dichloroacetate-treated rats. Drug Metab Dispos 1997;25:1223–1227.
59. Haber LT, Maier A, Gentry PR, Clewell HJ, Dourson ML. Genetic polymorphisms in assessing interindividual variability in delivered dose. Regul Toxicol Pharmacol 2002;35:177–197.
60. Bull RJ, Sanchez IM, Nelson MA, Larson JL, Lansing AJ. Liver tumor induction in B6C3F1 mice by dichloroacetate and trichloroacetate. Toxicology 1990;63:341–359.
61. DeAngelo AB, Daniel FB, Most BM, Olson GR. The carcinogenicity of dichloroacetic acid in the male Fischer 344 rat. Toxicology 1996;114:207–221.
62. Boorman GA. Drinking water disinfection byproducts: review and approach to toxicity evaluation. Environ Hlth Perspect 1999;107 (Suppl 1):207–217.
63. Krasner SW, McGuire MJ, Jacangelo JG, Patania NL, Reagan KM, Aieta EM. The occurence of disinfection by-products in U.S. drinking water. J Am Waterworks Assoc 1989;81:41–53.
64. Stacpoole PW, Henderson GN, Yan Z, James MO. Clinical pharmacology and toxicology of dichloroacetate. Environ Hlth Perspect 1998;106 (Suppl 4):989–994.
65. Stacpoole PW, Henderson GN, Yan Z, Cornett R, James MO. Pharmacokinetics, metabolism and toxicology of dichloroacetate. Drug Metab Rev 1998;30:499–539.
66. Cornett R, James MO, Henderson GN, Cheung J, Shroads AL, Stacpoole PW. Inhibition of glutathione S-transferase zeta and tyrosine metabolism by dichloroacetate: a potential unifying mechanism for its altered biotransformation and toxicity. Biochem Biophys Res Commun 1999;262:752–756.
67. Armstrong RN. Structure, catalytic mechanism, and evolution of the glutathione transferases. Chem Res Toxicol 1997;10:2–18.
68. Oakley AJ, Bello ML, Battistoni A, Ricci G, Rossjohn J, Villar HO, Parker MW. The structures of human glutathione transferase P1-1 in complex with glutathione and various inhibitors at high resolution. J Mol Biol 1997;274:84–100.
69. Anderson WB, Liebler DC, Board PG, Anders MW. Mass spectral characterization of dichloroacetic acid-modified human glutathione transferase zeta. Chem Res Toxicol 2002;15:1387–1397.
70. Curry SH, Lorenz A, Chu PI, Limacher M, Stacpoole PW. Disposition and pharmacodynamics of dichloroacetate (DCA) and oxalate following oral DCA doses. Biopharm Drug Dispos 1991;12:375–390.

71. Fernandez-Canon JM, Baetscher MW, Finegold M, Burlingame T, Gibson KM, Grompe M. Maleylacetoacetate isomerase (MAAI/GSTZ)-deficient mice reveal a glutathione-dependent nonenzymatic bypass in tyrosine catabolism. Mol Cell Biol 2002; 22:4943–4951.
72. Lantum HB, Cornejo J, Pierce RH, Anders MW. Perturbation of maleylacetoacetic acid metabolism in rats with dichloroacetic acid-induced glutathione transferase zeta deficiency. Toxicol Sci 2003;74:192–202.
73. Saghir SA, Schultz IR. Low-dose pharmacokinetics and oral bioavailability of dichloroacetate in naive and GST-zeta-depleted rats. Environ Hlth Perspect 2002; 110:757–763.
74. Schultz, IR, Sylvester SR. Stereospecific toxicokinetics of bromochloro- and chlorofluoroacetate: effect of GST-zeta depletion. Toxicol Appl Pharmacol 2001; 175:104–113.
75. Schultz IR, Merdink JL, Gonzalez-Leon A, Bull RJ. Dichloroacetate toxicokinetics and disruption of tyrosine catabolism in B6C3F1 mice: dose-response relationships and age as a modifying factor. Toxicology 2002;173:229–247.
76. Izumi M, Hirayama Y, Sugai K, et al. Adverse effects of dichloroacetate in a girl with mitochondrial disorder. No To Hattatsu 2003;35:54–58.

5

Glucuronidation of Fatty Acids and Prostaglandins by Human UDP-Glucuronosyltransferases

Anna Radominska-Pandya, Joanna M. Little, and Arthur Bull

Summary

This chapter summarizes methods and experimental approaches involved in the study of glucuronidation of several naturally occurring metabolites of the free fatty acids (FFAs), linoleic acid (LA), and arachidonic acid (AA). Data on FA glucuronidation from both human liver microsomes and human recombinant UDP-glucuronosyltransferase 2B7 (UGT2B7) are presented. Several unique methods for synthesis of FAs that are not commercially available are also described. Moreover, comprehensive methods for measurements of FA glucuronidation, isolation of biosynthesized glucuronides, and analysis by HPLC, HPLC–MS, and GC–MS are discussed in detail. The enzymatic assays presented in this chapter can also be used for studying glucuronidation of other hydrophobic endogenous compounds, including many drugs and environmental pollutants. The potential value of these methods is highlighted by the growing appreciation of the roles of FFA and FA-glucuronides in human health and disease.

Key Words

Arachidonic acid; eiconsanoids; epoxides; fatty acids; fatty acid derivatives synthesis; fatty acid glucuronides; gas chromatography–mass spectrometry; glucuronidation assays; high-performance liquid chromatography; high-performance liquid chromatography–mass spectrometry; human; linoleic acid; liquid chromatography–mass spectrometry; peroxisome proliferator-activated receptor; prostaglandins; thin layer chromatography; UDP-glucuronosyltransferases; UGT2B7.

1. INTRODUCTION

In this chapter, we describe the methods involved in the study of glucuronidation of several naturally occurring metabolites of the free fatty acids (FFAs), linoleic acid (LA), and arachidonic acid (AA). Multiple oxidative

From: *Methods in Pharmacology and Toxicology,*
Drug Metabolism and Transport: Molecular Methods and Mechanisms
Edited by: L. Lash © Humana Press Inc., Totowa, NJ

metabolites of LA exist. For example, when LA is metabolized by 15-lipoxygenase, 13-hydroxyoctadecadienoic (13-HODE) and 13-oxooctadecadienoic (13-OXO) acids are biosynthesized. The structures and metabolism of these LA derivatives are presented in Fig. 1. LA can also be metabolized by a variety of cytochrome P450 enzymes to form the 9,10- and 12,13-dihydroxyoctadecadienoic acids (LA 9,10- and 12,13- diols) via the intermediate LA-monoepoxides, as shown in Fig. 2. Both groups of oxidized LA derivatives have a number of important cellular effects.

Enzymatic oxidation of LA leads to the controlled production of at least two biologically active compounds, 13-HODE and 13-OXO (*see* Fig. 1). Both of these compounds serve as endogenous ligands for peroxisome proliferator-activated receptors (PPARs), although they appear to have differing biological activities *(1–3)*. For example, 13-HODE has been shown to be a mitogenic factor for hepatic tumors, whereas 13-OXO is linked to the differentiation of colon epithelial cells. In particular, the enzyme responsible for production of 13-OXO, 13-HODE dehydrogenase, and PPARγ are both found in more differentiated cells of the intestinal mucosa *(4,5)*. The opposing biological effects of these two compounds suggest that their metabolic disposition plays an important role in the control of cellular signaling.

In contrast, products of CYP450 metabolism, such as LA epoxides and LA diols, have been implicated in a number of pathophysiological processes in vivo. For example, LA monoepoxides (LA-epoxides) are produced at high levels during acute inflammation and are found in lavage fluid of patients with adult respiratory distress syndrome and in the serum of patients suffering from severe burns *(6,7)*. The LA 9,10- and 12,13-diols are significantly more cytotoxic than the corresponding LA-epoxides in several in vitro models *(8–10)*. These studies link the hydrolysis of LA-epoxides to cytotoxicity. It was reported that oxidized fatty acids (OFAs) can be incorporated into membrane phospholipids, resulting in the formation of novel secondary messengers involved in signal transduction pathways *(11–13)*.

Eicosanoids are products of biotransformation of AA via cyclooxygenases and lipoxygenases (structures and metabolites are presented in Fig. 3) and play a role in many processes in the body. For example, prostaglandins (PGs), the products of cyclooxygenases, participate in vascular, kidney, and reproductive functions *(14)*. The lipoxygenase system also converts AAs to hydroxylated metabolites (hydroxyeicosatetraenoic acids [HETEs] and LKB_4) that are vasoactive, angiogenic, tumorigenic, and are active in platelet activation and aggregation, immune responses, differentiation, and apoptosis *(15–19)*.

Recently, studies of the role of FA in modulation of cell signaling pathways *(20)* indicated that FAs such as phytanic acid (PA) and docosahexaenoic acid

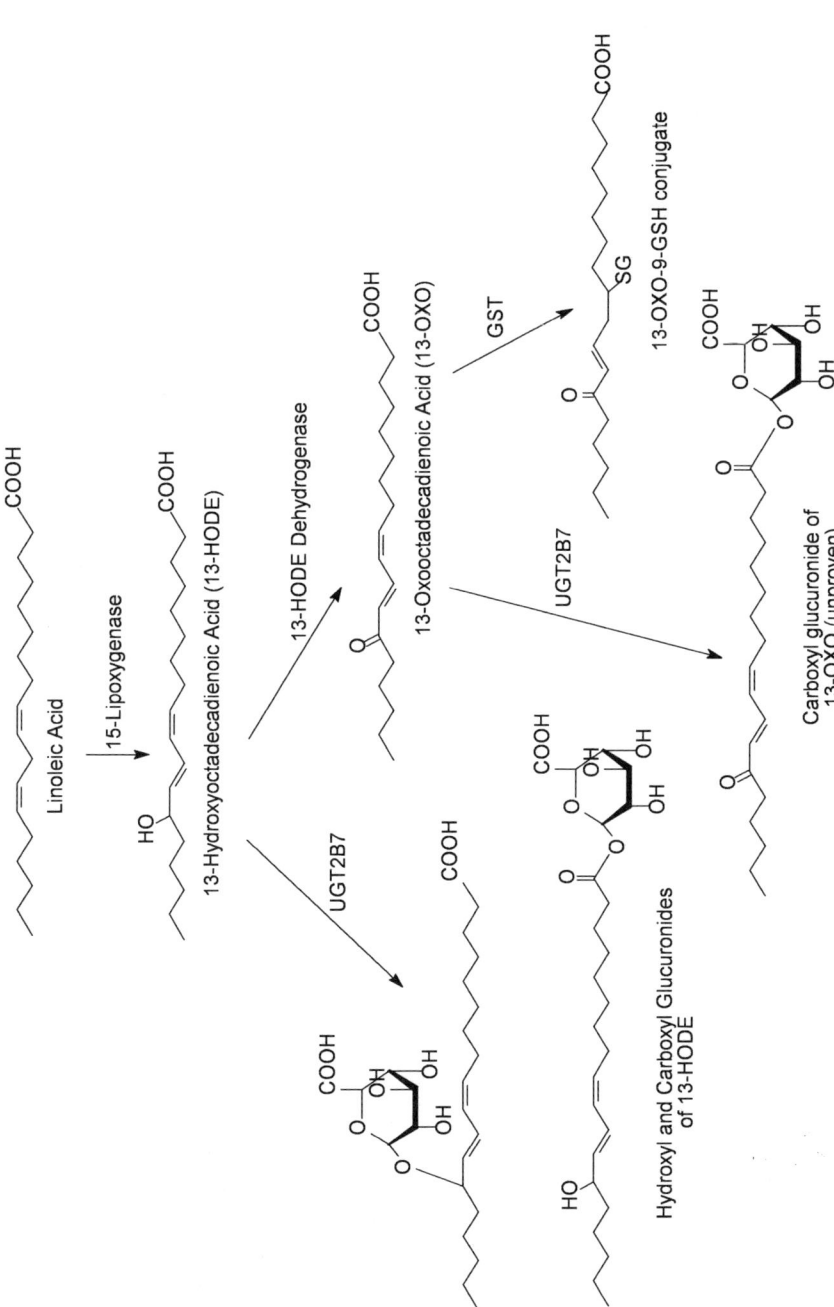

Fig. 1. Structures and metabolism of LA, 13-HODE and 13-OXO. (Reprinted from ref. *34* with permission from ASPET.)

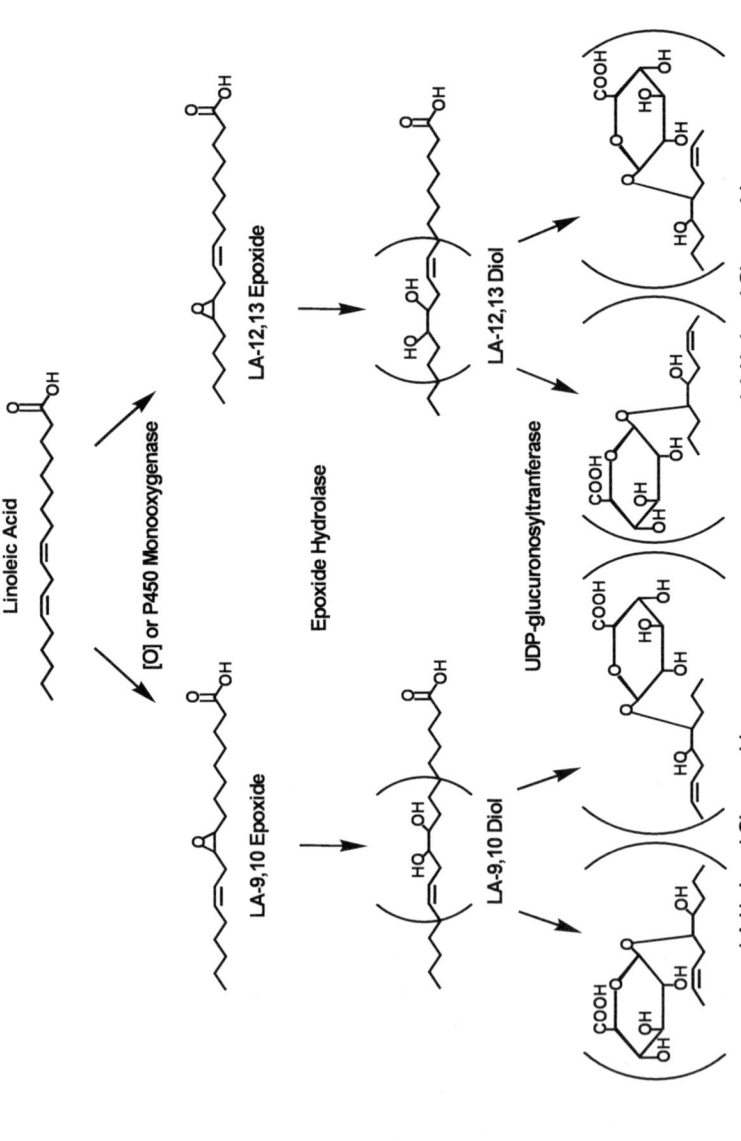

Fig. 2. Metabolic pathway for LA and its metabolites. LA is converted to individual positional monoepoxides during lipid peroxidation or by CYP-mediated reactions resulting in the formation of LA-9,10- and 12,13-epoxides. Each monoepoxide may be metabolized to the corresponding diol in the presence of soluble or microsomal epoxide hydrolase. The resulting diols may then be conjugated with glucuronic acid at the carboxyl (not shown) or individual hydroxyl positions by UGTs. (Reprinted from ref. 57. Copyright 2000, with permission from Elsevier.)

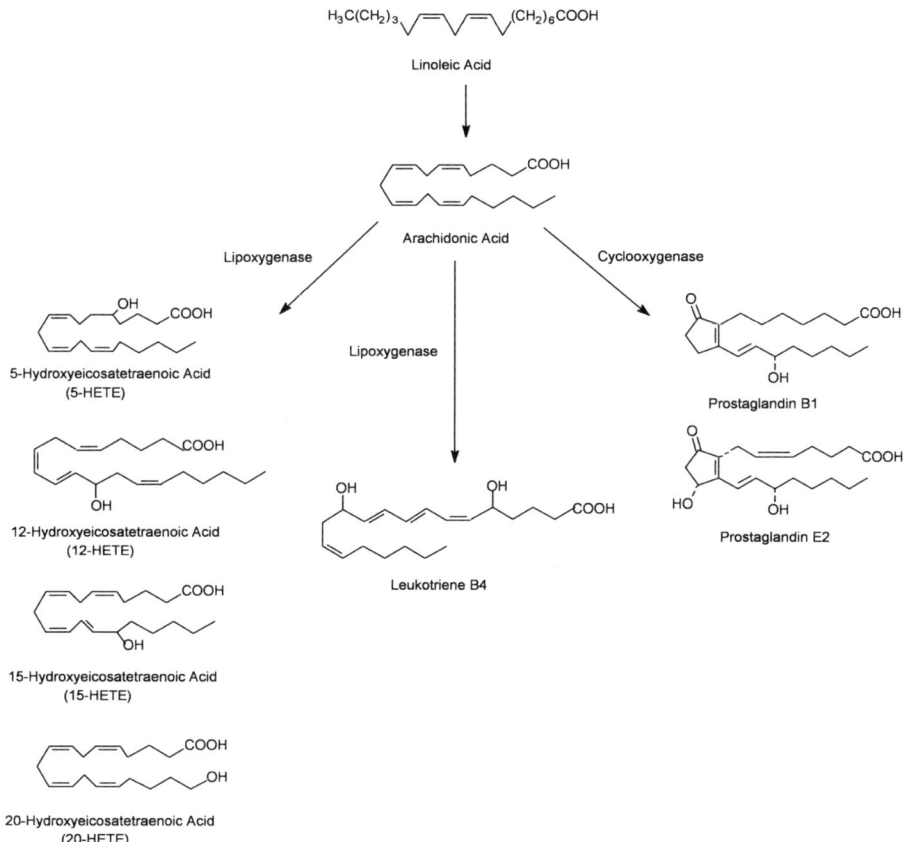

Fig. 3. Biotransformation of AA via cyclooxygenases and lipoxygenases to bioactive eicosanoids.

(DHA) activate the nuclear receptors, retinoid X receptor (RXR) and peroxisome proliferator-activated receptor (PPAR) *(21,22)*. PA is a branched-chain FA that is a constituent of dairy products, meat, and fish and has been shown to be a naturally occurring ligand for PPARα *(23)*. DHA is a constituent of the human diet, particularly fatty fish, and plays a physiological role in brain maturation and development and retinal development. Studies have demonstrated that DHA is a highly specific ligand for RXRα in mouse brain *(24)* and has been reported to be a ligand for PPARα *(25)*.

These critical functions of OFA could be regulated by glucuronidation; however, information on FA biotransformation via glucuronidation is limited. Glucuronidation is carried out by UDP-glucuronosyltransferases (UGTs), which comprise a family of enzymes involved in the metabolism of a variety of hydrophobic endogenous and exogenous compounds. This covalent modification generally renders the substrate less biologically active and more hydrophilic and thus more readily excreted in urine or bile. However, glucuronide conjugation may also produce derivatives with enhanced biological activity, promote transport to target tissues, and/or regulate concentration *(26)*.

The first glucuronides of OFAs were isolated from and identified in human urine *(27–29)* and primary human hepatocyte cultures *(30)*, thus demonstrating the role of UGTs in these reactions. The glucuronides of dihydroxy FA were first isolated from the urine of patients with generalized peroxisomal disorders and were considered detoxification products of these cytotoxic diols *(28)*. The major compounds isolated were LA-9,10 and -12,13-diol glucuronides (*see* Fig. 2). The monohydroxylated AA derivative, 20-HETE, was also isolated as a glucuronide from the urine of normal subjects and, at significantly higher levels, from patients with hepatic cirrhosis *(27,29)*. Finally, certain eicosanoids have been identified as substrates for UGTs. The biosynthesis of glucuronides of several eicosanoids by isolated human and rat hepatocytes has been described *(30,31)*.

Recently, our laboratory has become interested in the characterization of the glucuronidation of FFAs and their oxidized derivatives and reported the first in vitro studies demonstrating that OFA glucuronides can be biosynthesized by human liver and intestinal microsomes *(32–34)*. These studies demonstrated that LA, LA-diols, 13-HODE and 13-OXO, as well as AA, are conjugated with glucuronic acid in vitro *(32–35)*. It is noteworthy that both 13-HODE and 13-OXO are substrates for UGTs, while only 13-OXO is a substrate for glutathione transferase *(34,36)*. Thus, UGT activity could play a major role in the biological effects produced by the enzymatic oxidation and secondary metabolism of LA. The human UGT2B7 isoform has been identified as the only available UGT isoform with the ability to glucuronidate both the hydroxyl and carboxyl functions of LA and LA-diols.

We also investigated the glucuronidation of PA and DHA by human liver and intestinal microsomes and recombinant UGT2B7 *(37)*. The results showed that both PA and DHA were effectively glucuronidated in vitro by human liver and intestinal microsomes and recombinant UGT2B7. In our most recent studies, we carried out in vitro characterization of the glucuronidation of 15- and 20-HETE and two prostaglandins, PGE_1 and PGB_2, compounds with recognized physiological significance, and compared the results with the glucuronidation of AA, the parent compound *(38)*. All these compounds were efficiently glucuronidated by human UGTs. Belanger's group reported that leukotriene B_4, and 5- and 12-HETE are also glucuronidated by human UGT isoforms *(39)*. In summary, these glucuronidation studies provide overwhelming evidence that glucuronidation of FA is a physiologically significant process and an essential part of mammalian cell metabolism.

This chapter describes the most recent developments in the area of FA and OFA glucuronidation. Several unique syntheses of FA that are not commercially available are described. Moreover, comprehensive methods for FA glucuronidation, isolation of biosynthesized glucuronides and high-performance liquid chromatography–mass spectrometry (HPLC–MS) analysis are discussed in detail. The majority of the information presented was obtained in our laboratories.

2. MATERIALS

[^{14}C]Linoleic acid ([^{14}C]LA), [^{14}C]UDP-glucuronic acid ([^{14}C]UDPGlcUA), and [^{3}H]arachidonic acid ([^{3}H]AA) were from PerkinElmer Life Sciences (Boston, MA). Unlabeled free fatty acids, LA, AA, phytanic acid (PA, 3,7,11,15-tetramethylhexadecanoic acid) and *cis*-4,7,10,13,16,19-docosahexaenoic acid (DHA) (>95% pure), unlabeled UDPGlcUA, saccharolactone, and *N*-(2-hydroxyethyl) piperazine-*N'*-(2-ethane) sulfonic acid (HEPES) were from Sigma (St. Louis, MO). 5-, 12-, 15-, 20-HETE, prostaglandin (PG) E_2, and PGB_1 were from Cayman Chemicals (Ann Arbor, MI). All other chemicals were of the highest purity available.

3. METHODS

3.1. Synthesis of FA Substrates

The majority of FA and their oxidized derivatives are available commercially and their commercial sources are given in Subheading 2. However, several FA substrates for glucuronidation reactions were synthesized in our laboratories. The synthesis of 13*(S)*-hydroxyoctadecadienoic acid [13*(S)*-HODE] and 13-oxooctadecadienoic acid (13-OXO) in both unlabeled and radioactive form were chemically synthesized according to protocols presented in the following subheadings. Especially important was the elaboration of the synthesis and chiral-HPLC separation of the LA-9,10- and 11,13-diols. The protocols include all the FA intermediates essential for the preparation of the final products.

3.1.1. Synthesis of 13-Hydroperoxy-(z,e)-9,11-octadecadienoic Acid (13-HPODE)

The synthesis of 13-HPODE, a direct intermediate in the synthesis of 13*(S)*-HODE, was achieved using soybean lipoxygenase at elevated pH *(40)*. This reaction yields a single isomer, 13*(S)*-HPODE, which results in a single isomer of the final product being obtained. Alternative lipoxygenase enzymes can be used to produce other stereoisomers or photochemical oxygenation can be performed to obtain a mixture of all possible isomers *(41,42)*. All solutions should be kept on ice during the procedure to maximize yield and minimize product decomposition. 13*(S)*-HPODE was prepared by the soybean lipoxygenase-catalyzed oxygenation of LA, followed by reduction of the resulting hydroperoxide with sodium borohydride or triphenyl phosphine *(43)*. The reaction was carried out in 47 mM sodium borate buffer, pH 9.0, that was oxygenated by bubbling with oxygen for 15 min at 0°C. Sufficient LA was added from an 88 mM stock solution in 95% ethanol to yield a final concentration of 0.78 mM. The reaction was initiated by the addition of 2.1×10^3 units/mL of soybean lipoxygenase (Sigma). After incubation on ice for 5 min, the reaction was terminated by addition of concentrated HCl and immediately extracted three times with an equal volume of peroxide-free ether. The ether was back-washed with 0.5 vols of water and residual water removed by stirring with anhydrous $MgSO_4$. The ether was removed under vacuum and the residue dissolved in about 10 mL of ethanol. If residual water remains, it can be removed by co-distillation with absolute ethanol. Thin-layer chromatography (TLC) on silica gel developed with hexane–2-propanol–acetic acid (115:11:1) was be used to analyze product formation and ensure complete conversion of LA to 13-HPODE. The hydroperoxide was detected by either iodine or a ferrous thiocyanate spray reagent *(44)*.

3.1.2. Synthesis of 13(S)-Hydroxyoctadecadienoic Acid (13-HODE) and 1-[^{14}C]13-HODE

13*(S)*-HPODE, prepared as described in Subheading 3.1.1., was reduced with sodium borohydride or triphenyl phosphine *(43)*. The ethanolic solution of 13-HPODE was cooled on ice and one equivalent of solid sodium borohydride was added with stirring. After 15 min on ice, the reaction was stirred for another 15 min at room temperature, acidified, and extracted with ether, which was then dried with $MgSO_4$ and then removed under vacuum. If necessary, the product was purified by chromatography on silicic acid eluted with hexane containing from 3% to 20% ethyl acetate. The yield of product was quantitated by measuring the absorbance at 237 nm, using a molar absorptivity of 28,000 M^{-1} cm^{-1}. It is worthy of mention that there is some controversy in the literature concerning the appropriate value for the molar absorptivity, with values ranging from about 23,000 to 28,000 M^{-1} cm^{-1}, although the value determined in our laboratory is closer to the latter figure *(45)*. Radiolabeled 1-[^{14}C]13-HODE was prepared in the same manner using 1-[^{14}C]LA.

3.1.3. Synthesis of 13-Oxooctadecadienoic Acid (13-OXO) and 1-[^{14}C]13-OXO

To prepare 13-OXO, 100 mg of 13-HPODE was dissolved in anhydrous pyridine and cooled on ice *(46)*. Over a period of 10 min, 2.5 mL of acetyl chloride was added with stirring, and about 250 mL of water was added and the mixture was extracted several times with one volume of ethyl ether. The ether layer was washed with 200 mL of saturated $CuSO_4$ and dried with $MgSO_4$. Column chromatography on silicic acid eluted with 5% ethyl acetate in hexane was used to purify the product. After the appropriate fractions were pooled and the solvent removed, the product was dissolved in ethanol and quantitated by measuring the absorbance at 280 nm, using a molar absorptivity of 28,000 M^{-1} cm^{-1}. 1-[^{14}C]13-OXO was prepared in the same manner using 1-[^{14}C]LA.

3.1.4. Synthesis of 9,10-and 12,13-Dihydroxyoctadecadienoic Acids (LA-9,10 and LA-12,13 Diols)

3.1.4.1. SYNTHESIS OF METHYL ESTER LA-MONOEPOXIDES AND METHYL LA-DIOLS

LA methyl ester derivatives are very valuable compounds for studying the glucuronidation of oxidized derivatives of LA. Derivatization of the carboxyl function directs the glucuronidation reaction exclusively to the hydroxyl functions. Several methylated compounds were therefore synthesized.

The monoepoxides of methyl linoleate were chemically synthesized using *m*-chloroperoxybenzoic acid, as previously described *(9)*. Methyl ester monoepoxides (MeLA-epoxides) were separated from diepoxides and starting material by chromatography on a silica column using a mobile phase of methylene chloride–ethyl ether (98:2, v/v), and hydrolyzed to their corresponding methyl ester diols (MeLA-diols) by reacting with 5% perchloric acid in an equal volume of acetonitrile at 25°C for 1 h.

3.1.4.2. SYNTHESIS OF FREE ACID LA-EPOXIDES AND LA-DIOLS

To prepare the LA-epoxide, LA was dissolved in dichloromethane and 0.5 mol% methyltrioxorhenium was added, followed by 12 mol% pyridine. To this solution, 1.5 equivalents of 30% H_2O_2 were added dropwise over 5–10 min. During H_2O_2 addition, the solution was kept at 20–25°C with stirring for about 30 min. The reaction was terminated by adding a catalytic amount of MnO_2 to decompose excess H_2O_2. The mixture was then extracted with dichloromethane and purified by chromatography on silica gel eluted with dichloromethane–ethyl acetate–acetic acid (94.9:5:0.1). After TLC, LA-epoxides were visualized by iodine vapor.

LA-epoxides also can be chemically synthesized using peracetic acid. LA (1.5 mmol) was dissolved in 40 mL of methylene chloride. Peracetic acid (5.0 mmol) was added and stirred at 25°C for 2 h. The reaction mixture was dried under vacuum and stored at 4°C.

LA-diols were prepared by acid-catalyzed hydrolysis of LA-epoxides. For hydrolysis, 0.20 mmol of the purified LA-epoxides were dissolved in 1.0 mL of acetonitrile and stirred with an equal volume of 5% perchloric acid for 1 h at room temperature. The reaction was terminated by the addition of 1.5 mL of saturated NaCl and the mixture was extracted three times with ethyl ether. The organic phases were pooled, dried over sodium sulfate, filtered, dried under vacuum, and stored at 4°C until purified.

3.1.5. HPLC Purification of Methyl Ester and Free Acid Monoepoxides and Diols

Methyl ester and free acid LA monoepoxide and diol reaction products were analyzed by normal-phase HPLC (NP-HPLC) using a 4.6 × 250 mm, 5 µm silica column (Varian, Walnut Creek, CA) with a LC-600 chromatograph (Shimadzu, Japan) equipped with a SPD-6AV variable wavelength UV-VIS detector. Separation of positional isomers of the MeLA-epoxides and diols was achieved by eluting the column under isocratic conditions using mobile phases of isooctane–2-propanol (497.5:2.5, v/v) and hexane–2-propanol (485:15, v/v), respectively. Separation of free acid positional isomers was achieved by eluting the column under isocratic conditions using a mobile phase of hexane–2-propanol–acetic acid (496.25:3.75:0.5, by vol) for the monoepoxides and hexane–2-propanol–acetic acid (480.0:20.0:0.5, by vol) for the diols. A flow rate of 1.0 mL/min and a detection wavelength of 202 nm were used for all analytical separations. Sufficient quantities of each purified positional isomer of the methyl ester and free acid diols for enzyme assays were obtained by passing each reaction product through a Dynamax Silica 10.0 × 250 mm semi-preparative column (Varian) at a flow rate of 4.7 mL/min using the mobile phases and detection wavelength described earlier.

3.1.6. Methylation and GC-MS Analysis

Methyl esters were prepared by treating 6.0 µmol of each free acid positional isomer with 2.0 M (trimethylsilyl) diazomethane. Methylated products were analyzed by NP-HPLC using the conditions described in Subheading 3.1.5. and analyzed by gas chromatography–mass spectrometry (GC–MS). GC–MS was performed on a model TSQ 700 triple quadrupole instrument (Finnigan Corp., San Jose, CA) with a DB-5ms capillary column (30 m × 0.25 mm inner diameter × 0.25 µm film thickness) (J&W Scientific, Folsom, CA). The instrument was equipped with a model 3400 GC (Varian Instruments, Walnut Creek, CA) and a model CTC-A200S autosampler (Leap Technologies, Carrboro, NC). The GC injector was a Varian SPI (septum-equipped, temperature programmable injector) with helium as the carrier gas, set to 10 psi head pressure. The GC column was heated from 80°C to 300°C with a temperature ramp of 10°C/min with the final temperature being held for 2 min. The injector and transfer line was heated appropriately. The MS was operated in the electron ionization (EI) mode (70 V, 150°C) and the first quadrupole was scanned from *(m/z)* 50 to 450 with a 0.5-s cycle time. The calculation of purity was based on the integration of the peaks from the reconstructed ion chromatograms using ICIS software (Finnigan Corp.).

3.1.7. Chiral-HPLC Separation of LA-Diols

Enantiomers of the racemic LA-diols were isolated using a 4.6 × 250 mm Chiralcel OB column (Chiral Technologies Inc., Exton, PA). The 12,13-diol enantiomers were separated as free acids and the 9,10-diol enantiomers were separated as the methyl esters. Each separation was achieved using an isocratic mobile phase consisting of hexane–2-propanol (492.5:7.5, v/v). Acetic acid (0.1%) was added to the mobile phase for the separation of the LA-12,13-diol isomers. A flow rate of 1.0 mL/min and a detection wavelength of 202 nm were used. The enantiomers of the MeLA-9,10-diols were collected and converted to the corresponding free acid diols by sonication and incubation at 50°C for 1 h in 0.4 M KOH in methanol. The samples were subsequently mixed on a vortex mixer, sonicated, and incubated for an additional 30 min, after which the reaction mixture was adjusted to pH 7.0 with formic acid and extracted with ethyl ether. The resulting free acid enantiomers were collected by NP-HPLC as described in Subheading 3.1.5.

3.2. Glucuronidation Assays

Glucuronidation reactions are catalyzed by microsomal UGTs and require UDP-glucuronic acid (UDP-GlcUA) as an essential cofactor (47). Activity of UGTs is dependent on the presence of phospholipids in vivo and in vitro and is known to be influenced by multiple factors, such as the presence of detergents, sonication, the type of buffer, ionic strength, pH, and the presence of activators. The glucuronidation assays with FFA and their derivatives were carried out in our laboratories with human liver and intestinal microsomes and recombinant UGT isoforms as the enzyme sources. All of our assays were carried out under the same conditions so that experiments carried out with different FA substrates can be easily compared (Table 1). There are several major problems that occur with the glucuronidation assays. Because microsomal UGTs exhibit latency, microsomes are typically activated with membrane-disrupting procedures to achieve optimal UGT activity. In all of our microsomal assays, Brij 58 was used as the detergent, which plays a dual role in the assay. First, it activates the microsomes, and second, it solubilizes the hydrophobic FA substrates. Because detergent treatment of recombinant UGTs frequently results in significant inhibition of UGT activity, alamethicin treatment of the membrane preparations is the preferred method of activation and was used in all the experiments with recombinant UGTs.

3.2.1. Procedures for Enzymatic Assays

UGT activity in microsomes was determined using labeled substrate and UDP-GlcUA or unlabeled substrate and [^{14}C]UDP-GlcUA as the sugar donor, as described in detail previously *(48,49)*. In brief, substrates were solubilized in micelles with Brij 58 (micelle concentration, 0.12%; final concentration, 0.05%) *(50–52)*. Substrates (final concentration: 100–250 µM) were preincubated with protein (50 µg) in 100 mM HEPES-NaOH, pH 7.4, 5 mM MgCl$_2$, and 5 mM saccharolactone at room temperature for 10 min. Reactions were started by the addition of UDP-GlcUA (4 mM final concentration) and incubated at 37°C for 20 min. For assays carried out with recombinant UGTs, FA substrates were introduced to the reaction mixture in ethanol and UGTs were activated with alamethicin (final concentration, 60 µg/mg of protein), also dissolved in ethanol. The final concentration of ethanol in the incubation was less than 3%.

Reactions were stopped by the addition of 20 µL of ethanol, samples were mixed with a vortex mixer and placed on ice. Aliquots were applied to TLC plates and glucuronidated products and unreacted substrate were separated by development (once for LA, AA, PA, DHA and other FFAs, twice for 13-HODE and 13-OXO and three times for the LA diols) in chloroform–methanol–glacial acetic acid–water (65:25:2:4, by vol). These TLC conditions allowed for the separation of carboxyl- and hydroxyl-linked glucuronides. Radioactive compounds were localized on TLC plates by autoradiography for 3–4 days at –80°C. An autoradiograph of a representative TLC separation is shown in Fig. 4. Silica gel in zones corresponding to the glucuronide bands, or corresponding areas from control lanes, were scraped into scintillation vials and radioactivity was measured by liquid scintillation counting.

3.2.2. β-Glucuronidase Hydrolysis

Direct proof that a given FA substrate is glucuronidated comes from a comparison of the product of the glucuronidation reaction before and after treatment with β-glucuronidase. For β-glucuronidase hydrolysis, after the standard assay procedure, duplicate reactions were stopped with 1 mL of 0.1 M glycine–trichloroacetic acid buffer, pH 2.8, and samples were applied to BondElut C$_{18}$ cartridges (Varian, Palo Alto, CA), primed as recommended by the manufacturer. The cartridges were washed with 5 mL of glycine–trichloroacetic acid buffer and 5 mL of water and eluted with 3 mL of methanol; the methanol was evaporated. For each set of duplicate samples, one was dissolved in 30 mM sodium phosphate buffer, pH 7.4, containing 50 U of *E. coli* β-glucuronidase, and the other sample was dissolved in buffer alone (60 µL). Both samples were incubated for 4 h at 37°C after which reactions were stopped with ethanol. The samples were then handled as for a standard assay.

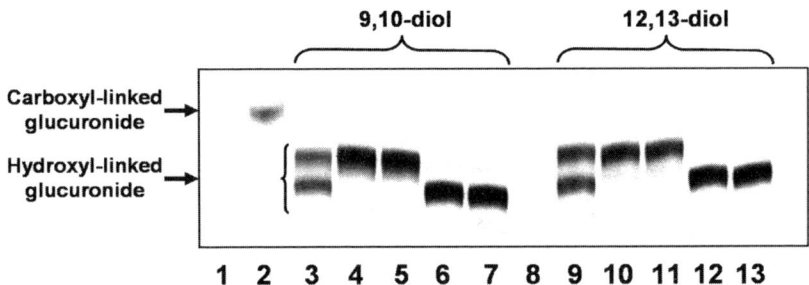

Fig. 4. TLC analysis of biosynthesized LA and LA-diol glucuronides. Control assays performed in the absence of substrate *(lanes 1* and *8)*, carboxyl-linked glucuronide of LA *(lane 2)*, hydroxyl-linked glucuronides of racemic LA-9,10-diol *(lane 3)*, and individual hydroxyl-linked glucuronides of the (−) enantiomer *(lanes 4* and *5)* and (+) enantiomer *(lanes 6* and *7)* of LA-9,10-diol. Similar results are seen for hydroxyl-linked glucuronides of racemic LA-12,13-diol *(lane 9)* and individual hydroxyl-linked glucuronides of the (−) enantiomer *(lanes 10* and *11)* and (+) enantiomer *(lanes 12* and *13)* of LA-9,10-diol. The autoradiograph shown is representative of two identical experiments. (Reprinted from ref. *57*. Copyright 2000, with permission from Elsevier.)

3.2.3. TLC Characterization of Biosynthesized Glucuronides

Initial identification of the position of glucuronide conjugation (carboxyl- or hydroxyl-linked) was determined by TLC. TLC separation of glucuronides of FA and their derivatives provides a useful method for identification of the position where the glucuronic acid moiety is attached. Because carboxyl-linked glucuronides are alkali-labile, whereas hydroxyl-linked glucuronides are not, comparison of the recovery of product from TLC in acidic and basic solvent systems (hydroxyl- and carboxyl-linked glucuronides from the acidic system; only hydroxyl-linked glucuronides from the basic system) allows for an assignment of the glucuronide as either a carboxyl (ester) or a hydroxyl (ether) linkage. For this analysis, identical reaction mixtures were chromatographed in the acidic solvent system described in Subheading 3.2.1. and in a basic solvent consisting of ethyl acetate–ethanol–30% NH_4OH (45:45:15, by vol). Following development, the plates were subjected to autoradiography and handled as described in Subheading 3.2.1.

3.2.4. Kinetic Analyses

Kinetic constants (apparent K_m and V_{max}) are calculated graphically by assumption of a particular kinetic model or by model fitting. When the Michaelis–Menten equation or other nonbisubstrate kinetic models are used to calculate kinetic parameters for glucuronide formation, the concentration of

Table 1
Glucuronidation of FAs and Their Oxidized Derivatives by Human Liver and Recombinant UGT2B7

Substrate	Glucuronide formed	Enzymatic activity (nmol/mg protein × min)	
		Human liver microsomes	UGT2B7[c]
AA	Carboxyl	1.1	0.9
LA[a,b]	Carboxyl	2.4	1.3
13-HODE[a]	Carboxyl	2.1	9.8
13-HODE[a]	Hydroxyl	8.6	0.4
13-OXO[a]	nd	3.4	1.4
LA-9,10-diol(+)[b]	Hydroxyl	7.0	4.5
LA-9,10-diol(–)[b]	Hydroxyl	6.8	3.4
LA-12,13-diol(+)[b]	Hydroxyl	9.2	5.4
LA-12,13-diol(–)[b]	Hydroxyl	7.9	3.9
15-HETE	Carboxyl	0.5	0.1
20-HETE	Hydroxyl	1.4	0.8
20-HETE	Carboxyl	0.2	0.1
PGB1	Carboxyl	3.1	1.2
PGE2	Carboxyl	2.3	0.4

Values are the mean of two or four separate duplicate determinations.
[a]Data taken from ref. *33*.
[b]Data taken ref. *32*.
[c]Human recombinant UGT2B7 was expressed in HK293 cells, as described in Experimental Procedures.
nd, Not determined.

cofactor (UDPGA) or aglycon (FA) in the incubation should be 10 times the apparent K_m of the other compound. The time of the incubation for kinetic analysis is routinely 10 min.

For the glucuronidation of FA and derivatives by human liver microsomes, enzymatic activities were determined as described in Subheading 3.2.4. with varying concentrations of FA substrate (25–750 µM) at a constant concentration of [^{14}C]UDP-GlcUA (4 mM). The data were analyzed and Michaelis–Menten kinetic parameters were determined using EnzymeKinetics software (Trinity Software, Campton, NH). See Table 2.

3.3. Preparative Synthesis of FA Glucuronides

The conventional methods of identification of enzymatic reaction products, such as nuclear magnetic resonance and MS, have been successfully applied to

Table 2
Apparent Kinetic Parameters for Glucuronidation of Fatty Acid Substrates by Recombinant UGT2B7

Substrate (position of glucuronide)	K_m (µM)	V_{max} (nmol/mg of protein × min)	V_{max}/K_m (µL/mg × min)
LA (carboxyl)[a]	124 ± 19.5	2.78 ± 0.01	25.0 ± 8.8
AA (carboxyl)[a]	182.7 ± 37.6	1.67 ± 0.5	9.0 ± 1.4
13-HODE (carboxyl)[b]	26	1.30	500.0
13-HODE (hydroxyl)[b]	75, 7	0.8, 0.4	10.7, 57.1
13-OXO (nd)[b]	32, 12	1.1, 1.02	34.4, 83.3
LA-9,10-diol(+)[c]	43.3 ± 4.6	4.5 ± 0.2	111.4 ± 13.6
LA-9,10-diol(−)[c]	74.0 ± 3.0	5.5 ± 0.2	74.6 ± 2.1
LA-12,13-diol(+)[c]	60.2 ± 15.4	5.4 ± 0.2	94.3 ± 8.3
LA-12,13-diol(−)[c]	72.2 ± 4.0	5.4 ± 0.2	76.3 ± 5.2
20-HETE (carboxyl)[d]	27	0.9	33.3
PGB1 (carboxyl)[d]	34	1.2	35.3
PGE2 (carboxyl)[d]	86	0.9	10.5

[a]Values are presented as the means ± standard deviations of at least two separate duplicate determinations and are taken from are taken from ref. 34 and Little, J. M., *unpublished data.*
[b]Values are presented as the means of one or two separate duplicate determinations and are taken from ref. 33.
[c]Values are presented as the means ± SE of at least five separate determinations and are taken from ref. 34.
[d]Values are presented as the means of duplicate determinations and are taken from ref. 38.

glucuronides of certain classes of compounds, for example, bile acids (53–55). These methods of identification require standard reference compounds, such as chemically synthesized glucuronide. There are very few glucuronide standards available for rigorous product identification and, so far, no single chemically synthesized FA glucuronide is commercially available. There are several indirect approaches utilized by investigators to identify a given compound as a glucuronide. For example, TLC, HPLC, and MS are frequently used to compare the enzymatic products of assays carried out with UDP-GlcUA and, especially, with and without β-glucuronidase treatment, as described in Subheading 3.2.2. In our laboratory, we have developed preparative glucuronide synthesis, using enlarged glucuronidation assays. This method of glucuronide biosynthesis has several of advantages. Only specific glucuronides are produced, the glucuronide molecule does not need to be derivatized for analytical analysis, and only naturally occurring isomers are produced. The disadvantage of this method results from the fact that only small amounts of a product can be obtained. However, several examples of biosynthesis of FA glucuronides and their analysis by HPLC–MS are presented in the subheadings that follow.

3.3.1. Preparation of Individual Glucuronide Conjugates for HPLC–MS and MS/MS

Multiple standard analytical incubations were usually performed with human liver microsomal preparation from donors exhibiting the highest glucuronidating activity. The glucuronides were isolated by TLC with multiple developments as described in Subheading 3.2.1. After separation by TLC, the relatively hydrophobic glucuronide bands were visualized by spraying the plate with water. The plates were dried and the silica gel from each glucuronide band was transferred to a Pasteur pipet containing glass wool. The glucuronides were eluted with 6 × 0.5 mL of methanol and the eluates were dried and analyzed.

Alternatively, large preparative incubations are carried out, containing up to 10 mg of microsomal proteins and supplemented with additional unlabeled UDP-GlcUA during incubations of 2 h, as described in ref. 54. Following incubation, the reactions were stopped by the addition ice-cold 0.1 M glycine–trichloroacetate buffer, pH 2.8. Partial purification of products was accomplished by solid-phase extraction on BondElut C_{18} cartridges (Varian), followed by preparative TLC, either in underivatized form or as the methyl ester acetate derivatives, as previously described (51).

4. MASS SPECTRAL ANALYSIS OF THE GLUCURONIDES OF THE COMPOUNDS DISCUSSED IN SUBHEADING 3.2.

There are several publications describing the isolation, identification, and characterization of OFA and their glucuronides from the urine of patients with generalized peroxisomal disorders or biosynthesized in cell culture studies *(27–31)*. Typically, fast atom bombardment (FAB)–MS GC–ECMS, and GC–MS were utilized for those studies. It is anticipated that the analysis of glucuronide conjugates by mass spectrometry will be greatly assisted by the use of relatively new LC–MS and atmospheric pressure ionization techniques (API).

Prior to the advent of LC–MS, the identification of glucuronide conjugates required the synthesis of derivatives of the conjugates; in many cases methylation was used to confer the necessary volatility for analysis by GC–MS techniques. The disadvantage of this approach is that the derivatization was often incomplete, leading to complex spectral data. Thus, the older methods will soon be replaced by LC–MS approaches involving API.

The practicality of LC–MS for the study of glucuronide conjugates is well established for a number of drugs and a recent comparison of ionization techniques clearly demonstrates that electrospray ionization (ESI) is superior for the detection of glucuronide conjugates as compared to other ionization techniques, including atmospheric pressure photoionization and atmospheric pressure chemical ionization *(56)*.

4.1. Mass Spectral Analysis of the Glucuronides of 13-HODE and 13-OXO

We used FAB analysis to confirm the existence of the glucuronides of 13-HODE and 13-OXO *(34)*. Although this analysis did not yield information with respect to the site of glucuronidation, it did confirm that monoglucuronides were the major products produced. Molecular ions for each species were detected. The molecular ion for the carboxyl-linked 13-HODE glucuronide and its methyl ester, produced after treatment with trimethylsilyldiazomethane, were observed at m/z 472 and 486 respectively. The hydroxyl-linked 13-HODE glucuronide showed ions at m/z 472 for the underivatized compound and 542 for the permethylated compound.

The FAB mass spectrum for the 13-OXO glucuronide treated with trimethylsilyldiazomethane showed ions of equal intensity at m/z 469 (M++H) and 471 (M+–H) in a glycerol matrix and an ion at 470 in nitrobenzyl alcohol.

4.2. ESI HPLC-MS and MS/MS and Analysis of LA Diol Glucuronides

Glucuronidation products were analyzed by C_{18} reverse-phase HPLC–MS and MS/MS using a Brownlee MicroGradient pumping system, a Rheodyne 8125 micro-HPLC injector, and a Finnigan LCQ™ quadrupole ion trap mass spectrometry system. A 1 × 100 mm C_{18} ODS Hypersil column was used with 0.5% aqueous ammonium acetate, pH 7.5, in 25% acetonitrile as the mobile phase at a flow rate of 50 µL/min. The column outlet was connected directly to the electrospray ion source of the mass spectrometer. The following ion source settings were used: negative ESI, heated capillary 240°C, nitrogen sheath gas 80%, auxillary gas off. The system was autotuned during direct infusion (50 µL/min) of a solution containing LA-9,10-diol glucuronides in the mobile phase. Alternate MS scans from m/z 100–600 and collision-induced, decomposition MS/MS product ions were acquired throughout these analyses. The precursor ion for the product ion scans was the [M-H]$^-$ ion (m/z 489.3) for LA-diol glucuronides. A collision energy of 28% and isolation width of 2.0 units was used. For the methyl linoleate diol glucuronides, the molecular ion at m/z 489 was readily detected, as was a fragment at m/z 313 owing to loss of the glucuronide moiety.

Representative MS and MS/MS product ion spectra and predicted structures for the precursor and product ions obtained with the MeLA-diol glucuronides are shown in Fig. 5. In general, electron impact ionization mass spectra yield fragments corresponding to the loss of the glucuronide moiety and MS/MS experiments frequently display an ion of m/z 176, derived from the glucuronic acid moiety. This ion can often be the major daughter ion observed in MS/MS experiments.

4.3. Analysis of Glucuronides of LTB$_4$, 5-, 12-, and 15-HETE and 13-HODE by LC-MS

One other published example of eicosanoid MS is the report by Turgeon et al. (39) identifying the biosynthesisis of glucuronides of LTB$_4$, several HETEs and 13-HODE by human microsomal and recombinant UGT isoforms. In brief, HPLC was used to isolate metabolites biosynthesized in glucuronidation assays. An Alliance 2690 HPLC system (Waters, Milford, MA) with a Phenomenex Colombus C$_{18}$ column (50 × 3.2 mm, 5 µm particle size, Phenomenex, Torrance, CA) was used with a two-solvent gradient system: 1 mM ammonium formate in water (A) and 1 mM ammonium formate in methanol (B). Products were separated using a flow rate of 0.7 mL/min with a linear gradient from 15% to 95% B in A for 6 min, followed by a hold for 2 min, and finally returned to 15% B over 2 min. The HPLC column was coupled to a Finnigan LCQ ion trap MS using negative ion ESI.

5. GENERAL CONCLUSIONS AND FUTURE APPLICATIONS OF GLUCURONIDATION METHODS

The enzymatic assays presented in this chapter can be employed for glucuronidation of other hydrophobic endogenous compounds, as well as drugs and environmental pollutants. As demonstrated in Table 1, the FFAs, AA, and LA, and their oxidized derivatives, including PGs, can be glucuronidated by both human liver microsomes and human recombinant UGT2B7 with very

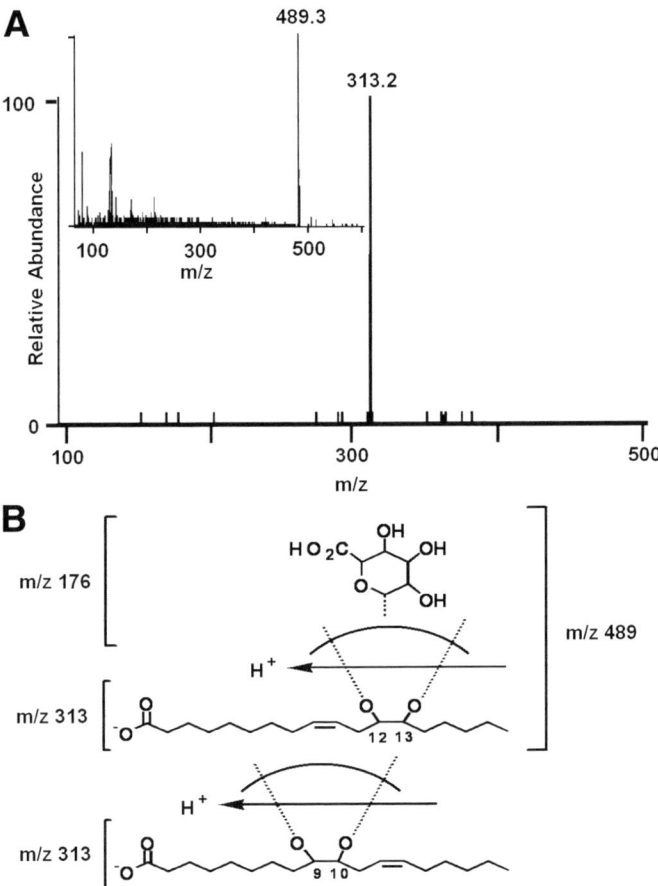

Fig. 5. ESI HPLC-MS and MS/MS spectra of the biosynthesized LA-9,10- and -12,13-diol glucuronides. MS analysis (**A**, inset) revealed a parent ion (m/z 489.3) corresponding to a LA-diol monoglucuronide. MS/MS analysis (**A**) of the parent ion produced a single product ion corresponding to LA-diol (m/z 313.2). (**B**) Product ions observed by MS/MS analysis of the m/z 489 ion and an illustration of the possible positions of glucuronic acid conjugation for 9,10- and 12,13-LA-diols. The spectrum shown is representative of those obtained from all four LA-diol glucuronide products biosynthesized by human liver microsomes (HLMs).

high activity. Based on our experience, we recommend that each FA substrate should be efficiently solubilized, preferably by the formation of mixed micelles with mild detergents such as Brij 58. For experiments with membrane preparations of recombinant isoforms, the use of alamethicin is recommended. For each new substrate, optimization of the assays in terms of protein concentration, time of incubation, pH, and substrate concentration is required.

UGT2B7 was the only isoform investigated in the glucuronidation of FFAs and OFAs in our studies. However, there is evidence that other isoforms from the UGT1A family are also involved *(39)*. The enzymatic activities toward OFAs, which vary from low to high nanomoles per milligram of protein per min, are among the highest observed for glucuronidation of endogenous substrates. It is also obvious that the hydroxyl function is a much better glucuronic acid acceptor than the carboxyl group. The K_m values presented in Table 2 show that human recombinant UGT2B7 has a very high affinity for OFA derivatives. K_m values for glucuronidation of the carboxyl groups of LA and AA are much higher than those for the OFAs, which indicates that they are poorer substrates for human UGTs. Other classes of FA, such as short-chain and medium-chain FAs and their oxidized derivatives, are potential substrates for glucuronidation catalyzed by human UGT isoforms.

There are several methods for the separation and identification of glucuronidated conjugates and the unreacted substrate. Here we presented TLC, HPLC, and HPLC–MS approaches routinely used in our laboratories and those of other investigators. It is anticipated that, in the near future, new approaches, such as LC–MS and API techniques will be more widely used. However, these are relatively time-consuming and expensive techniques and will probably be used only for identification and rigorous characterization of new glucuronide conjugates. TLC and HPLC are relatively inexpensive and sufficient for multiple sample processing. It is anticipated that these techniques will still be used for a while longer.

ACKNOWLEDGMENTS

This work was supported in part by NIH Grants DK51971, DK56226, and DK60109 and tobacco settlement funds (A. R-P.).

REFERENCES

1. Eling TE, Glasgow WC. Cellular proliferation and lipid metabolism: importance of lipoxygenases in modulating epidermanl growth factor-dependent mitogenesis. Cancer Metast Rev 1994;13:397–410.
2. Nagy L, Tontonoz P, Alvarez JGA, Chen H, Evans RM. Oxidized LDL regulates macrophage gene expression through ligand activation of PPAR gamma. Cell 1998;93:229–240.
3. Sauer LA, Dauchy RT, Blask De, Armstrong BJ, Scalici S. 13-Hydroxyoctadecadienoic acid is the mitogenic signal for linoleic acid-dependent growth in rat hepatoma 7288CTC in vivo. Cancer Res 1999;59:4688–4692.
4. Bronstein JC, Bull AW. The correlation between 13-hydroxyoctadecadienoate dehydrogenase (13-HODE dehydrogenase) and intestinal cell differentiation. Prostaglandins 1993;46:387–395.

5. Mansen A, Guardiola-Diaz A, Rafter J, Branting C, Gustafsson J-A. Expression of the peroxisome proliferator-activated receptor (PPAR) in the mouse colonic mucosa. Biochem Biophys Res Commun 1996;222:844–851.
6. Kosaka K, Suzuki K, Hayakawa M, Sugiyama S, Ozawa T. Leukotoxin, a linoleic epoxide: its implication in the late death of patients with extensive burns. Mol Cell Biochem 1994;139:141–148.
7. Ozawa T, Hayakawa M, Kosaka K, et al. Leukotoxin, 9,10-epoxy-12-octadecenoate, as a burn toxin causing adult respiratory distress syndrome. Adv Prostaglandin Thromboxane Leuk Res 1991;21B:569–572.
8. Moghaddam MF, Grand DF, Cheek JM, Greene JF, Williamson KC, Hammock BD. Bioactivation of leukotoxins to their toxic diols by epoxide hydrolase. Nat Med 1997;3:562–566.
9. Moran JH, Weise R, Schnellmann RG, Freeman JP, Grant DF. Cytotoxicity of linoleic acid diols to renal proximal tubular cells. Toxicol Appl Pharmacol 1997; 146:53–59.
10. Stimers JR, Dobretsov M, Hastings SL, Jude AR, Grant DF. Effects of linoleic acid metabolites on electrical activity in adult rat ventricular myocytes. Biochim Biophys Acta 1999;1438:359–368.
11. Cho Y, Ziboh VA. Incorporation of 13-hydroxyoctadecadienoic acid (13-HODE) into epidermal ceramides and phospholipids: phospholipase C-catalyzed release of novel 13-HODE-containing diacylglycerol. J Lipid Res 1994;35:255–262.
12. Liu B, Khan WA, Hannun YA, et al. 12(S)-Hydroxyeicosatetraenoic acid and 13(S)-hydroxyoctadecadienoic acid regulation of protein kinase C-α in melanoma cells: role of receptor-mediated hydrolysis of inositol phospholipids. Proc Natl Acad Sci USA 1995;92:9323–9327.
13. Pongracz J, Lord JM. The lipoxygenase product 13-hydroxyoctadecadienoic acid (13-HODE) is a selective inhibitor of classical PKC isoenzymes. Biochem Biophys Res Commun 1999;256:269–272.
14. Vane JR, Bakhle YS, Botting RM. Cyclooxygenases 1 and 2. Annu Rev Pharmacol Toxicol 1998;38:97–120.
15. Funk CD. The molecular biology of mammalian lipoxygenases and the quest for eicosanoid functions using lipoxygenase-deficient mice. Biochim Biophys Acta 1996;1304:65–84.
16. Ghosh J, Myers CE. Inhibition of arachindonate 5-lipoxygenase triggers massive apoptosis in human prostate cancer cells. Proc Natl Acad Sci USA 1998;95: 13182–13187.
17. Kelavkar UP, Nixon JB, Cohen C, Dillehay D, Eling TE, Badr KF. Overexpression of 15-lipoxygenase-1 in PC-3 human prostate cancer cells increases tumorigenesis. Carcinogenesis 2000;22:1765–1773.
18. Nie D, Tang K, Diglio C, Honn KV. Eicosnaoid regualtion of angiogenesis: role of endothelial arachidonate 12-lipoxygenase. Blood 2000;95:2304–2311.
19. Payan DG, Goetzl EJ. Specific suppression of human T lymphocyte function by leukotriene B4. J Immunol 1998;131:551–553.

20. Hwang D, Rhee SH. Receptor-mediated signaling pathways: potential targets of modulation by dietary fatty acids. Am J Clin Nutr 1999;70:545–556.
21. Kitareewan S, Burka LT, Tomer KB, et al. Phytol metabolites are circulating dietary factors that activate the nuclear receptor RXR. Mol Biol Cell 1996;7:1153–1166.
22. Lemotte PK, Keidel S, Apfel CM. Phytanic acid is a retinoid X receptor ligand. Eur J Biochem 1996;236:328–333.
23. Zomer AW, van der Burg B, Jansen GA, Wanders RJA, Poll-The BT, van der Saag PT. Pristanic acid and phytanic acid: naturally occurring ligands for the nuclear receptor peroxisome proliferator-activated receptor α. J Lipid Res 2000;41:1801–1807.
24. de Urquiza AM, Liu S, Sjoberg M, et al. Docosahexaenoic acid, a ligand for the retinoid X receptor in mouse brain. Science 2000;290:2140–2144.
25. Keller H, Dreyer C, Medin J, Mahfoudi A, Ozato K, Wahli W. Fatty acids and retinoids control lipid metabolism through activation of peroxisome proliferator-activated receptor-retinoid X receptor heterodimers. Proc Natl Acad Sci USA 1993;90:2160–2164.
26. Radominska-Pandya A, Czernik P, Little JM, Battaglia E, Mackenzie PI. Structural and functional studies of UDP-glucuronsyltransferases. Drug Metab Rev 1999;31:817–900.
27. Prakash C, Zhang JY, Falck JR, Chauhan K, Blair JA. 20-Hydroxyeicosatetraenoic acid is excreted as a glucuronide conjugate in human urine. Biochem Biophys Res Commun 1992;185:728–733.
28. Street JM, Evans JE, Natowicz MR. Glucuronic acid-conjugated dihydroxy fatty acids in the urine of patients with generalized peroxisomal disorders. J Biol Chem 1996;271:3507–3516.
29. Sacerdoti D, Balazy M, Angeli P, Gatta A, McGiff JC. Eicosanoid excretion in hepatic cirrhosis. Predominance of 20-HETE. J Clin Invest 1997;100:1264–1270.
30. Wheelan P, Hankin JA, Bilir B, Guenette D, Murphy RC. Metabolic transformation of leukotriene B_4 in primary cultures of human hepatocytes. J Pharmacol Exp Ther 1999;288:326–334.
31. Hankin JA, Wheelan P, Murphy RC. Identification of novel metabolites of prostaglandin E2 formed by isolated rat hepatocytes. Arch Biochem Biophys 1997;340:317–330.
32. Jude AR, Little JM, Freeman JP, Evans JE, Radominska-Pandya A, Grant DF. Linoleic acid diols are novel substrates for human UDP-glucuronosyltransferases. Arch Biochem Biophys 2000;380:294–302.
33. Jude AR, Little JM, Czernik P, Tephly TR, Grant DF, Radominska-Pandya A. Glucuronidation of linoleic acid diols by human microsomal and recombinant UDP-glucuronosyltransferases: identification of UGT2B7 as the major isoform involved. Arch Biochem Biophys 2001;389:176–186.
34. Jude AR, Little JM, Bull AW, Podgorski I, Radominska-Pandya A. 13-Hydroxy- and 13-oxooctadecadienoic acids: novel substrates for human UDP-glucuronosyltransferases. Drug Metab Dispos 2001;29:652–655.

35. Radominska-Pandya A, Czernik PJ, Little JM. Human UDP-glucuronosyltransferase 2B7. Curr Drug Metab 2001;2:283–298.
36. Bull AW, Seeley SK, Geno JL, Mannervik B. Conjugation of the linoleic acid oxidation product, 13-oxooctadecadienoic acid, a bioactive endogenous substrate for mamalian glutathione transferase. Biochim Biophys Acta 2002;1571:77–82.
37. Little JM, Williams L, Xu J, Radominska-Pandya A. Glucuronidation of the dietary fatty acids, phytanic acid and docosahexaenoic acid, by human UDP-glucuronosyltransferases. Drug Metab Dispos 2002;30:531–533.
38. Sonka J, Little JM, Samokyszyn V, Radominska-Pandya A. Glucuronidation of arachidonic acid, 20-HETE and prostaglandin E2 by human hepatic and intestinal UDR-glucuronosyltransferases and recombinant UGT2B7. Drug Metab Rev 2002; 34(Suppl 1):194.
39. Turgeon D, Chouinard S, Belanger P, Picard S, Labbe JF, Borgeat P, Belanger A. Glucuronidation of arachidonic and linoleic acid metabolites by human UDP-glucuronosyltransferase. J Lipid Res 2003;44:1182–1191.
40. Funk MO, Isaac R, Porter NA. Preparation and purification of lipid hydroperoxides from arachidonic and γ-linolenic acids. Lipids 1976;11:113–117.
41. Gardner HW. Lipoxygenase as a versatile biocatalyst. JAOCS 1979;73:1347–1357.
42. Porter NA, Logan J, Kontoyiannaidou V. Preparation and purification of arachidonic acid hydroperoxides of biological importance. J Org Chem 1979;44:3177–3181.
43. Bull AW, Nigro ND, Golembieski WA, Crissman JD, Marnett LJ. *In vivo* stimulation of DNA synthesis and induction of ornithine decarboxylase in rat colon by fatty acid hydroperoxides, autooxidation products of unsaturated fatty acids. Cancer Res 1984;44:4924–4928.
44. Abraham MH, Davies AG, Llewellyn DD, Thain EM. The chromatographic analysis of organic peroxides. Anal Chim Acta 1957;17:499–503.
45. Graff G, Anderson LA, Jaques LW. Preparation and purification of soybean lipoxygenase-derived unsaturated hydroperoxy and hydroxy fatty acids and determination of molar absorptivities of hydroxy fatty acids. Anal Biochem 1990;188: 38–47.
46. Porter NA, Wujek JS. Allylic hydroperoxide rearrangement: β-scission or concerted pathway. J Org Chem 1987;52:5085–5089.
47. Dutton GJ. Glucuronidation of Drugs and Other Compounds. Boca Raton, FL: CRC Press, 1980.
48. Little JM, Lehman PA, Nowell S, Samokyszyn V, Radominska A. Glucuronidation of all trans-retinoic acid and 5,6-epoxy-all trans-retinoic acid: Activation of rat liver microsomal UDP-glucuronosyltranferase activity by alamethicin. Drug Metab Dispos 1997;25:5–11.
49. Little JM, Radominska A. Application of photoaffinity labeling with [11,12-^{3}H] all *trans*-retinoic acid to characterization of rat liver microsomal UDP-glucuronosyltransferase(s) with activity toward retinoic acid. Biochem Biophys Res Commun 1997;230:497–500.
50. Radominska-Pyrek A, Zimniak P, Chari M, Golunski E, Lester R, Pyrek JS. Glucuronides of monohydroxylated bile acids: specificity of microsomal glucuronyl-

transferase for the glucuronidation site, C-3 configuration, and side chain length. J Lipid Res 1986;27:89–101.
51. Radominska-Pyrek A, Zimniak P, Irshaid YM, Lester R, Tephly TR, Pyrek JS. Glucuronidation of 6α-hydroxy bile acids by human liver microsomes. J Clin Invest 1987;80:234–241.
52. Radominska-Pandya A, Little JM, Pandya JT, et al. UDP-Glucuronosyltransferases in human intestinal mucosa. Biochim Biophys Acta 1998;1394:199–208.
53. Panfil I, Lehman PA, Zimniak P, Ernst B, Franz T, Lester R, Radominska A. Biosynthesis and chemical synthesis of carboxyl-linked glucuronide of lithocholic acid. Biochim Biophys Acta 1992;1126:221–228.
54. Radominska A, Little JM, Pyrek JS, et al. A novel UDP-Glc-specific glucosyltransferase catalyzing the biosynthesis of 6-O-glucosides of bile acids in human liver microsomes. J Biol Chem 1993;268:15127–15135.
55. Zimniak P, Radominska A, Zimniak M, Lester R. Formation of three types of glucuronides of 6-hydroxy bile acids by rat liver microsomes. J Lipid Res 1988;29: 183–190.
56. Keski-Hynnilä H, Kurkela M, Elovaara E, et al. Comparison of elctrospray, atmospheric pressure chemical ionization, and atmospheric pressure photoionization in the identification of apomorphine, dobutamine, and entacapone phase II metabolites of biological samples. Anal Chem 2002;74:3449–3457.
57. Jude A, Little J, Gall W, Evans J, Grant D, Radominska-Pandya A. Linoleic acid diols: novel substrates for human liver UDP-glucuronosyltransferases. 1999 ASBMB Satellite Meeting, San Francisco, CA, 1999.

6

Transcriptional Regulation of UDP-Glucuronosyltransferases

Anna Radominska-Pandya, Peter I. Mackenzie, and Wen Xie

Summary

Recent evidence has been provided that five nuclear receptors (NRs), (pregnane X receptor [PXR], constitutive androstane receptor [CAR], farnesoid X receptor [FXR] and peroxisome proliferator-activated receptor [PPARα and γ]) regulate the expression of *UGT1A* loci. This chapter presents an overview of the most recent developments in our understanding of transcriptional regulation of UDP-glucuronosyltransferase (UGT) genes, and specifically focuses on the regulation of UGTs via NRs, with a strong emphasis on the biochemical and molecular techniques applied to this area of investigation. Procedures are described for the isolation and analysis of UGT proximal and distal promoters. The use of transgenic animals in the study of the mechanism of regulation of UGT expression is described, as is the assessment of the effects of various gene inducers on expression of UGTs in HepG2 and Caco-2 cell culture. Techniques for transient transfection of HepG2 and Caco-2 cells with NRs and UGT promoter constructs are presented. In addition, general methods are provided for various molecular and biochemical methods used in the isolation and characterization of UGT promoters.

Key Words

Aryl hydrocarbon receptor; bile acids; bilirubin; (bio)flavonoids; CaCo-2 cells; constitutive androgen receptor; cytochrome P450; DNase 1 footprinting; electrophoretic mobility shift assay; glucuronidation assays; HepG2 cells; luciferase reporter constructs; mouse: "humanized"; mouse: transgenic; Northern blot hybridization; peroxisome proliferator-activated receptor; pregnane X receptor; retinoids; reverse transcriptase-polymerase chain reaction; steroid hormones; transfection: transient; UDP-glucuronosyltransferase; UGT promoter constructs; UGT transcriptional regulation; xenobiotic response element.

1. INTRODUCTION

This chapter presents an overview of the most recent developments in our understanding of transcriptional regulation of UDP-glucuronosyltransferase

From: *Methods in Pharmacology and Toxicology, Drug Metabolism and Transport: Molecular Methods and Mechanisms*
Edited by: L. Lash © Humana Press Inc., Totowa, NJ

(UGT) genes. A recent detailed review *(1)* summarizes all the newest developments in both constitutive and transcriptional regulation of UGT genes. Therefore, we discuss here information on the regulation of UGTs via nuclear receptors (NRs), with a strong emphasis on the biochemical and molecular techniques applied to this area of investigation. Recently, evidence has been provided that four nuclear receptors (pregnane X receptor [PXR], constitutive androstane receptor [CAR], peroxisome proliferator-activated receptors [PPARα and γ) regulate the expression of *UGT1A* loci *(2–4)*. Specifically, our preliminary studies and published work have shown that *UGT1A1, 1A3, 1A4*, and *1A6* are regulated by PXR *(4,5)*. *UGT1A1* and *1A6* are regulated by CAR *(3,4)* and *UGT1A9* is regulated by PPARα and γ *(2)*. It is also well documented that regulation of *UGT1A1* is mediated by the arylhydrocarbon receptor (AhR) *(6)*. The nuclear response elements (NRE) in the promoters of *UGT1A1* and *UGT1A9* that bind PXR and the PPARs, respectively, have been identified *(2,4)*. Very recently, Barbier et al. showed that, in human hepatocytes, *UGT2B4* is induced by FXR *(7)*.

Taking into consideration the number of physiologically important human UGTs and the accumulated information on NR-mediated expression of drug-metabolizing enzyme (DME) genes, progress in the area of UGT regulation is relatively modest. Although a mechanistic understanding of transcriptional regulation of other DMEs has not yet been fully achieved, it has been propelled in the last 10 yr by advances in the generation of transgenic animals and extensive tissue culture studies. Compared to CYP450 investigations, progress in the regulation of UGT genes is relatively limited. There are several reasons for this modest development. First, UGTs do not demonstrate significant induction by typical CYP450 inducers. Next, because UGTs are membrane-bound proteins, their purification was relatively difficult, and protein sequences were not obtained nor were specific antibodies generated. All of this has hampered the development of gene regulation studies. Moreover, there was relatively less interest in these phase II detoxification enzymes because their physiological significance was not considered exciting. UGTs were considered to be strictly detoxification enzymes, carrying out the final step of solubilization of hydrophobic compounds, created to a large extent by oxidative metabolism catalyzed by CYP450s.

However, there has been a dramatic change in our recent understanding of the significance and functions of UGTs, which emphasizes that, in addition to the detoxification role, UGTs are also involved in other important cellular processes. UGTs can synthesize derivatives that are biologically active, some of which demonstrate increased toxicity *(8–10)*. In addition, mounting evidence indicates that UGTs, like other DMEs, are involved in controlling the steady-state concentrations of NR ligands, thus limiting the duration of action of the receptor *(11,12)*. Therefore, UGTs appear to be very important regulators of the biological activity of many signaling molecules.

Historically, development of studies on regulation of UGT gene expression began with experiments investigating the effect of different inducers in animal and tissue culture models. The *UGT1A* genes are induced by xenobiotics, especially polycyclic aromatic hydrocarbons, barbiturates, and several hormones *(1)*. Expression of the human *UGT1A6* gene is also induced by dioxin and several antioxidants and, recently, it was demonstrated that bioflavonoids are very strong regulators of UGTs from the 1A family *(1)*. Exposure of cell cultures to various concentrations of inducers has been used to detect increases in the levels of UGT proteins and enzymatic activities. In parallel, investigations of changes in *UGT* mRNA levels have been carried out. Two different approaches, including Northern blot analysis and/or reverse transcriptase-polymerase chain reaction (RT-PCR) using specific primers, were the major methods of choice. Such techniques are very effective and are the final methods applied to experiments carried out both in tissue culture and in vivo in animals. All these approaches are discussed in detail.

The crucial step in the study of the transcriptional regulation of genes is the identification of the molecular mechanism involved in this process. Understanding of the mechanism of upregulation or suppression of UGT genes involves isolation and analysis of UGT proximal and distal promoters. This approach has been successfully implemented recently in identification of NREs of *UGT1A1, 1A6*, and *1A9*. The human *UGT1A* gene locus and several genes from the *UGT2B* family have been cloned and analyzed for potential regulatory elements. These investigations were followed by cloning of fragments of regulatory sequences into specific vectors, to generate a series of luciferase reporter constructs. The function of these elements was analyzed by DNA–protein binding electrophoretic mobility shift assays (EMSA). Finally, mutations in regulatory sequences were used for the absolute confirmation of the involvement of these sequences in the regulatory process.

Generation of transgenic animals is now revolutionizing the investigation of the functions of both DMEs and the NRs involved in their regulation. Actually, the use of knockout PXR/SXR and humanized PXR mice provided the first direct evidence that some isoforms of the *UGT1A* family are targets for PXR. These experiments are also discussed in detail.

All these procedures, which are routinely carried out in our laboratories, will be discussed here, with special emphasis on their application to *UGT* gene regulation. In principle, the general strategies for our approach, which have been successfully applied to studies of gene regulation of some UGTs, can be applied to other UGTs and DMEs.

2. MATERIALS AND METHODS

2.1. Background

Studies of human UGT induction have shown that several human isoforms are inducible by hormones and exogenous compounds in cell cultures *(1)*. The largest amounts of data have been collected for *UGT1A1*, which is induced by phenobarbital (PB) and has also been shown to be inducible by 3-methylcholanthrene (3-MC) and oltipraz in human hepatocytes *(13)*. Recent studies demonstrated a high level of induction of *UGT1A1* by flavonoids in human HepG2 cells *(14)* and by chrysin in Caco-2 cells *(15)*. Expression of the human *UGT1A6* gene is also induced by dioxin via binding of the Ah receptor to a xenobiotic response element (XRE) located about 1.5 kbp upstream of the transcription start site *(16)*. Antioxidants, such as *tert*-butylhydroquinone (*t*-BHQ), 2,3,7,8-tetrachlorodibenzo-*p*-dioxin (TCDD), and quercetin, also induce *UGT1A6* expression but the mechanism mediating this effect is unknown *(17,18)*. *UGT1A6* is also inducible by β-naphthoflavone (βNF) in human hepatocytes and Caco-2 cells *(19,20)*. *UGT1A3* and *1A9* are also induced by βNF in Caco-2 cells and *UGT1A9* is inducible by TCDD and *t*-BHQ *(18,19)*. UGTs from the *2B* family are much less inducible and the only data available demonstrate that *UGT2B15* in LNCaP cells responds to several agents, including interleukin-1α, epidermal growth factor (EGF), dihydrotestosterone, and biochanin *(21)*.

Information concerned with the identification of the NRs involved in UGT gene regulation has been recently collected. Our preliminary data and published work have shown that *UGT1A1, 1A3, 1A4,* and *1A6* are regulated by PXR. *UGT2B7* is regulated by the farnesoid X receptor (FXR), and *UGT1A9* is regulated by PPARα and γ. Barbier et al. recently showed that, in human hepatocytes, *UGT2B4* is induced by FXR *(7)*. As compared to the studies on CYP450, these are very limited and at present we are working on the development of this topic. The information presented above describes all the available data on induction of UGTs and the role of NRs mediating this process that has been published during the past several years. The biochemical and molecular biological methods described in the following subheadings have been elaborated in our laboratories and some of the data presented here have not yet been published.

2.2. General Approach

Recently, our laboratories have studied the effect of various gene inducers on expression of *UGT1A* and *2B* family isoforms in Caco-2 and HepG2 cells. These cells were selected because they contain both UGT genes and several relevant NRs, including hPXR and hFXR. Our experiments showed that, in HepG2 cells, the endogenous levels of both mRNA and protein of *UGT1A* family isoforms were relatively low. However, when the cells were exposed to proper inducing agents, very significant increases (2- to 10-fold) of UGT mRNA were obtained. Caco-2 cells contain reasonable levels of *UGT1A* isoforms, with *UGT1A6* being the predominant enzyme. On the other hand, both cell lines contain significant levels of *UGT2B7* and therefore are an excellent model for the *UGT2B7* regulation (induction and suppression) studies. It is recommended that the results from HepG2 and Caco-2 studies be confirmed with human hepatocytes and, when available, enterocytes. These cells contain the whole set of hepatic and intestine-specific UGTs, as well as relevant NRs. Several experiments from other laboratories have demonstrated that the primary human hepatocyte model could be successfully applied to studies of UGT gene regulation *(7,20)*.

In our experiments, we used several inducing and suppressing agents, such as rifampicin (RIF) and phenobarbitol (PB) (ligands for PXR and CAR), and various endogenous compounds, such as fatty acids (FAs), bile acids (BAs), steroid hormones, and bioflavonoids, which are both substrates for UGTs and ligands for NRs. It is essential to optimize the conditions for the studies of the effects of inducers and suppressors. Time of the exposure, concentration of the regulators and the effects of vehicle, and cell density should be investigated in individual, preliminary experiments. Besides the effects of various inducers, the effect of expression of relevant NRs has also been examined. For example, the induction via RIF was carried out in the presence and absence of hPXR variants. The effect of BA and retinoic acid (RA) on the regulation of UGT2B7 protein levels and activity was studied in the presence and absence of FXR. Besides the UGT induction studies, experiments were designed to identify the NRs involved in upregulation and/or suppression of UGT genes by natural compounds. Detailed experimental protocols, including the induction of UGT genes and the effect of transient transfection with NRs, such as hPXR variants and FXR, are presented in Subheading 2.3.

2.3. Specific Methods for Studying the Effect of Inducer/Suppressors on UGT Expression

2.3.1. Induction of UGT Genes by Chemicals in HepG2 and Caco-2 Cells

The human hepatocellular carcinoma cell line HepG2 (ATCC HB-8065) and human adenocarcinoma cells (Caco-2, ATCC HTB-37) were obtained from the American Type Culture Collection (Manassas, VA). Both cell lines were maintained at 37°C, 5% CO_2 in high glucose Dulbecco's modified Eagle's medium (DMEM) with L-glutamine supplemented with 1% nonessential amino acids, 1 m*M* sodium pyruvate, and 10% fetal bovine serum (all from Invitrogen, Carlsbad, CA). The culture medium was changed twice weekly during maintenance. When cells were 60–80% confluent, they were washed in DMEM and replacement medium containing various concentrations of chemicals and vehicle (0.1% dimethyl sulfoxide [DMSO]) was added. Untransfected cells used for isolation of control RNA were harvested when they neared confluence.

The concentrations of inducers or suppressors were initially evaluated. For RIF, PB (obtained from Sigma, St. Louis, MO), and other drugs, concentrations from 5 to 100 μM were checked. Initial concentrations of the endogenous compounds, such as BA and FA, were in a range of 5–25 μM. The concentrations of hormones and signaling molecules such as RA and its derivatives were very low (0.01–5.0 μM). Both short (0–3 h) and long (6–48 h) times of exposure to the inducers were checked. The viability of the cells was evaluated microscopically. Isolation of mRNA and subcellular fractions for evaluation of protein levels and enzymatic activities were routinely carried out as described in Subheadings 3.2., 3.7., and 3.9.

Experiments with human hepatocytes and enterocytes can be carried out according to the protocols described for HepG2 and Caco-2 cells. Primary cultures of human hepatocytes are available from a number of commercial sources (Gentest, Woburn, MA; Clonetics, San Diego, CA; In Vitro Technology, Baltimore, MD) or can be obtained from the Liver Tissue Procurement and Distribution System, University of Pittsburgh. These suppliers can provide the hepatocytes in multiwell plates, individual plates, or flasks. In most cases, primary cultures of human hepatocytes can be maintained in culture by following protocols established by the supplier and other investigators, before initiating experiments with test agents. Prior to use for studies, the overall metabolic function, synthetic capability (e.g., albumin synthesis and secretion), viability (~75%), and morphological integrity (e.g., mitochondrion integrity, cell polarity) of each preparation of hepatocytes should be assessed by established procedures.

Enterocyte cultures can be prepared and maintained following published methods *(22)*. Our laboratory has access to fresh human intestinal tissue that will allow for preparation of large amounts of enterocytes. The protocol for enterocyte isolation is as follows: segments of human small intestine are washed thoroughly in buffer, cut into small pieces, and incubated with buffer containing dispase type I (Roche Molecular Biochemicals) and collagenase type XI (Sigma) at room temperature for 30 min. The digest is dispersed by vigorous pipetting and sedimented under gravity for 1 min. The supernatant is mixed with the appropriate medium and centrifuged at approx 5g (350 rpm) for 3 min. The pellet is washed with the same medium and resuspended in growth medium and placed in tissue culture dishes. Initial experiments should establish optimum conditions for growth and determine a time frame for cell growth and viability before one proceeds with the studies.

2.3.2. Transient Transfection of HepG2 and Caco-2 Cells With NR Plasmids and UGT Promoter Constructs

Both types of cells can be transiently transfected with NR plasmids, and the effect of this transfection in the presence and absence of inducers or suppressors can be evaluated for mRNA, protein, and glucuronidation activity. Moreover, the same system can be used for transfection with various promoters and promoter constructs for measuring luciferase activity in the presence and absence of specific inducers or suppressors.

For transient transfection, HepG2 or Caco-2 cells are seeded in 6- or 12-well plates at 1×10^6 and 2.5×10^5 cells per well, respectively. Transfections are performed in triplicate using 5 µg of expression plasmid or empty parent vector and 10 µL of LipofectAMINE™ 2000 Reagent (Invitrogen, LF2000), according to the manufacturer's instructions. At 6–7 h after transfection, the cells are washed in DMEM and replacement medium containing appropriate concentrations of inducers, suppressors, or vehicle (0.1% DMSO) is added. At 24 h posttransfection, the cells are treated again with inducers, suppressors, or vehicle in fresh DMEM. After a total of 40 h, the transfected cells are washed with phosphate-buffered saline and harvested for RNA extraction. The cloning and characterization of UGT promoters will be described in detail in Subheadings 4. and 5. Here, some of the details of the cell culture experiments in relation to the promoter transfection analysis are given. To measure promoter activity, cells are transfected with a UGT promoter/luciferase construct and/or NR expression vectors in the presence and absence of the inducers or suppressors. Cells are grown in six-well plates and the assay conditions are optimized with respect to cell density, concentration range of the UGT promoter/luciferase vector, concentration of inducers and time of exposure. After transfection with NRs, cells are treated with the required concentration of inducers, suppressors, or vehicle (0.1% DMSO) for 48 h and luciferase activity is assayed using standard protocols.

3. GENERAL METHODS
3.1. Plasmids and Cloning of NR

A majority of the plasmids for UGTs and NRs are already available in our laboratories or from other investigators. The expression vectors for constitutively active versions of the PXR variant T1, pCMX-VP-hPXR, and CAR, pCMX-VP-CAR, have been described previously *(23,24)*. Here, we provide an example of the synthesis of hPXR variants carried out in our laboratories. In brief, plasmids for expression of hPXR variants T1, T2, and T3 were constructed by insertion of PCR-amplified cDNAs (described in Subheading 3.4.) into the *Xba*I and *Hind*III sites of pCMV5. Each cDNA was confirmed by sequencing and subsequently transferred to the pCMX plasmid by *Bam*HI/ *Hind*III restriction to generate vectors corresponding to the constitutively active T1, T2, and T3 constructs. The pCMV5- and pCMX-based vectors showed no discernible difference in expression of the PXR variants. The detailed synthesis and the use of these PXR plasmids for UGT transcriptional regulation studies have been published in *(4)*.

3.2. RNA Isolation

Cell culture samples were harvested directly into 2 mL of Trizol reagent (Invitrogen) and stored at −80°C until required for RNA isolation. RNA was further purified using the RNeasy Midi Kit (Qiagen, Valencia, CA). Alternatively, total RNA from transfection experiments was directly harvested using the RNeasy Mini Kit (Qiagen GmbH, Germany). To avoid any contamination of the RNA by genomic DNA, cells were treated with RNase-free DNase I (Promega, Madison, WI). Total RNA samples were then quantified using the RiboGreen RNA Quantitation reagent kit (Molecular Probes, Eugene, OR). Ribo-Green RNA Quantitation reagent is an ultrasensitive fluorescent nucleic acid stain, specifically designed for the quantification of RNA in solution.

3.3. Primers for UGTs

Primer pairs were designed to amplify specifically across exon boundaries in mRNA from UGTs from both the *UGT1A* and *UGT2B* families (Table 1). For *UGT1A* and *UGT2B7* amplification, each reaction was paused at 72°C with 18 cycles remaining and 50 ng of both β-actin 1 primers were added as an internal reference. For the remainder of the semiquantitative reactions, control PCR for β-actin 2 was performed as a separate reaction. The specificity of all primer pairs was confirmed by sequencing or restriction analysis of the PCR products. Semiquantitative analysis of each PCR by densitometry was carried out using NIH Image software (NIH, Bethesda, MD).

3.4. Semiquantitative RT-PCR

cDNA was synthesized by mixing 1 µL of total RNA from each sample with 100 pmol of random hexamers in 50 mM Tris-HCl, pH 8.3, 75 mM KCl, 3 mM MgCl$_2$, 10 mM dithiothreitol (DTT), 100 U of MMLV reverse transcriptase, 20 U of RNase inhibitor, and 1 mM of each dNTP in a total volume of 20 µL (Promega). Semiquantitative hPXR PCR reactions were performed as follows: a 10-µL cDNA aliquot was added to a reaction mixture containing 10 mM Tris-HCl buffer, pH 8, 20 mM KCl, 0.1% Triton X-100, 1.5 mM MgCl$_2$, 0.2 mM of each dNTP, 50 pmol of each primer, and 2 U of *Taq* DNA polymerase (Promega), in a total volume of 50 µL. The mixture was subjected to 34 cycles consisting of a 45-s denaturing step at 94°C, a 45-s annealing step at 59°C, and

Regulation of UGTs

a 45-s elongation step at 72°C in a thermal cycler (MJ Research, Reno, NV). Amplification of the ubiquitously expressed β-actin cDNA was performed under the same conditions in separate experiments. Amplification products were resolved by agarose gel (2%) electrophoresis and detected by ethidium bromide staining. The bands were visualized under UV light and photographed with a computer-assisted camera. Quantification of each band was performed by densitometric analysis using NIH Image software. Figure 1 is representative of a typical semiquantitative RT-PCR experiment.

3.5. Real-Time PCR

It is recommended that the final gene expression experiments be carried out using real-time quantitative PCR. The strength of this method lies in the fact that the amplification efficiency is determined for each assay and is optimized to 100%, thus ensuring that the fluorescence of the measured PCR product is directly representative of the original mRNA. This method requires using specific primers, some of which have been described for UGTs *(7)*. There are several protocols for real-time PCR and an example of a protocol to be used in our laboratory is given here.

We use the standard protocols, chemistries, and the Prism 7700 amplification and detection systems from Applied Biosystems (ABI). For each sample, cDNA is synthesized from total RNA using Taqman Reverse Transcription Reagents from ABI. Primer sequences are selected from sequences in the NCBI database using the Taqman Probe and Primer Design function (ignoring the probe) of the Primer Express v. 1.5 software. PCR reactions are assembled using the SYBR Green PCR Master Mix. Control reactions are run lacking template. This is a check for reagent contamination and to determine the melting temperature of the specific product of interest as compared to possible PCR artifacts. For assay optimization and sample comparison, standard curves are produced using a pool containing each sample cDNA. Data points are generated using fourfold serial dilutions of cDNA, that is, a two-PCR cycle difference in detection between each data point. Individual samples are then compared using the standard curve method described in Applied Biosystems User Bulletin No. 2. In addition, a method for real-time PCR, which was utilized for the measurement of *UGT2B4* and *UGT1A6* gene expression, has been described in detail by Barbier et al. *(7)*.

3.6. Northern Blot Analysis

Experiments were performed according to established protocols *(23)*. In brief, total RNA was isolated using TRIzol® Reagent (Invitrogen) as described in Subheading 3.2. Twenty micrograms of total RNA was separated on 1.25% agarose–6% formaldehyde gels in 1X 3-(*N*-morpholino) propanesulfonic acid

Table 1
PCR Primers and Conditions for Semiquantitative Analysis of UGTs

Target transcript	Primer set F: Forward primer R: Reverse primer	Anneal. temp (°C)	Amplicon size (bp)	No. of cycles on HepG2 cDNA	No. of cycles on Caco-2 cDNA
UGT1A	F: tgaaagcatatgcaatggcgt R: tcaatgggtcttggatttgtg	50	466	30	27
UGT1A1	F: atgctgtggagtcccagggc R: ccattgatcccaaagagaaaacc	50	932	30	30
UGT1A3	F: atggcaatgttgaacaatatg R: ggtctgaattggttgttagtaatc	58	247	35	35
UGT1A4	F: acgctgggctacactcaagg R: gacaggtacttagccagcacc	66	200	40	35
UGT1A6	F: cttttcacagaccagccttac R: tatccacatctcttgaggacag	58	289	42	25
UGT1A7	F: tggctcgtgcagggtggactg R: ttcgcaatggtgccgtccagc	63	310	nd	35
UGT1A8	F: ctgctgacctggcttgct R: ccattgagcatcggcgaaat	63	248	nd	35
UGT1A9	F: gaggaacatttattatgccaccg R: ccattgatcccaaagagaaaacc	50	281	34	32
UGT1A10	F: cctcttcctatgtcccaatga R: gcaacaaccaaattgatgtgtg	63	205	nd	35

UGT2B	F: aagttctaggaagacccactac R: caccacaaccacattttctcca	58	205	30	na
UGT2B4	F: tctactcttaaatttgaagtttatcctgt cR1: tcagcccagcagctcaccacaggg	58	278	30	na
UGT2B7	F: agttggagaatttcatcatgcaacaga cR1: tcagcccagcagctcaccacaggg	58	232	26	30
β-Actin1	F: ctggcggcaccaccatgtaccct R: ggaggggccggactcgtcatact	50	205	18	18
β-Actin2	F: cgtaccactggcatcgtgat R: gtgttggcgtacaggtcttt	58	452	18	18

Two common primers are used for the *UGT2B* isoform PCR: cR1 has two mismatches to *UGT2B4*, and one mismatch to *UGT2B7*. The nucleotide sequences for *UGT1A4F*, *UGT1A6F*, and R, *UGT1A10R* and all *UGT2B* primers were obtained from Congiu et al. (25). The sense primer for *UGT1A10* was designed by Strassburg (26).
nd; Not detected, na; not attempted.

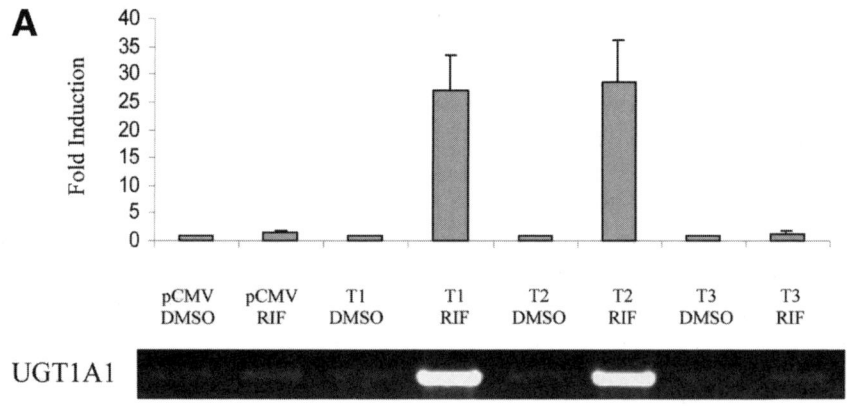

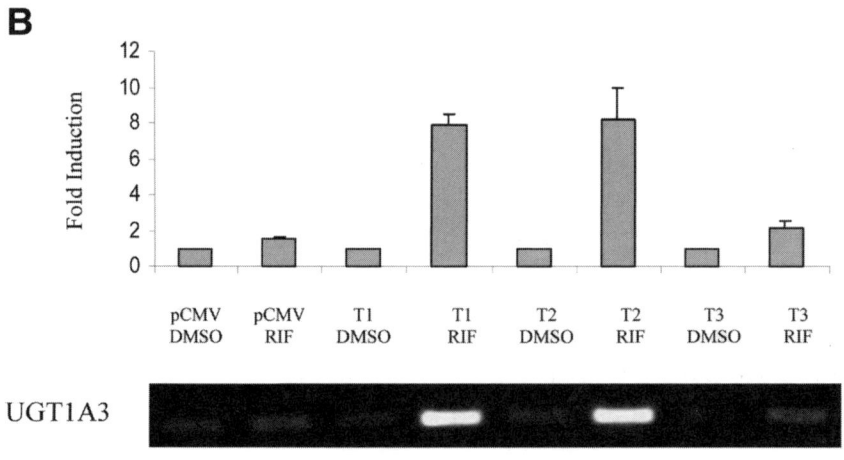

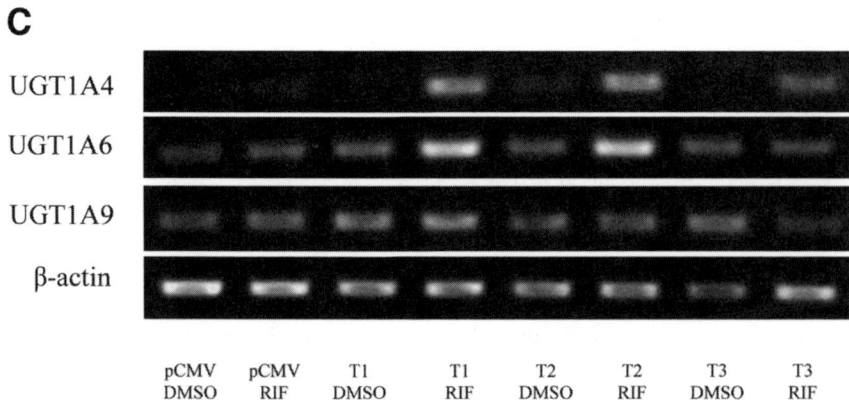

(MOPS) buffer and transferred to a Hybond-N+ nylon membrane (Amersham) in 10X saline–sodium citrate (SSC) (0.75 M NaCl, 0.075 M Na citrate). After UV crosslinking, membranes were probed with ^{32}P-labeled cDNA using the Random Labeling Kit (Roche Applied Science, Indianapolis, IN). The membranes were cohybridized or subsequently rehybridized with a plasmid containing the murine GAPDH cDNA for normalization of loading.

For Northern hybridization, membranes were prehybridized in prehybridization buffer (50% formamide, 5X SSC, 10 mM Na$_3$PO$_4$, 1 mM EDTA, 0.5% sodium dodecyl sulfate [SDS], 10X Denhardt's solution, (Ficoll), polyvinylpyrrolidone, and bovine serum albumin [BSA], 2 mg/mL each) and 20 µg/mL of denatured salmon sperm DNA (Sigma) at 42°C for 2 h. The prehybridization solution was then replaced with hybridization solution (50% formamide, 5X SSC, 10 mM Na$_3$PO$_4$, 1 mM EDTA, 0.5% SDS, 10X Denhardt's solution, 200 µg/mL of denatured salmon sperm DNA, and 5% dextran sulfate) containing 1×10^6 cpm/mL radiolabeled probe. The hybridization was performed at 42°C for 12–16 h. After hybridization, the membranes were washed using standard stringent washing conditions. In brief, the membranes were washed twice with buffer I (2X SSC, 0.1% SDS) at room temperature, twice with buffer II (1X SSC, 0.1% SDS) at 65°C, and twice with buffer III (0.1X SSC, 0.1% SDS) at 65°C. The membranes were then wrapped in Saran Wrap® and subjected to autoradiography at –80°C for the appropriate amount of time.

3.7. Cell Harvest and Preparation of Subcellular Fractions

When harvesting cells for the isolation of subcellular fractions (microsomes and cytosolic fraction) for enzyme analyses and Western blots, cells from each treatment group were rinsed twice with ice-cold Hank's balanced salt solution

---

Fig. 1. *(see opposite page)* Variable regulation of UGT1A isoforms by hPXR variants T1, T2, and T3. HepG2 cells transfected with constructs containing hPXR variants T1, T2, or T3 were exposed to DMSO or RIF (10 µM). HepG2 cells were seeded in six-well plates at 1×10^6 and 2.5×10^5 cells per well, respectively. Transfections were performed in triplicate using 5 µg of expression plasmid or empty parent vector and 10 mL of LipofectAMINE 2000 according to the manufacturer's instructions. At 6–7 h after transfection, the cells were washed in DMEM and replacement medium containing 10 mM RIF (Sigma-Aldrich, St. Louis, MO) or vehicle (0.1% DMSO) was added. At 24 h posttransfection, the cells were treated again with RIF or solvent in fresh DMEM. After a total of 40 h, all transfections were washed in PBS and harvested for RNA extraction. Following exposure, transcriptional regulation by PXR isoforms was assessed by semiquantitative RT-PCR for: (**A**) *UGT1A1*, (**B**) *UGT1A3*, and (**C**) *UGT1A4*, *UGT1A6*, and *UGT1A9*. Where graphs are presented, the results are presented as the means ± SD ($n = 3$).

(HBSS). Homogenization buffer (50 mM Tris-HCl, pH 7.0, 150 mM KCl, 2 mM EDTA) was added to each dish (2–3 mL total volume per group) and cells were scraped with a rubber policeman. Harvested cells from each treatment were pooled and sonicated with a Vibra-Cell probe sonicator at 40 W for 15–20 s. Cell lysates were centrifuged at 9000g for 20 min at 4°C. Supernatants were collected and centrifuged at 100,000g for 60 min at 4°C. The final microsomal pellets were resuspended in 100–300 µL of 0.25 M sucrose with the aid of a Potter–Elvehjem tissue grinder fitted with a Teflon pestle. An aliquot (5 µL) was removed for protein determination.

3.8. Western Blots

Western blot analysis was carried out using anti-UGT1A-peptide and anti-UGT2B7-peptide antibodies (antihuman-UGT2B7-peptide and antihuman-UGT1A-peptide antibodies were obtained from Gentest). Monoclonal (mouse) anticalnexin antibody (IgG) was from Affinity Bioreagents (Golden, CO). For analysis of PXR, anti-PXR (N-16) and anti-PXR (N-19) antibodies were used (polyclonal goat anti-PXR N-16 and N-19 antisera were from Santa Cruz Biotechnology, Santa Cruz, CA). Equal amounts of protein from each sample (30 µg) were separated by SDS-polyacrylamide gel electrophoresis (SDS-PAGE) on 10% gels and transferred to nitrocellulose. Prior to immunostaining, the nitrocellulose was stained with Ponceau S, a reversible protein stain, to ensure equal protein loads between lanes and to visualize the molecular weight standards. Immunoreactive protein was detected by enhanced chemiluminescence (ECL) using SuperSignal West Femto reagents from Pierce (Rockford, IL). A typical Western blot analysis is shown in Fig. 2.

3.9. Glucuronidation Assays

Glucuronidation assays were performed to examine whether changes in UGT expression coincided with changes in glucuronidation. HepG2 and Caco-2 cells were harvested and cell membranes, which contain UGTs, were prepared and glucuronidation assays, in general, were carried out as described previously *(27)*. Membrane-bound UGTs require activation, usually with detergent, to obtain maximal enzymatic activity. However, detergent treatment of membrane fractions obtained from cell cultures frequently results in significant inhibition of recombinant UGT activity. It has been demonstrated that treatment with alamethicin, a channel-forming agent, results in a significant activation of the majority of recombinant UGT isoforms *(28)*. Therefore, this treatment is routinely used with experiments involving recombinant UGTs.

UGT activity in cell membrane fractions were determined using labeled substrate and UDP-glucuronic acid (UDP-GlcUA) or unlabeled substrate and [^{14}C]UDP-GlcUA as the sugar donor. For assays carried out with recombinant

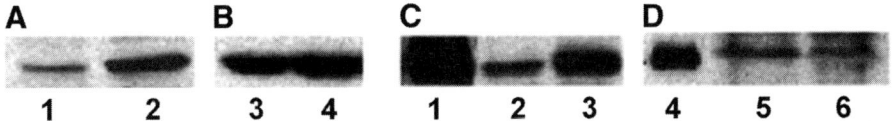

Fig. 2. Western blot analysis of hPXR and UGTs in HepG2 and Caco-2 cells. Western blot analysis of (**A**), HepG2 cells visualized with anti-PXR 16 antibody; (**B**), Caco-2 cells visualized with anti-PXR 16 antibody; (**C**) CaCo-2 protein visualized with anti-pan-UGT1A antibody; and (**D**), anti-UGT2B7 antibody. Ten micrograms of total cell lysate (A1) and cytosol (A2) from HepG2 cells were separated by SDS-PAGE and transferred to nitrocellulose and exposed to anti-hPXR16 antibody. Ten micrograms of total cell lysate (B3) and cytosols (B4) from Caco-2 cells were separated by SDS-PAGE and transferred to nitrocellulose and exposed to anti-hPXR16 antibody. Total membranes from CaCo-2 cells treated with the DMSO or 25 μM concentration of chrysin were exposed to anti-UGT1A-peptide antibody; (C1) standard of recombinant UGT1A1, (C2) untreated and (C3) chrysin-treated cells. Total membranes from CaCo-2 cells treated with the DMSO or 25 μM concentration of chrysin were exposed to anti-UGT2B7-peptide antibody; (D1) standard of recombinant UGT2B7, (D2) untreated, and (D3) chrysin-treated cells.

UGTs, all substrates were introduced to the reaction mixture in ethanol and UGTs were activated with alamethicin (final concentration, 60 μg/mg of protein), also dissolved in ethanol with a final ethanol concentration of <3%. Substrates (final concentration, 100 μM) were preincubated with 20 μg of cell membranes in 100 mM N-(2-hydroxyethyl)piperazine-N'-(2-ethanesulfonic acid) (HEPES)–NaOH, pH 7.4, 5 mM MgCl$_2$, and 5 mM saccharolactone at room temperature for 10 min. Reactions were started by the addition of UDP-GlcUA (final concentration, 4 mM) and incubated at 37°C for 15 min. Reactions were then stopped by the addition of 20 μL of ethanol. Samples were mixed on a vortex mixer, placed on ice, and aliquots were applied to thin-layer chromatography (TLC) plates (Baker Si250, 19C(PA); VWR, Irving, TX). Glucuronidated products and unreacted substrate were separated by development in chloroform–methanol–glacial acetic acid–water (65:25:2:4, by vol). Radioactive compounds were localized on TLC plates by autoradiography for 3–4 d at –80°C. Silica gel in zones corresponding to the glucuronide bands, or corresponding areas from control lanes, were scraped into scintillation vials and radioactivity was measured by liquid scintillation counting.

A variety of known UGT1A substrates were examined, including β-estradiol (a 1A1 preferred substrate), acetaminophen (a 1A6 preferred substrate), the xenobiotics, 4-nitrophenol and 4-hydroxy-2-amino-1-methyl-6-phenylimidazo [4,5-b]pyridine (4-OH-PhIP), phenolic corticosteroids (cortisol, cortisone, and corticosterone), and thyroid hormones (reverse triiodothyronine [rT_3] and thyroxine [T_4]). For analysis of the enzymatic activity of isoforms from the UGT2B family, steroid hormones and retinoids were used as the primary substrates. Glucuronidation assays carried out with ER isolated from human donors and transgenic animals required somewhat different assay conditions than those for cell membrane assays. UGTs in ER preparations are, in general, much less sensitive to detergent than membrane preparations of recombinant enzymes. In all of our microsomal assays, Brij 58 was used as the activating detergent and also served to solubilize hydrophobic substrates. UGT activity in ER was determined using labeled substrate and UDP-GlcUA or unlabeled substrate and [^{14}C]UDP-GlcUA as the sugar donor, as described previously in detail *(29,30)*. In brief, substrates were solubilized in micelles with Brij 58 (micelle concentration, 0.12%; final concentration, 0.05%) *(27,31,32)*. Substrates (final concentration, 100–250 μ*M* substrate) were preincubated with protein (50 μg) in 100 m*M* HEPES–NaOH, pH 7.4, 5 m*M* $MgCl_2$, and 5 m*M* saccharolactone at room temperature for 10 min. Reactions were started by the addition of UDP-GlcUA (final concentration, 4 m*M*) and incubated at 37°C for 20 min. The isolation and measurement of biosynthesized glucuronides were carried out as described for recombinant UGTs.

4. ISOLATION AND CHARACTERIZATION OF UGT PROMOTERS
4.1. Background

The transcription of genes is controlled by the assembly of a transcription initiation complex containing DNA polymerase and various accessory factors on or near the transcription start site, which is contained within the gene promoter *(33)*. Promoters are defined as the DNA upstream from the transcribed sequence and may include part of the first exon. The initiation complex directs the polymerase to begin transcribing at the correct start site. The binding of the initiation complex and the rates of transcription initiation are in turn controlled by transcription factors (*trans* factors) that bind to the promoter to enhance or inhibit recruitment of the transcription initiation complex, usually via interactions with coregulatory proteins and proteins in the initiation complex. The promoter is the central component that integrates these protein–protein interactions to facilitate gene expression and, hence, is crucial to the regulation of the gene. To begin to define the mechanisms that regulate a specific gene, the promoter must be characterized. This involves determining the transcription start site and the site of assembly of the transcription initiation complex, and identifying the nuclear proteins (*trans* factors) that regulate transcription initiation and the DNA elements (*cis* factors) to which they bind. The focus of this section is the use of in vitro methods and cell culture to aid in UGT promoter characterization. However, the data from these studies ideally

Regulation of UGTs

require careful evaluation in in vivo models of gene regulation. Furthermore, gene expression is controlled by the coordinated action of many *cis* and *trans* elements, some of which may not be found in the promoter but nevertheless act through the promoter. These factors include locus control regions, matrix attachment regions, enhancers, and silencers. DNA methylation is also important in the control of gene expression. Strategies to investigate these factors are not described here.

4.2. General Approach

To define the 3′-end of a UGT promoter, it is necessary to determine the transcription start site. Several methods can be used for this purpose, including primer extension, S1 mapping, and RNA ligase mediated-rapid amplification of cDNA ends (RLM-RACE) *(34)*. The latter method is more suitable for the detection of transcription start sites in low abundant transcripts as it incorporates an amplification step. We have used this method to define the transcription start site of UGT genes, which is described in Subheading 5.1.

The 5′-end of the promoter is more difficult to define, as theoretically, it should be upstream from all the transcription factor binding sites that support the normal expression of the gene. If the next gene upstream is known, then the beginning of the promoter can be established. If this information is unavailable, then the length of the promoter is usually limited by the amount of DNA that can be cloned into the gene reporter plasmids and transfected into cultured cells. This is usually up to 18 kb in length. The promoter is cloned by PCR from genomic DNA or, more generally, from appropriate clones in a library of genomic DNA. Lambda, cosmid, and BAC (bacterial artificial chromosomes) libraries are used for this purpose. The cloned promoter is then inserted into vectors containing a reporter gene and its capacity to drive transcription of the reporter is tested in cell culture. The reporter genes are usually chosen because they are absent in the cell line to be transfected and highly sensitive techniques to measure their expression are available. They include the firefly luciferase and bacterial chloramphenicol acetyl transferase genes. The choice of cell line depends on the gene promoter under study. However, to be confident that the *trans* factors necessary for regulation of the promoter are present in the recipient cell line, the cell line should exhibit appropriate endogenous expression of the gene whose promoter is being investigated. Details on the cloning of UGT promoters, their transfection into liver and gastrointestinal cell lines, and assays to test their capacity to drive the transcription of reporter genes are described in Subheadings 5.2. and 5.3.

Having established that the promoter is active, serial deletions from the 5′-end are made to define the regions in the promoter that are important for its activity. These regions are generally composed of 10–30 nucleotides and are sites of binding of transcription factors. The binding of nuclear proteins to these DNA elements is detected in footprint assays and gel electrophoretic mobility shift assays, as described in Subheadings 5.4. and 5.5., respectively. The identity of the DNA binding proteins can be established with antibodies or the use of in vitro synthesized protein in EMSA. Identity of transcription factors and their binding sites is also guided by consultation of the transcription factor databases such as TRANSFAC *(35)* and NUBIScan *(36)*. Unknown factors may be isolated by screening of cDNA expression libraries with concatenated DNA containing the *cis* element of interest. Alternatively, the transcription factors can be purified on resin-bound DNA and identified with mass spectrometric techniques.

Confirmation of the importance of a *cis* element is provided by its mutation in the promoter and consequent alteration of promoter activity. Confirmation of the importance of a particular *trans* factor is provided by alterations in promoter activity when expression plasmids encoding the factor are cotransfected with promoter reporter constructs. The principle underlying the latter approach is that the transcription factor of interest is not present in saturating amounts in the cell and so effects can be measured by the expression of extra factor synthesized from the expression vector. If this is not the case, it may be necessary to construct dominant-negative mutants of the transcription factor and look for changes in promoter activity when expression plasmids containing these mutants are cotransfected with the promoter–reporter constructs.

In general, the above strategy should be sufficient to identify the *cis* and *trans* factors most important in regulating the expression of a specific UGT gene. As mentioned earlier, however, the significance of these factors in controlling gene expression in vivo requires careful evaluation.

5. METHODS FOR THE ANALYSIS OF UGT PROMOTERS

5.1. Determination of Transcription Start Sites

Transcription start sites were mapped using RLM-RACE, provided in the First Choice kit (Ambion AS, Austin, TX, USA). In brief, RNA was decapped, ligated to an RNA adaptor oligonucleotide and used as a template in sequential PCR reactions. The final PCR product contained the 5′-end of the mRNA (the decapped base), which was identified by DNA sequencing. The protocol was designed to amplify cDNA only from full-length capped RNA, which avoids false positives caused by RNA degradation.

Total RNA was isolated from cells using the Qiagen RNAeasy midi kit (Qiagen GmbH, Hilden, Germany). Five micrograms of total RNA were treated with calf intestinal phosphatase (CIP) to prevent subsequent ligation and purified by phenol–chloroform extraction. Capped mRNA was protected from the action of the phosphatase. The cap was subsequently removed with tobacco acid pyrophosphatase, according to the manufacturer's protocol. The resulting full-length RNA was ligated with the 5′-RACE adapter provided and used as template for reverse transcription. The UGTs of interest were amplified by PCR using a reverse primer specific to the UGT and the 5′-RACE outer primer provided, under the following conditions: 94°C for 4 min followed by 35 cycles of 94°C for 30 s, 55°C for 30 s, 72°C for 1 min, and then 72°C for 10 min. Nested PCR with a UGT-specific primer and the 5′-RACE inner primer provided was carried out. The PCR products were purified with the QIAquick PCR purification kit (Qiagen) and cloned into the pCR Blunt vector (Invitrogen Corp., Carlsbad, CA) according to the manufacturer's protocol. Several clones were selected and sequenced to identify the decapped base, which is the transcription start site.

5.2. Isolation of UGT Promoters and Preparation of Reporter Constructs

Clones containing UGT promoters can be isolated from commercial human λ or cosmid genomic libraries after several rounds of screening. In brief, DNA fragments from the 5′-ends of the cDNAs encoding the UGTs of interest were labeled with [^{32}P]dATP by random priming using the DECAprime II DNA labeling kit (Ambion). The DNA on Hybond-N membranes (Amersham Biosciences) from plaque lifts was denatured, neutralized, and crosslinked to the membrane by UV irradiation. Prehybridization of the membranes was carried out in a solution of 5X SSC, 0.5X Denhardt's (5% [w/v] each of Ficoll 400, polyvinylpyrrolidone, and bovine serum albumin, fraction V, Sigma) and 0.5% SDS for 4 h at 42°C before hybridization overnight with 1×10^6 cpm/μL of probe. Membranes are washed twice in 2X SSC, 0.1% SDS for 5 min at room temperature, and twice in 0.1X SSC, 0.1% SDS for 30 min at 65°C followed by exposure to autoradiography film with intensification screens at −70°C overnight. Positive plaques were picked and screened by restriction digestion and sequencing for appropriate UGT promoter inserts. UGT promoters of various lengths were amplified from these clones or from human genomic DNA by PCR, using primers designed with information from the sequencing of the genomic clones and/or from the human genome databases. The primers contain different restriction sites for directional cloning into the pGL3 luciferase reporter vector (Promega). To generate the series of 5′ deletion constructs, appropriate restriction enzymes, PCR or the Erase-a-Base® system (Promega) may be used. For example, the proximal *UGT2B7* promoter region and a series of 5′ deletion constructs were generated by the Erase-a-Base® system. In brief, a forward primer with a flanking *Sma*I restriction endonuclease site and a reverse primer with *Sma*I restriction endonuclease site was used to amplify the proximal 1.3 kbp *UGT2B7* region and subcloned into corresponding sites in pGL3-Baic vector. The plasmid containing the insertion was digested by *Nhe*I and *Kpn*I. The linear fragment was digested by exonuclease III and aliquots were removed at different times to obtain the series of 5' deletions. S1 nuclease was added to remove the remaining 5' overhang and resulting blunt ends were linked by adding Klenow fragment, dNTPs, and T4 DNA ligase. Positive clones containing *UGT2B7* promoter insertion were sequence-verified per standard protocols. Sequencing should always be performed to confirm that the correct promoter deletion construct has been synthesized.

5.3. Expression of UGT Promoter–Luciferase Reporter Constructs

The UGT promoter constructs were tested in transient transfections using pRL-null (expressing *Renilla* luciferase protein in low levels) to normalize for transfection efficiency. In brief, cells were split the day prior to transfection to reach approx 80% confluency before transfection. Transient transfections were performed in 24-well plates using LipofectAMINE 2000 Reagent (LF2000) with 0.5–1.0 μg of promoter construct plus 0.01–0.05 μg of pRL-null and 2–3 μL of LF2000 per well following the manufacturer's protocol. Transient transfections were carried out in the presence of fetal calf serum and in the absence of antibiotic. The cells were harvested 2 d after transfection. The harvested cells were washed twice in 1X phosphate-buffered saline (PBS) (137 mM NaCl, 2.7 mM KCl, 10 mM Na$_2$HPO$_4$, 1.8 mM K$_2$HPO$_4$, pH 7.4) and lysed in 1X passive lysis buffer (PLB) for 15 min at room temperature. Twenty microliters of the lysate was used in the dual luciferase activity assay. Luciferase activity was measured in a top counter following the manufacturer's protocol (Promega).

5.4. DNase 1 Footprint Analysis

The identification of transcription factor binding sites by DNase 1 footprint analysis relies on the protection of these sites from nuclease digestion when bound to transcription factor. The protected sites are revealed as "footprints" on denaturing polyacrylamide gels. The site of assembly of the transcription initiation complex can also be identified with this procedure. To detect transcription factor sites on UGT promoters, a solid-phase DNase I footprinting protocol using Dynabeads M-280 Streptavidin-coated beads (Dynal, Oslo, Norway) may be used *(37)*. In this procedure, the promoter fragment to be assessed for transcription factor binding sites is amplified by PCR with biotinylated oligonucleotide primers. The PCR products are bound to magnetic beads, incubated with nuclear extract or purified transcription factor, treated with DNase 1, and the digested fragments analyzed by gel electrophoresis.

In a typical experiment, the promoter region of interest was amplified in two separate reactions with forward biotinylated primer and reverse primer in one reaction and forward primer and reverse biotinylated primer in the second reaction. This detects transcription factor binding sites on the sense and antisense DNA strands, respectively. Each PCR was carried out in 20 µL containing 1X *Pfu* buffer, 250 µM (each) dNTP, 2 ng each forward and reverse primer, 10 ng of template (genomic-clone containing the UGT promoter of interest), and 1 U of *Pfu Turbo* DNA polymerase. After amplification, the PCR products were purified with the Qiagen PCR purification kit and mixed with Dynabeads that have been washed twice with coupling buffer (2 M NaCl, 10 mM Tris, pH 8, 1 mM EDTA). After incubation at room temperature for 60 min with constant mixing, the beads were washed twice in TE (10 mM Tris-HCl, 1 mM EDTA, pH 8.0) before resuspension in 15 µL Tris-HCl buffer, pH 8.5. Following the addition of 2 µL of 10X T4 polynucleotide kinase buffer, 2 µL of [$^{32}\gamma$]ATP (3000 Ci/mmol) and 1 µL of T4 polynucleotide kinase, the solution is incubated at 37°C for 1 h with occasional mixing. The excess label is removed by washing twice with 200 µL of coupling buffer.

For the footprint reaction, the beads containing the radiolabeled DNA were mixed with 10 µL nuclear extract (0–50 µg) and 1 µg of poly dI-dC in binding buffer (20 mM HEPES, pH 7.9, 2 mM MgCl$_2$, 1 mM dithiothreitol (DTT), 20% glycerol). After incubation for 30 min on ice, 1–5 µL of DNase 1 (1 U/µL in binding buffer) was added and digestion was stopped after a predetermined time (between 10 s and 5 min) with 100 µL of stop buffer (50 mM Tris-Cl, 2% SDS, 10 mM EDTA). The beads were washed once with 100 µL of wash solution (10 mM EDTA, 2 M NaCl), once with 100 µL of TE and then boiled for 5 min in formamide loading buffer. The DNA fragments were separated on 6% sequencing gels. Sequencing ladders were generated with the same sense and antisense primers used for footprinting and electrophoresed on the same gel as the footprint reactions. This permits direct determination of the sequence that binds nuclear proteins. The nuclear extracts used in the footprint reaction were prepared essentially according to ref. *38*. Purified transcription factors may also be used. A typical experiment is shown in Fig. 3.

5.5. Gel Electrophoretic Mobility Shift Assay

Gel electrophoretic mobility shift assay (EMSA) is a sensitive method to detect the binding of proteins to duplex DNA. In essence, a small radiolabeled, double-stranded DNA fragment is incubated with nuclear protein and the protein–DNA complexes are resolved by electrophoresis on polyacrylamide gels. The specificity of the DNA–protein binding can be assessed by mutating the DNA binding site or by competition with unlabeled DNA. The protein in the DNA–protein complex can be identified with specific antibodies, which retard migration of the protein–DNA complex to cause a "supershift."

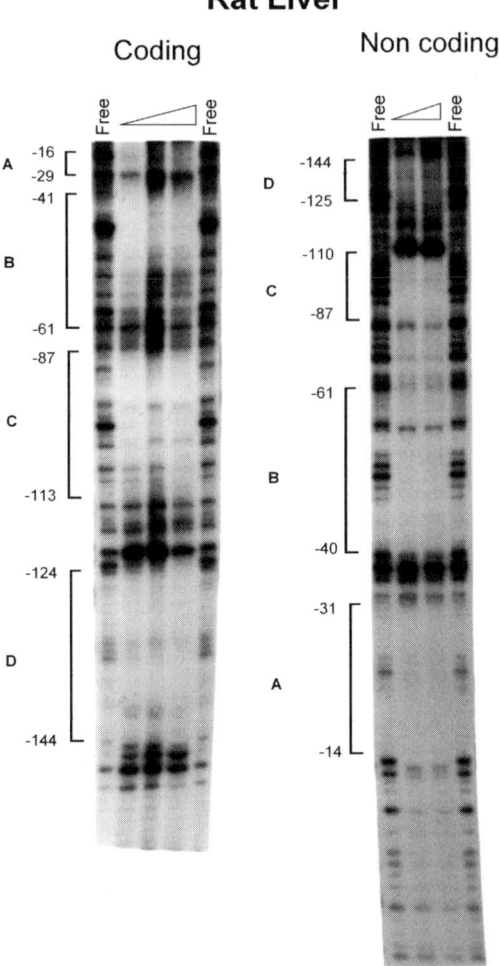

Fig. 3. Footprint analysis of the UGT2B1 gene promoter. The coding and noncoding strands spanning nucleotides −205 to +14 of the UGT2B1 gene promoter were end-labeled with ^{32}P and incubated with 0 (free), 25, 50, and 100 μg of rat liver nuclear extracts. Areas protected from DNase 1 digestion (i.e., the footprints) are denoted A–D. (Reprinted from ref. *37* with permission from Mary Ann Liebert Inc., Publishers.)

The sense and antisense oligonucleotides (5 μg each) were annealed in 1X annealing buffer (40 m*M* Tris-HCl, pH 7.5, 20 m*M* MgCl$_2$, 50 m*M* NaCl) in a total volume of 100 μL by incubating for 5 min at 95°C, followed by 5 min at 65°C and then cooling to room temperature. One microliter of the annealed oligonucleotides was end-labeled by the addition of 1 μL of [γ-^{32}P]ATP and

0.5 U of polynucleotide kinase (PNK) in a total volume of 10 μL of 1X PNK buffer, and incubated for 1 h at 37°C. Excess [γ-^{32}P]ATP was removed by column purification using MicroSpin™ G-25 columns (Amersham) following addition of 90 μL of 1X TE. Radiolabeled oligonucleotides were diluted to approx 50,000 cpm and 1 μL was added to a mixture containing 1 μL of nuclear extract (~5 μg) or 1 μL of in vitro transcribed transcription factor, 1 μg of poly dI-dC and 12 μL of TM-1 buffer (25 mM Tris-HCl, pH 7.6, 100 mM KCl, 5 mM MgCl$_2$, 0.5 mM EDTA, 10% glycerol) on ice. The transcription factors were synthesized with the TNT-coupled reticulocyte lysate system (Promega). If required, unlabeled annealed oligonucleotide at 25–100 times molar excess was added for competition studies or 1 μL of antibody was added for supershift assays. The mixture was incubated at room temperature for 30 min before electrophoresis on a 4% nondenaturing acrylamide gel for 2 h at 4°C in 0.5X TBE (45 mM Tris-borate, pH 8.3, 1 mM EDTA) at 250 V. The gel was subsequently dried and exposed to X-ray film to reveal protein–DNA complexes. A typical experiment is shown in Fig. 4.

6. ANIMAL STUDIES

6.1. Background

6.1.1. Current Models to Assess Xenobiotic Enzyme Inducibility and Their Limitations

To date, there has been no reliable in vivo system outside of the human to assess directly and quantitatively human drug-induced xenobiotic enzyme production. Primary cultures of human hepatocytes represent a unique in vitro system to evaluate the induction of phase I and phase II DMEs. Many investigators have successfully used human hepatocyte cultures to investigate the effect of various agents on the induction of DMEs *(41–43)* and reviewed in refs. *44,45*). Accordingly, in current pharmaceutical development, a majority of assessment of induction of CYP3A4 and phase II enzymes has been performed using primary human hepatocytes. While valuable, the utility of human hepatocytes is compromised by interindividual variability, limited tissue sources, as well as the high cost.

In addition to human hepatocytes, rodents have been standard components in the assessment of potential toxicity in the development of candidate human drugs for many decades. However, it is well known that the xenobiotic induction of many DMEs exhibits clear species specificity. The species difference is probably best exemplified in drug induction of the CYP3A enzymes. For example, the antibiotic RIF is a specific CYP3A inducer in humans, whereas the antiglucocorticoid, pregnenolone-16α-carbonitrile (PCN), is a rodent-specific

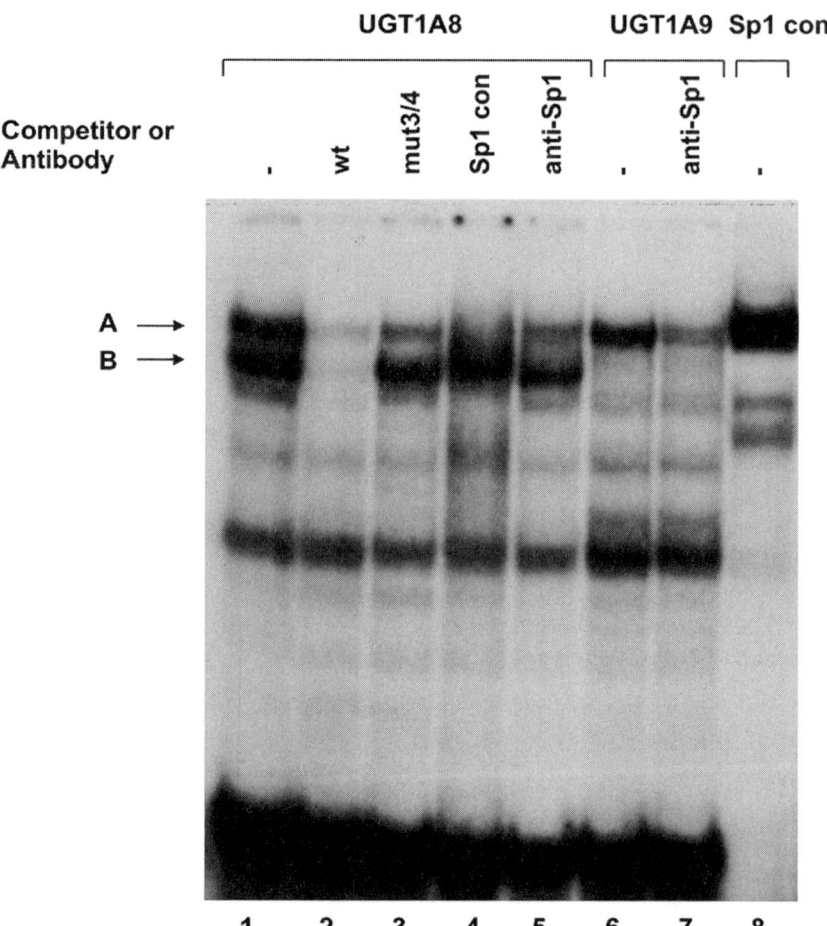

Fig. 4. Electrophoretic mobility shift assay (EMSA) of the UGT1A8, 1A9 and 1A10 Sp1/initiator-like region. Double-stranded oligonucleotide probes (50,000 cpm) corresponding to wild-type and mutant *UGT1A8, 1A9,* and *1A10* Sp1/initiator-like regions (−34/+8 of *UGT1A8*) were incubated with 5 μg Caco-2 nuclear extracts and resolved on a 4fi nondenaturing polyacrylamide gel. The two major complexes, A and B, are indicted with arrows and the minor complexes are bracketed (labeled with an *asterisk*). (Reprinted from ref. *38*, with permission from ASBMB.)

CYP3A inducer *(46–50)*. Pharmacologic studies in primary cultures of hepatocytes suggest that it is not the structure of the CYP3A genes that dictates the pattern of CYP3A inducibility, but rather, there must be a species-specific cellular factor(s) *(51)*.

6.1.2. PXR-Mediated and Mechanism-Based Prediction of Enzyme Inducibility

The establishment of PXR as a xenosensor has made it possible to design receptor-based bioassay to assess drug-induced activation of PXR in vivo, thereby inferring enzyme inducibility by these drugs. The effects of pharmaceuticals on PXR transcriptional activity should be an important factor to be considered in drug development and clinical practice to avoid adverse drug–drug interactions (for reviews, see refs. *52–54*). On the one hand, activation of PXR by agonistic drugs leads to accelerated drug metabolism and/or clearance by upregulating many DMEs, rendering the treatment ineffective. On the other hand, inadvertent inhibition of PXR may cause suppression of enzymes, leading to heightened drug toxicity. However, in some cases, activation of PXR and the resultant induction of DMEs may be beneficial to eliminate toxic stimuli that may cause pathological conditions. For example, the secondary bile acid, licotholic acid (LCA), is hepatotoxic and has been implicated in cholestatic liver diseases *(55–57)*. A recent report showed that sustained activation of hPXR and induction of CYP3A in transgenic mice are sufficient to confer resistance to LCA hepatotoxicity *(58)*. Therefore, a great need has developed for cost-effective screening of compounds that activate PXR, potentially leading to increased enzyme expression.

6.1.3. Use of hPXR "Humanized" Mouse Models to Study the Regulation of DMEs

Rodents have been standard components in the assessment of drug metabolism and toxicity. At the same time, they may not be reliable predictors of the human DME inducibility owing to the species-specificity of xenobiotic responses. In spite of those limitations, however, very important information has already been generated. For example, using both transfection and transgenic approaches, we have demonstrated that the species origin of the PXR receptor, rather than the promoter structure of enzyme-coding genes, dictates the species-specificity of enzyme inducibility, such as that of CYP3A *(23)*. The species-specific ligand specificity is largely due to the divergence of amino acid sequences in the ligand-binding domains of the human and mouse receptors and the resulting differences in crystal structures *(59)*. These findings led us to create "humanized" mice, in which the mouse PXR was genetically replaced in the liver by its human homolog, resulting in a "humanized" hepatic xenobiotic response profile. These mice readily responded to the human-specific inducer RIF in a concentration range equivalent to the standard oral dosing regimen in humans *(23)*. The same mice can be used to study the pharmacological regulation of UGT enzymes (*see* Subheading 6.3.). The creation of these mice represents a major step toward generating a humanized rodent toxicological model that is continuously renewable and completely standardized (for a review, *see* ref. *54*).

6.2. Creation of Transgenic Mice With Altered Activity of Xenobiotic Receptors

6.2.1. Creation of PXR Knockout Mice

The creation of PXR knockout mice provided a loss-of-function model to examine the function of the PXR receptor in UGT regulation. Figure 5A illustrates the strategy to create the PXR knockout mice. Mouse PXR genomic DNA was isolated by screening a 129/Sv library (Stratagene, La Jolla, CA) using PXR cDNA as a probe *(60)*. A targeting vector was generated by replacing the second and third exons of PXR with a PGK-Neo selection marker. The resulting mutant allele has a deletion of two exons spanning nucleotides 339–660 (including amino acids 63–170 of the DNA binding domain) *(58)*. A negative selection marker (PGK-TK) was introduced at the 5′-end of the short arm. J1 ES cells (a gift from Dr. K-F Lee, the Salk Institute) were electroporated with *Not*I-linearized targeting vector, and selected in 200 µg/mL of G418 and 0.2 µM ganciclovir. Single clones resistant to G418 and ganciclovir were screened for the designated homologous recombination by Southern blotting. PXR+/– ES cells were microinjected into C57BL6/J blastocysts, which were transplanted into uteri of pseudopregnant ICR mice. Chimeric male progeny were crossed with C57BL6/J females. Germline transmission of the disrupted allele was detected in agouti progeny by Southern blot and PCR using the following three oligonucleotides: common, 5-AGAAACACATAGAAACCCATC-CATG-3′, wild-type-specific, 5′-AGTCCACCAAGCCTGAGCCTCCTAC-3′, and mutant-specific, 5′-CTTGACGAGTTCTTCTGAGGGGATC-3′. The sizes of PCR products are 521 bp and 472 bp for the mutant and wild-type alleles, respectively.

The disruption of PXR alleles was confirmed by the absence of PXR expression in the liver and small intestine, as determined by Northern blotting *(23)*. The PXR null mice are both viable and fertile. Loss of PXR does not alter the basal expression of *CYP3A*, a prototypical PXR target gene. However, the *CYP3A* gene is no longer induced in response to prototypic rodent *CYP3A* inducers PCN or dexamethasone (DEX) *(23)*. This establishes that PXR is an essential mediator of *CYP3A* xenoregulation in vivo.

6.2.2. Creation of Transgenic Mice Expressing the Activated hPXR

Having established PXR as a xenobiotic receptor that regulates the expression of DMEs and transporters, we predict that genetic activation of PXR will cause sustained induction of PXR target genes, including the UGTs. We went

Regulation of UGTs

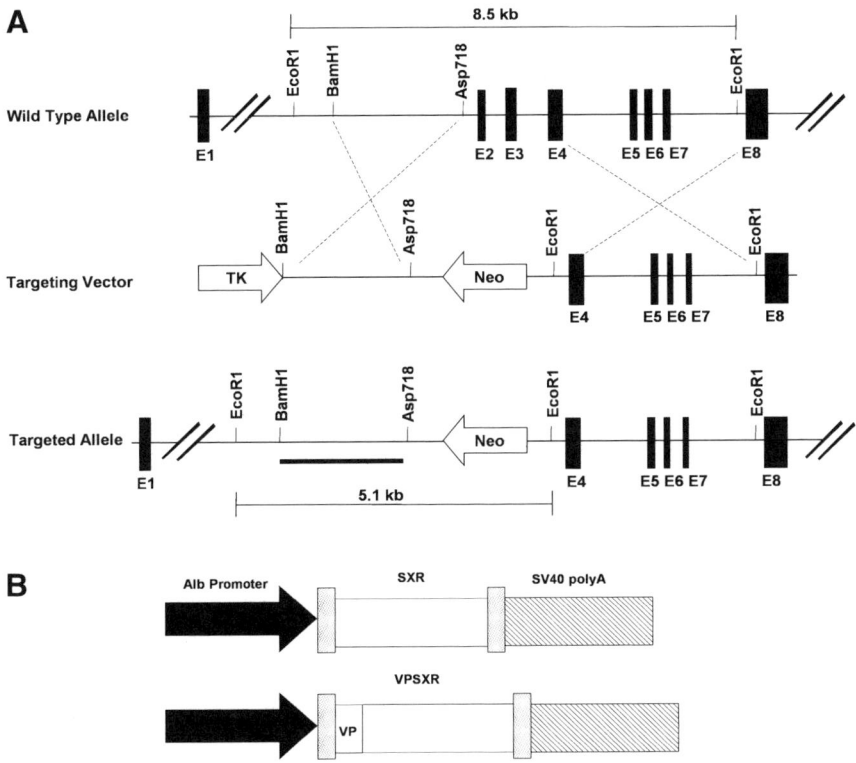

Fig. 5. Generation of PXR null and PXR transgenic mice. (**A**) Restriction map of the PXR gene and strategy to generate PXR mutant allele. (**B**) Schematic representations of the Alb-hPXR and Alb-VP-hPXR transgene constructs.

on to create "gain-of-function" transgenic mice expressing the constitutively activated hPXR, VP-hPXR. Sharing similar DNA binding specificity as its wild-type counterpart, VP-PXR was generated by fusing the VP16 activation domain of the herpes simplex virus to the amino-terminal of hPXR. Fig. 5B shows the schematic representation of the Alb-VP-hPXR transgene in which the cDNA of VP-hPXR is placed downstream of the mouse albumin promoter/enhancer (Alb) to achieve liver-specific expression of the transgene *(61)*. An SV40 intron/poly(A) sequence was subsequently placed downstream of VP-hPXR cDNAs. Transgenes were excised from the vector and purified using the QIAGEN Gel Extraction Kit (Qiagen) before microinjection into the pronuclei of fertilized mouse eggs. The injected eggs were implanted into the uteri of pseudopregnant females and the offspring were screened for the presence of the transgene by PCR. PCR was designed to be specific for the transgene with one oligonucleotide annealing to hPXR cDNA (5′-GAG CAA TTC GCC ATT ACT CTG AAG T-3′), and the other to the SV40 poly(A) sequences (5′-GTC CTT GGG GTC TTC TAC CTT TCT C-3′). The PCR was carried out in a DNA thermal cycler using the following program: 94°C for 1 min, 57°C for 2 min, and 72°C for 3 min. PCR products were analyzed by electrophoresis on a 1% agarose gel. Southern blot analysis was used to confirm the positivity, integrity and copy number of the transgene. For Southern blot, 8 µg of mouse tail genomic DNA was digested with the appropriate restriction enzymes and subjected to Southern blotting and hybridization using Hybond-N+ nylon membrane (Amersham), following the manufacturer's protocol. The probe used was the hPXR cDNA that is specific for human but not mouse PXR. We then bred the genetically positive founders to establish an individual transgenic line. The expression of VP-hPXR transgene was confirmed by Northern blotting *(23)*.

6.2.3. Creation of "Humanized" hPXR Transgenic Mice

First, transgenic mice expressing the wild-type hPXR in the liver were generated by using the albumin promoter as outlined in Fig. 5B *(23)*. Harboring both mPXR and hPXR, these mice exhibited a chimeric, or combined, *CYP3A* response to both human-specific RIF and rodent-specific PCN *(23)*. These results imply that mice expressing only hPXR could be fully humanized for the xenobiotic response. Mice bearing the fully humanized receptor in the liver were created by breeding the hPXR transgene into a mPXR knockout background (Fig. 6). In contrast to PXR knockout mice that were devoid of *CYP3A* induction by PCN and DEX, replacement of mPXR with hPXR restored xenobiotic regulation with a humanized response profile. Thus, the "humanized" mice were responsive to RIF, but not to PCN *(23)*. Expressing hPXR exclusively, the "humanized" mice represent a major step toward generating humanized toxicological models to predict xenobiotic enzyme inducibility and drug–drug interactions.

6.3. PXR-Mediated Genetic and Pharmacological Regulation of UGT Enzymes In Vivo

The creation of transgenic mice with heightened (VP-hPXR) or "humanized" hPXR activity allowed us to evaluate the genetic and pharmacological regulation of UGT gene expression in vivo. To evaluate whether individual isoforms of UGTs were transcriptional targets for PXR, we examined profiles of hepatic proteins and mRNAs isolated from transgenic mice harboring an activated hPXR in the liver *(4)*. Liver microsomal proteins were prepared and subjected to Western blot analysis using a pan-UGT1A antibody or a *UGT1A1* isoform-specific antibody (for details of the Western blot protocols, see Subheading 3.8.). As shown in Fig. 7A, the VP-hPXR mice had increased levels

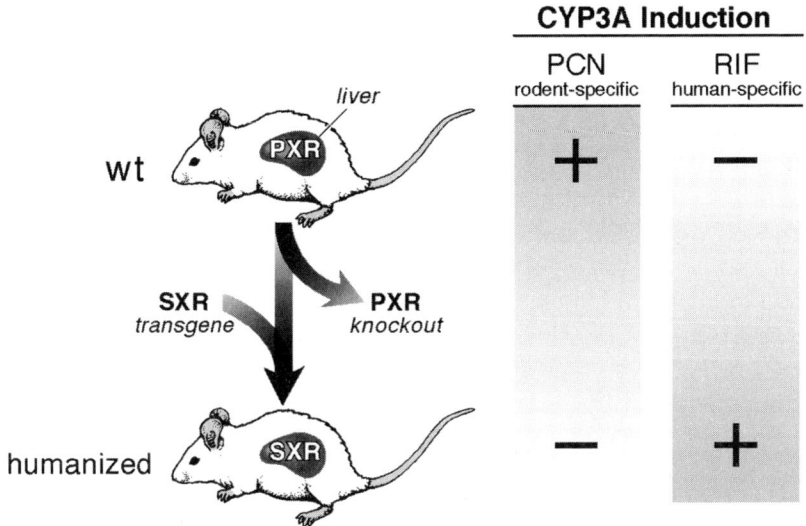

Fig. 6. Establishment of a humanized xenobiotic mouse. (Reprinted from ref. *51* with permission from the ASBMB.)

of both general UGT1A protein and the UGT1A1 isoform. Besides UGT1A1, Northern blot analysis (described in detail in Subheading 3.6.), revealed that *UGT1A6* mRNA was also upregulated (Fig. 7B). As expected, upregulation of general *UGT1A* mRNAs was observed when a probe containing the common exons 2–5 was used. This probe encompasses exons that are shared by all *UGT1A* family members, and thus measures combined regulation of the entire locus *(62)*. While the induction of UGT in VP-hPXR mice was clear, it was not as dramatic as that of *CYP3A11*, probably because not all UGT isoforms are PXR targets (Fig. 7B). The upregulation was liver-specific, as no change in UGT expression was seen in tissues that do not express the transgene, such as the small intestine (data not shown).

The PXR-mediated, pharmacological or ligand-dependent regulation of UGTs was evaluated in the humanized hPXR transgenic mice. As expected, treatment of these mice with RIF, a potent hPXR-specific activator, elevated UGT1A mRNA within 24 h of a single oral dose (Fig. 7C). This established that human PXR and its hormone specific ligands can regulate the UGT1A locus in vivo.

Presumably, increased UGT expression would be associated with increased glucuronidating activity. The preparation of microsomal fractions and details of the enzymatic assays were described in Subheading 3.9. Compared to wild-type littermates, liver microsomes prepared from VP-hPXR mice exhibit significantly higher glucuronidation activity toward β-estradiol, a known UGT1A1-selective

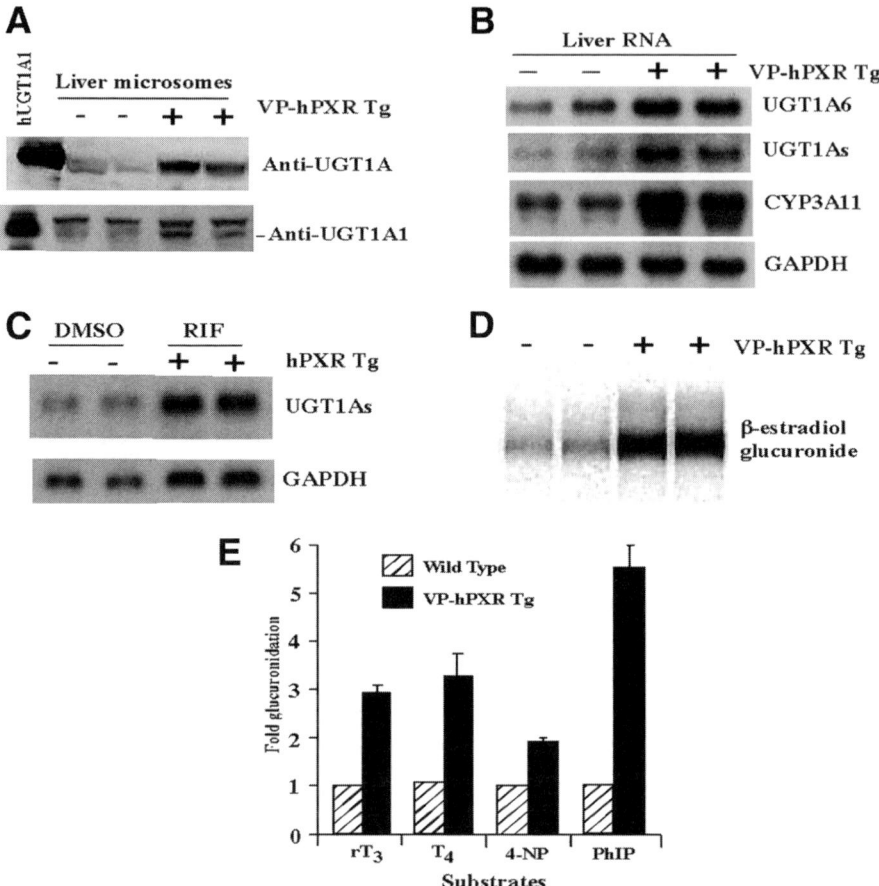

Fig. 7. Induction of UGT1A expression and glucuronidation. (**A**) Liver microsomes were prepared from wild-type and VP-hPXR transgenic mice and subjected to Western blot profiling by using a pan-anti-UGT1A antibody and a specific anti-UGT1A1 antibody. (**B**) Mouse liver total RNAs were subjected to Northern blot analysis. The membranes were probed for *UGT1A6*, *UGT1As*, *CYP3A11*, and GAPDH as a loading control. (**C**) Induction of *UGT1A* mRNA by RIF in hPXR transgenic mice. Wild-type or transgenic males were gavaged with a single dose of solvent or RIF (50 mg/kg) 24 h before they were killed. (**D**) Glucuronidation activity toward β-estradiol. An autoradiograph of a TLC separation is shown. (**E**) Glucuronidation activity toward thyroid hormones (rT3 and T4), and xenobiotics (4-nitrophenol and 4-OH-PhIP). Results are presented as fold increase in glucuronidation activity over wild type and represent the means ± SE.

substrate (Fig. 7D), thyroid hormones (rT_3 and T_4) classified as 1A1-preferred substrates *(63)* as well as the xenobiotic carcinogens 4-nitrophenol and 4-OH-PhIP, which are substrates for multiple 1A isoforms *(64)* (Fig. 7E).

6.4. Physiological Relevance of UGT Regulation In Vivo
6.4.1. Bilirubin Clearance

To examine the effect of PXR activation on bilirubin (BR) clearance, adult wild-type or VP-hPXR mice were subjected to a single dose of bilirubin (10 mg/kg) via tail vein injection. Bilirubin was purchased from Sigma and prepared in isotonic saline. One hour after injection, blood samples were collected via tail bleeding. Serum was separated and measured for levels of total BR and conjugated BR using diagnostic kits from Sigma or by a commercial service such as ANTECH Diagnostic (Lake Success, NY). An alternative method to induce hyperbilirubinemia was to treat mice with phenylhydrazine (PHZ). PHZ increases the plasma level of BR by increasing the rate of erythrocyte breakdown. The PHZ-induced hemolysis was carried out as previously described *(65)*. In brief, adult mice were injected intraperitoneally with a daily dose of 60 mg/kg of PHZ for 2 d. Blood samples were collected and analyzed for BR levels 48 h after the second injection. The results are shown in Fig. 8. We are currently using PXR knockout mice to determine whether loss of PXR affects BR clearance. Besides treatment with BR or PHZ in unchallenged PXR knockout mice, we also examined the effect of PCN-pretreatment on BR clearance and the effect of PXR status in this process. The PCN pretreatment was carried out as previously described *(58,66)*. In brief, mice were subjected to daily intraperitoneal injection of PCN (40 mg/kg) for 4 d prior to BR clearance experiment. PB pretreatment (40 mg/kg for 4 days) was included as a protection control, as PB has been shown to induce UGT1A1 in mice *(67)*.

Accumulation of BR in adult mice has been shown to cause liver injury as evidenced by elevated concentrations of serum alkaline phosphatase (ALP) and aspartate aminotransferase (AST) *(68)*. Experiments are in progress to measure both ALP and AST after induced hyperbilirubinemia, and compare BR toxicity between the wild-type, VP-hPXR transgenic, and PXR knockout mice.

6.4.2. Steroid Hormone Homeostasis

Besides xenobiotics, UGTs are essential for the metabolism and elimination of steroid hormones. The upregulation of UGT enzyme levels prompted us to assess a potential role for PXR in promoting steroid elimination and upregulating the adrenal axis. As shown in Fig. 9, liver microsomes of the VP-hPXR mice exhibited increased glucuronidation of several glucocorticoids, such as corticosterone, cortisol, and cortisone. To assess whether increased glucuronidation

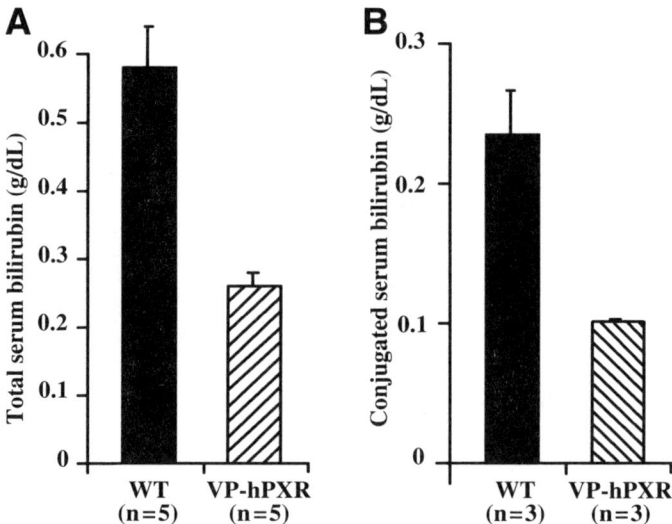

Fig. 8. Increased bilirubin clearance in VP-hPXR mice. Adult male wild-type and VP-hPXR mice were treated with a single dose of bilirubin (10 mg/kg), and serum levels of total (**A**) and conjugated (**B**) bilirubin were measured 1 h after injection.

was associated with increased levels of corticosterone, the principal glucocorticoid in rodents, its levels were measured. Mouse blood samples were collected in EDTA-coated tubes (Becton-Dickson, Bedford, MA) at 4:00 P.M. by retro-orbital eye bleeding within 1 min of initial disturbance. Plasma was obtained by centrifuging blood samples at $5200g$ (7000 rpm) for 4 min. The 24-h urine was collected using mouse metabolic cages (Nalgene, Medina, OH). Corticosterone levels in plasma or urine were measured with corticosterone [^{125}I] RIA Kit from ICN Biomedical, Irvine, CA). Statistical analysis was performed with InStat 2.03 software. The average plasma corticosterone concentration in wild-type

---

Fig. 9. *(see facing page)* Increased glucuronidation and output of corticosterone in VP-hPXR mice. (**A**) Increased glucuronidation of three corticosteroids—corticosterone, cortisone and cortisol—by liver microsomes of VP-hPXR mice. (**B**) Blood samples from 6-wk-old males were collected via retro-orbital eye bleeding, and plasma were prepared and subjected to corticosterone radioimmunoassay. Nonparametric Mann-Whitney test $p < 0.0001$. (**C**) Twenty-four-hour urine samples were collected from 8–10-wk old males, and subjected to corticosterone measurement. The p value is 0.5739 between wild-type and hPXR (not significant), 0.0004 between wild-type and VP-hPXR, and 0.0026 between hPXR and VP-hPXR, respectively.

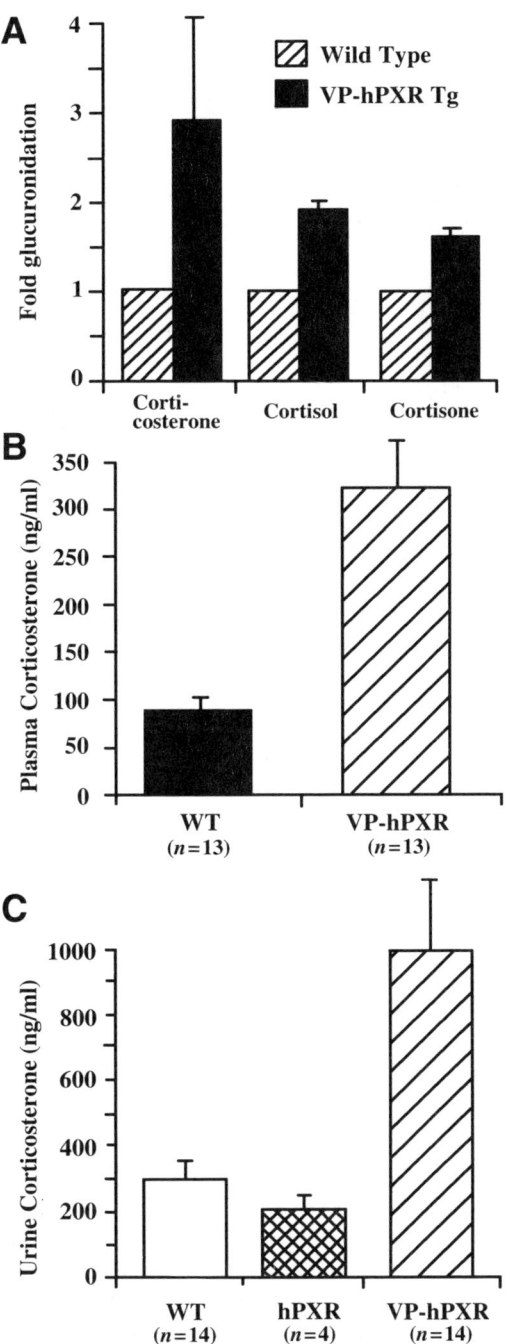

males was 88.8 ng/mL, similar to published results *(69)*, whereas the levels were elevated to 322 ng/mL in VP-hPXR mice (Fig. 9B), indicating an activation of the pituitary adrenal axis. A corresponding increase of urine corticosterone levels was seen in VP-hPXR mice (Fig. 9C), whereas no significant changes in urinary- (Fig. 9C) or blood- (data not shown) corticosterone levels were observed in the untreated hPXR transgenic mice. Thus, activation of PXR resulted in increased levels of steroid both in plasma and urine, consistent with the premise that PXR activation can promote steroid clearance, presumably via its induction of CYP and UGT protein synthesis.

7. SUMMARY

The methods described in this chapter, employing tissue culture, generation of transgenic animals and a variety of biochemical and molecular biology approaches can be applied to transcriptional regulation of a variety of DME genes. It became evident from the analysis of the techniques described in the most recent papers that there has been constant development and improvement of some of the described methods. For example, significant development of variations in the semiquantitative RT-PCR method allows efficient quantitation of cDNA levels. Although semiquantitative RT-PCR is still widely used for the preliminary evaluations of the cDNAs levels, it is recommended that quantitative QRT-PCR and real-time PCR be applied to those experiments that require rigorous cDNA quantitation. However, real-time PCR requires highly specific primers and is relatively expensive. In some instances, the instruments for this RT-PCR variation are only available in institutional core facilities or biotechnology companies. During the past 2 yr, the methods necessary for isolation and characterization of both distal and proximal gene promoters have also been significantly developed. The majority of the methods for UGT promoter analysis has come from our laboratories. It is also important to note that, recently, the focus of transcriptional regulation of DMEs and the role of the xenobiotic NRs has been shifted from their essential role in hepatic tissue to UGT regulation in extrahepatic tissues. Tissue-specific regulation may be dependent on a number of factors, such as relative affinity of ligands, exposure to complex mixtures of endogenous and exogenous compounds and levels of receptor expression in responsive tissues. Our comparative studies using HepG2 and Caco-2 cells demonstrated very significant differences in UGT expression between liver and intestine. Moreover, significant information on UGT regulation via nuclear receptors has been accumulated using transgenic animals. Future creation and characterization of transgenic animals targeted to the extrahepatic tissues will shed light on the regulation of expression of extrahepatic UGTs. It is anticipated that, in the very near future, significant new developments in UGT regulation will be reported that can be applied directly in both clinical and pharmacological settings.

ACKNOWLEDGMENTS

This work was supported in part by NIH Grants DK51971, DK56226, and DK60109 and tobacco settlement funds (A.R-P.) and ES12479 and CA107011 (W.X.). P.I.M is a National Health and Medical Research Council Senior Principle Research Fellow and is supported by grants from the Cancer Council of South Australia and the National Health and Medical Research Council of Australia. W.X. would also like to acknowledge support from the Competitive Medical Research Fund and the Central Research Development Fund from the University of Pittsburgh. Creation of the PXR transgenic mice was done by W.X. in the laboratory of Ronald M. Evans at the Salk Institute.

The authors would especially like to thank Joanna Little for her indispensable assistance in editing this chapter.

REFERENCES

1. Mackenzie PI, Gregory PA, Gardner-Stephen DA, et al. Regulation of UDP glucuronosyltransferase genes. Curr Drug Metab 2003;4:49–57.
2. Barbier O, Villeneuve L, Bocher V, et al. The UDP-glucuronosyltransferase 1A9 enzyme is a peroxisome proliferator-acivated receptor α and γ target gene. J Biol Chem 2003;278:13975–13983.
3. Sugatani J, Kojima H, Ueda A, et al. The phenobarbital response enhancer module in the human bilirubin UDP-glucuronosyltransferase *UGT1A1* gene and regulation by the nuclear receptor CAR. Hepatology 2001;33:1232–1238.
4. Xie W, Yeuh M-F, Radominska-Pandya A, et al. Control of steroid, heme and carcinogen metabolism by nuclear receptors PXR and CAR. Proc Natl Acad Sci USA 2003;100:4150–4156.
5. Gardner-Stephen DA, Heydel J-M, Goyal A, et al. Human PXR variants and their differential effects on the fegualtion of human UDP-glucuronosyltransferases. Drug Metab Dispos;32:340–347.
6. Yueh MG, Huang YH, Hiller A, Chen S, Nguyen N, Tukey RH. Involvement of the xenobiotic response element (XRE) in Ah receptor-mediated induction of human UDP-glucuronosyltransferase 1A1. J Biol Chem 2003;278:15001–15006.
7. Barbier O, Peneda Torra I, Sirvent A, et al. FXR induces the UGT2B4 enzyme in hepatocytes: a potential mechanism of negative feedback control of FXR activity. Gastroenterology 2003;124:1926–1940.
8. Bock KW. Metabolic polymorphisms affecting activation of toxic and mutagenic arylamines. TiPS 1992:223–226.
9. Oelberg DG, Chari MV, Little JM, Adcock EW, Lester R. Lithocholate glucuronide is a cholestatic agent. J Clin Invest 1984;73:1507–1514.
10. Vore M, Montgomery C, Meyers M. Steroid D-ring glucuronides: characterization of a new class of cholestatic agents. Drug Metab Rev 1983;14:1005–1019.

11. Nebert DW. Drug-metabolizing enzymes in ligand-modulated transcription. Biochem Pharmacol 1994;47:25–37.
12. Nebert DW. Proposed role of drug-metabolizing enzymes: regulation of steady state levels of the ligands that effect growth, homeostasis, differentiation, and neuroendocrine functions. Mol Endocrinol 1991;5:1203–1214.
13. Ritter JK, Kessler FK, Thompson MT, Grove AD, Auyeung DJ, Fisher RA. Expression and inducibility of the human bilirubin UDP-glucuronosyltransferase UGT1A1 in liver and cultured primary hepatocytes: evidence for both genetic and environmental influences. Hepatology 1999;30:476–84.
14. Walle UK, Walle T. Induction of human UDP-glucuronosyltransferase UGT1A1 by flavonoids-structural requirements. Drug Metab Dispos 2002;30:564–569.
15. Galijatovic A, Otake Y, Walle UK, Walle T. Induction of UDP-glucuronosyltransferase UGT1A1 by the flavonoid chrysin in Caco-2 cells-poteial role in carcinogen bioinactivation. Pharmaceut Res 2001;18:374–379.
16. Munzel PA, Lehmkoster T, Bruck M, Ritter JK, Bock KW. Aryl hydrocarbon receptor-inducible or constitutive expression of human UDP glucuronosyltransferase UGT1A6. Arch Biochem Biophys 1998;350:72–78.
17. Bock KW, Eckle T, Ouzzine M, Fournel-Gigleux S. Coordinate induction by antioxidants of UDP-glucuronosyltransferase UGT1A6 and the apical conjugate export pump MRP2 (multidrug resistance protein 2) in Caco-2 cells. Biochem Pharmacol 2000;59:467–470.
18. Munzel PA, Schmohl S, Heel H, Kälberer K, Bock-Hennig B, Bock KW. Induction of human UDP-glucuronosyltransferases (UGT1A6, UGT1A9, and UGT2B7) by t-butylhydroquinone and 2,3,7,8-tetrachlorodibenzo-p-dioxin in Caco-2 cells. Drug Metab Dispos 1999;27:569–573.
19. Sabolovic N, Magdalou J, Netter P, Abid A. Nonsteroidal anti-inflammatory drugs and phenols glucuronidation in Caco-2 cells. Identification of the UDP-glucuronosyltransferases UGT1A6, 1A3 and 2B7. Life Sci 2000;67:185–196.
20. Abid A, Sablovic N, Magdalou J. Expression and inducibility of UDP-glucuronosyltransferases 1-naphthol in human cultured hepatocytes and hepatocarcinoma cell lines. Life Sci 1997;60:1943–1951.
21. Hum DW, Belanger A, Levesque E, et al. Characterization of UDP-glucuronosyltransferases active on steroid hormones. J Steroid Biochem Mol Biol 1999;69:413–423.
22. Brandsch C, Friedl P, Lange K, Richter T, Mothes T. Primary culture and transfection of epithelial cells of human small intestine. Scand J Gastroenterol 1998;33:833–838.
23. Xie W, Barwick JL, Downes M, et al. Humanized xenobiotic response in mice expressing nuclear receptor SXR. Nature 2000;406:435–439.
24. Xie W, Barwick JL, Simon CM, et al. Reciprocal activation of xenobiotic response genes by nuclear receptors SXR/PXR and CAR. Genes Dev 2000;14:3014–3023.
25. Congiu M, Mashford ML, Slavin JL, Desmond PV. UDP-glucuronosyltransferase mRNA levels in human liver disease. Drug Metab Dispos 2002;30:129–134.

26. Strassburg CP, Oldhaffer K, Manns MP, Tukey RH. Differential expression of the UGT1A locus in human liver, biliary, and gastric tissue: identification of UGT1A7 and UGT1A10 transcripts in extrahepatic tissue. Mol Pharmacol 1997;52:212–220.
27. Radominska-Pyrek A, Zimniak P, Irshaid YM, Lester R, Tephly TR, Pyrek JS. Glucuronidation of 6α-hydroxy bile acids by human liver microsomes. J Clin Invest 1987;80:234–241.
28. Fisher MB, Campanale K, Ackermann BL, Vandenbranden M, Wrighton SA. In vitro glucuronidation using human liver microsomes and the pore-forming peptide alamethicin. Drug Metab Dispos 2000;28:560–566.
29. Little JM, Lehman PA, Nowell S, Samokyszyn V, Radominska A. Glucuronidation of all trans-retinoic acid and 5,6-epoxy-all trans-retinoic acid: activation of rat liver microsomal UDP-glucuronosyltranferase activity by alamethicin. Drug Metab Dispos 1997;25:5–11.
30. Little JM, Radominska A. Application of photoaffinity labeling with [11,12-^{3}H]all *trans*-retinoic acid to characterization of rat liver microsomal UDP-glucuronosyl-transferase(s) with activity toward retinoic acid. Biochem Biophys Res Commun 1997;230:497–500.
31. Radominska-Pyrek A, Zimniak P, Chari M, Golunski E, Lester R, Pyrek JS. Glucuronides of monohydroxylated bile acids: specificity of microsomal glucuronyltransferase for the glucuronidation site, C-3 configuration, and side chain length. J Lipid Res 1986;27:89–101.
32. Radominska-Pandya A, Little JM, Pandya JT, et al. UDP-Glucuronosyltransferases in human intestinal mucosa. Biochim Biophys Acta 1998;1394:199–208.
33. Lemon B, Tijian R. Orchestrated response: a symphony of transcription factors for gene control. Genes Dev 2001;14:2551–2569.
34. Shaefer B. Revolution in rapid amplification of cDNA ends: new strategies for polymerase chain reaction cloning of full length cDNA ends. Anal Biochem 1995;227:255–276.
35. Heinemeyer T, Wingender E, Reuter I, et al. Databases on transcriptional regulation: TRANSFAC, TRRD, and COMPEL. Nucleic Acids Res 1998;26: 364–370.
36. Podvinec M, Kaufamm MR, Handschin C, Meyer UA. NUBIScan, an in silico approach for prediction of nuclear receptor response elements. Mol Endocrinol 2002;16:1269–1279.
37. Hansen AJ, Lee YH, Gonzalez FJ, Mackenzie PI. HNF1 alpha activates the rat UDP glucuronosyltransferase UGT2B1 gene pomoter. DNA Cell Biol 1997;16:207–214.
38. Gregory PA, Gardner-Stephen DA, Lewinsky RH, Duncliffe KN, Mackenzie PI. Cloning and characterization of the human UDP-glucuronosyltransferase 1A8, 1A9 and 1A10 gene promoters. Differential regulation through an initiator-like region. J Biol Chem 2003; 278:36107–36114.
39. Kroeger KM, Abraham LJ. Magnetic bead purification of specific transcription factors using mutant competitor oligonucleotides. Anal Biochem 1997;250: 127–129.

40. Schreiber E, Matthias P, Muller MM, Schaffner W. Rapid detection of octamer binding proteins with "mini-extracts" prepared from a small number of cells. Nucleic Acid Res 1989;17:6419–6420.
41. Kostrubsky VE, Lewis LD, Strom SC, et al. Induction of cytochrome P4503A by taxol in primary cultures of human hepatocytes. Arch Biochem Biophys 1998;355: 131–136.
42. Kostrubsky VE, Strom SC, Wood SG, Wrighton SA, Sinclair PR, Sinclair JF. Ethanol and isopentanol increase CYP3A and CYP2E in primary cultures of human hepatocytes. Arch Biochem Biophys 1995;322:516–520.
43. Strom SC, Pisarov LA, Dorko K, Thompson MT, Schuetz JD, Schuetz EG. Use of human hepatocytes to study P450 gene induction. Methods Enzymol 1996;272: 388–401.
44. Li P. Primary hepatocyte cultures as an in vitro experimental model for the evaluation of pharmacokinetic drug–drug interactions. Adv Pharmacol 1997;43: 103–130.
45. Maurel P. The CYP3A family. In: Ioannides C, ed. Cytochrome P450: Metabolic and Toxicological Aspects. Boca Raton, FL: CRC Press, 1996:241–270.
46. Kocarek TA, Schuetz EG, Strom SC, Fisher RA, Guzelian PS. Comparative analysis of cytochrome P4503A induction in primary cultures of rat, rabbit, and human hepatocytes. Drug Metab Dispos 1995;23:415–421.
47. Schuetz EG, Schinkel AH, Relling MV, Schuetz JD. P-glycoprotein: a major determinant of rifampicin-inducible expression of cytochrome P4503A in mice and human. Proc Natl Acad Sci USA 1996;93:4001–4005.
48. Schuetz EG, Schuetz JD, Strom SC, et al. Regulation of human liver cytochromes P-450 in family 3A in primary and continuous culture of human hepatocytes. Hepatology 1993;18:1254–1262.
49. Watkins PB, Wrighton SA, Maurel P, Identification of an inducible form of cytochrome P-450 in human liver. Proc Natl Acad Sci USA 1985;82:6310–6314.
50. Wrighton SA, Schuetz EG, Watkins PB, et al. Demonstration of multiple species of inducible hepatic cytochromes P-450 and their mRNAs related to the glucocorticoid-inducible cyrochrome P-450 of the rat. Mol Pharmacol 1985;28: 312–321.
51. Barwick JL, Quattrochi LC, Mills AS, Potenza C, Tukey RH, Guzelian PS. Transspecies gene transfer for analysis of glucocorticoid-inducible transcriptional activation of transiently expressed human CYP3A4 and rabbit CYP3A6 in primary cultures of adult rat and rabbit hepatocytes. Mol Pharmacol 1996;50:10–16.
52. Sonoda J, Xie W, Rosenfeld JM, Barwick JL, Guzelian PS, Evans RM. Regulation of a xenobiotic sulfonation cascade by nuclear pregnane X receptor (PXR). Proc Natl Acad Sci USA 2002;99:13801–13806.
53. Xie W, Evans RM. Orphan nuclear receptors: the exotics of xenobiotics. J Biol Chem 2001;276:37739–37742.
54. Xie W, Evans RM. Pharmaceutical use of mouse models humanized for the xenobiotic receptor. Drug Discov Today 2002;7:509–517.

55. Guicciardi ME, Gores GJ. Bile acid-mediated hepatocyte apoptosis and cholestatic liver disease. Digest Liver Dis 2002;34:387–392.
56. Kullak-Ublick GA, Meier PJ. Mechanisms of cholestasis. Clin Liver Dis 2000;4: 357–385.
57. Radominska A, Treat S, Little J. Bile acid metabolism and the pathophysiology of cholestasis. Semin Liver Dis 1993;13:219–234.
58. Xie W, Radominska-Pandya A, Shi Y, et al. An essential role for SXR/PXR in detoxification of cholestatic bile acids. Proc Natl Acad Sci USA 2001;98:3375–3380.
59. Watkins RE, Wisely GB, Moore LB, et al. The human nuclear xenobiotic receptor PXR: structural determinants of directed promiscuity. Science 2001;292:2329–2333.
60. Blumberg B, Sabbagh W Jr, Juguilon H, et al. SXR, a novel steroid and xenobiotic-sensing nuclear receptor. Genes Dev 1998;12:3195–3205.
61. Pinkert CA, Ornitz DM, Brinster RL, Palmiter RD. An albumin enhancer located 10 kb upstream functions along with its promoter to direct efficient, liver-specific expression in transgenic mice. Genes Dev 1987;1:268–276.
62. Ritter JK, Chen F, Sheen YY, et al. A novel complex locus *UGT1* encodes human bilirubin, phenol, and other UDP-glucuronosyltransferase isozymes with identical carboxyl termini. J Biol Chem 1992;267:3257–3261.
63. Findlay KA, Kaptein E, Visser TJ, Burchell B. Characterization of the uridine diphosphate-glucuronosyltransferase-catalyzing thyroid hormone glucuruonidaion in man. J Clin Endocrinol Metab 2000;85:2879–2883.
64. Nowell S, Massengill J, Williams S, et al. Glucuronidation of 2-amino-1-methyl-6-phenylimidazo[4,5-b]pyridine (PhIP) by human microsomal proteins: Identification of the UGT1A isoforms involved. Carcinogenesis 1999;20:101–108.
65. Broudy VC, Lin NL, Priestley GV, Nocka K, Wolf NS. Interaction of stem cell factor and its receptor c-kit mediates lodgment and acute expansion of hematopoietic cells in the murine spleen. Blood 1996;88:75–81.
66. Brock WJ, Durham S, Vore M. Characterization of the interaction between estrogen metabolites and taurocholate for uptake into isolated hepatocytes. Lack of correlation between cholestasis and inhibition of taurocholate uptake. J Steroid Biochem 1984;20:1181–1185.
67. Garcia-Allen C, Lord PG, Loughlin JM, Orton TC, Sidaway JE. Identification of phenobarbitone-modulated genes in mouse liver by differential display. J Biochem Mol Toxicol 2000;14:65–72.
68. Kikuchi S, Hata M, Fukumoto K, et al. Radixin deficiency causes conjugated hyperbilirubinemia with loss of Mrp2 from bile canalicular membranes. Nat Genet 2002;31:320–325.
69. Smith GW, Aubry JM, Dellu F, et al. Corticotropin releasing factor receptor 1-deficient mice display decreased anxiety, impaired stress response, and aberrant neuroendocrine development. Neuron 1998;20:1093–1102.

7

Phenotypic and Genotypic Characterization of N-Acetylation

Craig K. Svensson and David W. Hein

Summary

Variation among the human population in the ability to acetylate drugs has been known since the observations on individual variations in isoniazid toxicity in the 1950s. The genetic basis for this was soon appreciated and has come to be known as the *N*-acetylation polymorphism. This chapter provides as background a description of some key studies that showed that acetylation was variable in the human population, that it is inherited, and the molecular basis for this phenomenon. Since accurate determination of acetylator phenotype is critical to testing a number of important hypotheses, including the link between disease risk and acetylator phenotype, limitations and potential problems with various methods of phenotype determination are discussed. Similarly, procedures and approaches for determination of *NAT1* and *NAT2* genotype are described. The final section brings phenotype and genotype together by examining the relationship between variant alleles and disease incidence. Increasingly, these studies have relied solely on the measurement of genotype, with the assumption that phenotype may be accurately deduced from genotype. There is a fairly wide degree of variability in the frequency of discordance between genotype and phenotype, however, especially when caffeine is used as a probe for phenotype determination. The potential consequences of this discordance are discussed.

Key Words

NAT alleles; *p*-aminosalicylate; aromatic amines; caffeine; cancer risk: bladder; dapsone; genotype; hydrazines; isoniazid; *N*-acetyltransferase (NAT); NAT1; NAT2; phenotype; polymorphisms; single nucleotide polymorphism; sulfamethazine.

1. DISCOVERY OF *N*-ACETYLATION POLYMORPHISM

Soon after the introduction of isoniazid for the treatment of tuberculosis, the development of toxicity in patients receiving extended treatment with the drug threatened to jeopardize its continued use *(1,2)*. Studies by Hughes et al. *(3)*

From: *Methods in Pharmacology and Toxicology,
Drug Metabolism and Transport: Molecular Methods and Mechanisms*
Edited by: L. Lash © Humana Press Inc., Totowa, NJ

demonstrated that acetylisoniazid was the primary metabolite of isoniazid excreted in urine and that patients were distributed into groups that excreted either a high or low amount of acetylisoniazid. Moreover, they found that patients who excreted a low amount of acetylisoniazid were more likely to develop peripheral neuritis when treated with isoniazid.

The first evidence that variation in acetylation was a heritable trait was provided by a study examining the variability in isoniazid excretion in identical and fraternal twins (4). The variability in isoniazid content excreted in 24-h urine in identical twins, fraternal twins, and unrelated subjects was 0.58, 5.34, and 10.4, respectively. As identical twins possess a common genome, the small variation noted in them suggests that environmental factors make only a small contribution to the overall variability in isoniazid disposition.

Further evidence for the role of inheritance in governing the variability of isoniazid metabolism was provided by a study of 484 subjects conducted by Evans et al. (5). Following a dose of 9.8–10 mg/kg, a frequency–distribution plot of the 6-h plasma isoniazid concentration exhibited a polymorphic pattern with an identifiable antimode of 2.5 μg/mL. The heterogeneity in the plasma isoniazid concentration could not be explained by race, presence or absence of tuberculosis, gender, or age. Analysis of data in 267 subjects from 53 complete families indicated that the slow acetylator phenotype was a heritable trait that was autosomal recessive. The frequency of the slow acetylator phenotype was found to be 52% in the population studied.

Several studies have suggested that the frequency distribution for isoniazid plasma concentrations may be more accurately described as trimodal (6,7), suggesting that rapid and slow acetylators are homozygous for nondominant alleles. Parkin et al. (8) provided evidence that tuberculosis patients receiving isoniazid can be distinguished by three phenotypes via analysis of isoniazid elimination rate constant or plasma area under the curve. Genotype analysis suggested a lack of allelic dominance and that heterozygote combinations result in an intermediate metabolism of isoniazid.

Subsequent to studies demonstrating the polymorphic metabolism of isoniazid, it was found that some other compounds metabolized by acetylation exhibited the same inheritance pattern observed with isoniazid, while still other compounds exhibited an acetylation pattern that did not appear to be governed by a heritable trait. For example, Evans and White (9) examined the acetylation of sulfamethazine in subjects whose acetylator phenotype was determined by isoniazid. Slow acetylators of isoniazid excreted 40–55% of sulfamethazine as the acetyl metabolite, while rapid acetylators of isoniazid excreted 60–90% of the dose as acetylsulfamethazine. Further studies demonstrated that the

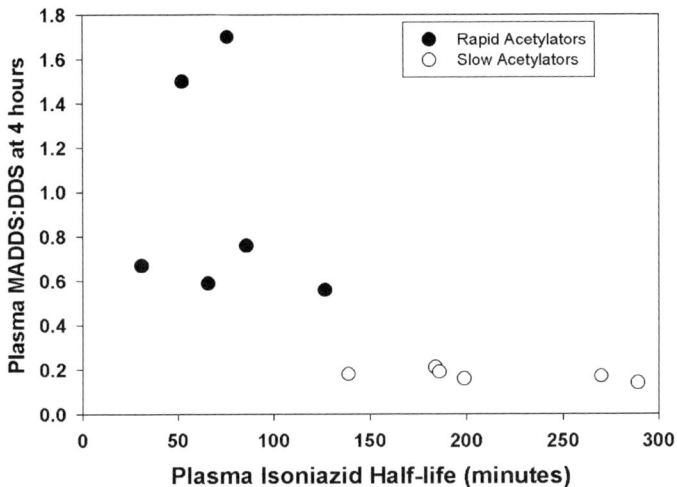

Fig. 1. Cosegregation in the acetylation of isoniazid and dapsone. Subject acetylator status was determined via isoniazid. DDS, Dapsone; MADDS, monoacetyldapsone. (Data from Gelber et al. [11]).

acetylation capacity of hydralazine and phenelzine cosegregates with isoniazid (9,10). Gelber and colleagues (11) examined the acetylation of isoniazid, dapsone, and sulfamethazine in patients with leprosy and normal volunteers. The acetylation of all three compounds was found to cosegregate. Figure 1 illustrates the relationship between the acetylation of isoniazid and dapsone observed in their subjects. The demarcation between fast and slow acetylators using either measure is not inherently obvious from visual inspection of the data (as is often the case with thiopurine methyltransferase and CYP2D6) and must be identified statistically. Importantly, it should be noted that while the ratio of acetylated metabolite to dapsone concentration varied less than fourfold in the subjects, the variation in plasma isoniazid half-life varied almost 10-fold. The half-life of dapsone did not differ between slow and rapid acetylators, most likely because of metabolic interconversion through acetylation–deacetylation, which does not occur to a measurable extent with other substrates exhibiting polymorphic acetylation.

Table 1 lists various compounds whose acetylation in man displays a polymorphic frequency distribution, as well as several compounds for whom frequency distribution plots of acetylation display a monomorphic pattern. In addition, there are several compounds (e.g., caffeine, nitrazepam) that are metabolized to metabolites that subsequently undergo polymorphic N-acetylation. The

**Table 1
Polymorphic and Monomorphic Substrates
Subject to N-Acetylation in Humans**

Polymorphic substrates	Monomorphic substrates
Dapsone	p-Aminobenzoic acid
Hydralazine	p-Aminosalicylic acid
Isoniazid	Sulfamethoxazole
Phenelzine	
Procainamide	
Sulfamethazine	
Sulfapyridine	

observation that arylamines could be metabolized to N-acetylated products in either a mono- or polymorphic fashion led to speculation as to the cause of these two patterns for a biotransformation that was dependent on the same cosubstrate and presumably similar catalytic process. Several decades passed before the tools of molecular biology provided the means to test these varied hypotheses.

2. MOLECULAR BASIS FOR N-ACETYLATION POLYMORPHISMS

The observation that the N-acetylation of drugs such as isoniazid are polymorphic in human populations whereas the N-acetylation of other drugs such as p-aminosalicylic acid yield apparently monomorphic distributions results from the substrate selectivity and molecular genetics of two N-acetyltransferase (NAT) isozymes, NAT1 and NAT2. The concept that separate enzymes were responsible for the N-acetylation of "polymorphic" and "monomorphic" substrates was introduced by Jenne (12), and subsequently confirmed in humans (13) and rodents (14). Human NAT1 and NAT2 are cytoplasmic enzymes that transfer an acetyl group from acetyl-coenzyme A (acetyl-CoA) to acceptor substrates (15). Both are products of single, intronless protein-coding exons of 870 base pairs (bp) encoding 290 amino acids (16,17). Human *NAT1* and *NAT2* coding exons are separated by less than 200 kbp on chromosome 8. In addition, a genomic pseudogene, designated *NATP*, is located between them (18,19). *NAT1* and *NAT2* share 87% nucleotide homology in the coding region, yielding less than a 20% difference in their amino acids. The protein structure of NATs was recently reviewed (20). Site-directed mutagenesis studies established a critical cysteine (Cys[68]) within the catalytic site that participates directly in acetyl transfer between the acetyl-CoA cofactor and acceptor substrates (21). Furthermore, site-directed mutagenesis revealed three amino acids (at positions 125, 127, and 129) that are very important for substrate selectivity (22). Although the crystallographic structure of eukaryotic NAT1 or NAT2 have yet to be resolved, molecular modeling of human NAT1 *(23)* and NAT2 *(24)* from prokaryotic NAT crystal structures reveals the importance of a catalytic triad (Cys^{68}-His^{107}-Asp^{122}) similar to that common in cysteine proteases.

Aromatic amines and hydrazines (*N*-acetylation) and *N*-hydroxy-aromatic and -heterocyclic amines (*O*-acetylation) are examples of acceptor substrates that, in general, are deactivated (*N*-acetylation) or activated (*O*-acetylation) by NAT1 and/or NAT2 *(15)*. NAT1 and NAT2 also catalyze the intramolecular *N,O*-acetyltransfer of *N*-hydroxy-*N*-acetyl-aromatic amines *(25)*. In Syrian hamsters *(26,27)*, extrahepatic *N*- and *O*-acetyltransferase expression is comparable to that in the liver, suggesting a significant role in extrahepatic tissues. Because both NAT1 and NAT2 catalyze the metabolic activation (via *O*-acetylation) of aromatic and heterocyclic amine carcinogens *(28–30)*, genetic polymorphism in NAT1 and/or NAT2 may modify cancer risk related to exposures to these carcinogens. *NAT1*4* and *NAT2*4* have traditionally been designated the "wild-type" human *NAT1* and *NAT2* alleles, respectively *(31)*. Because they are the most commonly occurring alleles in some, but not all, ethnic groups, the designation of the "wild-type" allele is somewhat arbitrary. An international *N*-acetyltransferase nomenclature committee is responsible for updating and publishing up-to-date listings of NAT alleles *(32)*. The website is: http://www.louisville.edu/medschool/pharmacology/NAT.html. Human *NAT1* and *NAT2* alleles can be written in uppercase, lowercase, or a combination of upper- and lowercase. Alleles are always italicized. Protein products of the alleles are not italicized and the asterisk is omitted. For example, the allele *NAT2*4* encodes the protein NAT2 4.

Reference *NAT1*4* and 25 variant *NAT1* alleles have been identified in human populations (Table 2). Some of the variant *NAT1* alleles have been expressed and characterized in *Escherichia coli* *(33–38)*, yeast *(39)* and COS-1 cells *(38)*. Some studies suggest that *NAT1*10* may be a rapid acetylator allele because it has been associated with slight increases in NAT activity in bladder and colon *(40,41)* and increased carcinogen–DNA adduct binding in urinary bladder *(41)*. However, recombinant expression studies have failed to confirm this conclusion *(38)*. The instability of human NAT1 *(13,29)* and its possible modification by substrate *(42)* is a problem for investigations in human tissues.

To better understand the functional effects of each individual single nucleotide polymorphism (SNP), human *NAT1*4* and 12 variant *NAT1* alleles possessing nucleotide polymorphisms in the coding region were expressed in yeast *(39)*. Five of the recombinant human NAT1 allozymes (NAT1 14B, 15, 17, 19, and 22) catalyzed both *N*-acetylation and *O*-acetylation at rates substantially below that of NAT1 4 and the other NAT1 allozymes *(39)*. Substantially lower levels of NAT1 protein were expressed by these same variant *NAT1* alleles. The reduced level of NAT1 17 and NAT1 22 protein and catalytic

Table 2
Human *NAT1* Alleles

Allele	Nucleotide change(s)	Amino Acid change(s)
*NAT1*3*	1095C>A	None
*NAT1*4*	None	None
*NAT1*5*	350,351G>C	R117T
	497-499G>C	R166T
	884A>G	E167Q
	Δ^{976}	
	Δ^{1105}	
*NAT1*10*	1088T>A	None
	1095C>A	
*NAT1*11A*	−344C>T	V149I
	−40A>T	S214A
	445G>A	
	459G>A	
	640T>G	
	Δ 9 between 1065 and 1090	
	1095C>A	
*NAT1*11B*	−344C>T	V149I
	−40A>T	S214A
	445G>A	
	459G>A	
	640T>G	
	Δ 9 between 1065 and 1090	
*NAT1*11C*	−344C>T	S214A
	−40A>T	
	459G>A	
	640T>G	
	Δ 9 between 1065 and 1090	
	1095C>A	
*NAT1*14A*	560G>A	R187Q
	1088T>A	
	1095C>A	
*NAT1*14B*	560G>A	R187Q
*NAT1*15*	559C>T	R187Stop
*NAT1*16*	[AAA] immediately after 1091	None
	1095C>A	
*NAT1*17*	190C>T	R64W

Table 2 *(continued)*

Allele	Nucleotide change(s)	Amino Acid Change(s)
NAT1*18A	Δ 3 between 1065 and 1087 1088T>A 1095C>A	None
NAT1*18B	Δ3 between 1065 and 1090	None
NAT1*19	97C>T	R33Stop
NAT1*20	402T>C	None
NAT1*21	613A>G	M205V
NAT1*22	752A>T	D251V
NAT1*23	777T>C	None
NAT1*24	781G>A	E261K
NAT1*25	787A>G	I263V
NAT1*26A	[TAA] insertion between 1065 and 1090 1095C>A	None
NAT1*26B	[TAA] insertion between 1065 and 1090	None
NAT1*27	21T>G 777T>C	None
NAT1*28	[TAATAA] deletion between 1065 and 1090	None
NAT1*29	1088T>A 1095C>A Δ^{1025}	None

(From http://www.louisville.edu/medschool/pharmacology/NAT.html)

activities appear to be related to decreased stability *(39)*. Further studies are needed to understand the role of SNPs outside the coding region.

Reference *NAT2*4* and more than 30 variant *NAT2* alleles have been identified in human populations (Table 3). The most common allele in Caucasian populations is *NAT2*5B*, whereas *NAT2*4* is the most common in Asian populations *(43)*. The *NAT2*14* cluster has so far been found predominantly within individuals of African descent *(43,44)*. Differences in *NAT2* allele frequency among various ethnic groups yield corresponding differences in frequency of rapid and slow acetylator phenotypes. Thus, Asian populations are primarily rapid acetylators, whereas most Caucasian and African populations have slightly higher proportions of slow than rapid acetylators *(45)*.

The basis for slow NAT2 acetylator phenotype appears to be reduction(s) in the amount of NAT2 protein *(17,46–48)*. These findings are supported by

Table 3
Human *NAT2* Alleles

Allele	Nucleotide change(s)	Amino acid change(s)
NAT2*4	None	None
NAT2*5A	341T>C	I114T
	481C>T	
NAT2*5B	341T>C	I114T
	481C>T	K268R
	803A>G	
NAT2*5C	341T>C	I114T
	803A>G	K268R
NAT2*5D	341T>C	I114T
NAT2*5E	341T>C	I114T
	590G>A	R197Q
NAT2*5F	341T>C	I114T
	481C>T	K268R
	759C>T	
	803A>G	
NAT2*5G	282C>T	I114T
	341T>C	K268R
	481C>T	
	803A>G	
NAT2*5H	341T>C	I114T
	481C>T	K268R
	803A>G	I287T
	859T>C	
NAT2*5I	341T>C	I114T
	411A>T	L137F
	481C>T	K268R
	803A>G	
NAT2*5J	282C>T	I114T
	341T>C	R197Q
	590G>A	
NAT2*6A	282C>T	R197Q
	590G>A	
NAT2*6B	590G>A	R197Q
NAT2*6C	282C>T	R197Q
	590G>A	K268R
	803A>G	

Table 3 (continued)

Allele	Nucleotide change(s)	Amino acid change(s)
NAT2*6D	111T>C	R197Q
	282C>T	
	590G>A	
NAT2*6E	481C>T	R197Q
	590G>A	
NAT2*7A	857G>A	G286E
NAT2*7B	282C>T	G286E
	857G>A	
NAT2*10	499G>A	E167K
NAT2*11A	481C>T	None
NAT2*11B	481C>T	S287 Frameshift
	859Del	
NAT2*12A	803A>G	K268R
NAT2*12B	282C>T	K268R
	803A>G	
NAT2*12C	481C>T	K268R
	803A>G	
NAT2*12D	364G>A	D122N
	803A>G	K268R
NAT2*13	282C>T	None
NAT2*14A	191G>A	R64Q
NAT2*14B	191G>A	R64Q
	282C>T	
NAT2*14C	191G>A	R64Q
	341T>C	I114T
	481C>T	K268R
	803A>G	
NAT2*14D	191G>A	R64Q
	282C>T	R197Q
	590G>A	
NAT2*14E	191G>A	R64Q
	803A>G	K268R
NAT2*14F	191G>A	R64Q
	341T>C	I114T
	803A>G	K268R
NAT2*14G	191G>A	R64Q
	282C>T	K268R
	803A>G	
NAT2*17	434A>C	Q145P
NAT2*18	845A>C	K282T
NAT2*19	190C>T	R64W

(From http://www.louisville.edu/medschool/pharmacology/NAT.html)

Table 4
Functional Effects of SNPs in NAT2[a]

SNP	Amino acid change	Sulfamethazine NAT catalytic activity[b]	NAT2 protein expression[b]	NAT2 protein stability[b]
T111C	None	+++	+++	+++
C190T	R64W	+	+	+
G191A	R64Q	+	++	+
C282T	None	+++	+++	+++
T341C	I114T	+	+	+++
G364A	D122N	+	+	ND[c]
A411T	L137F	+	+	ND[c]
A434C	E145P	+	+	+++
C481T	None	+++	+++	+++
G590A	R197Q	++	+	+
G759T	None	+++	+++	+++
A803G	K268R	+++	+++	+++
A845C	K282T	+++	+++	+
G857A	G286E	+++	+++	+

[a]Recombinant human NAT2 allozymes expressed in yeast or COS-1 cells. (Adapted from refs. 55,56).
[b]Relative to NAT2 4. +, 0–35%; ++, 36–70%; +++, >70%.
[c]Not determined.

recombinant expression of slow acetylator *NAT2* alleles in COS-1 *(17)*, Chinese hamster ovary *(49)*, and yeast *(50–52)* cells. Recombinant expressions of human *NAT2* alleles in COS-1 cells *(17)*, bacteria *(53,54)* and yeast *(51,52)* also point to differences in protein stability as a factor in NAT2 slow acetylator phenotype.

As shown in Table 2, a number of human *NAT2* alleles have been identified. They are arranged in clusters consistent with a signature SNP. Thus, *NAT2*4* is defined as the "wild-type" and represents the reference allele. Each allele in the *NAT2*5* cluster possesses a C341T mutation; each allele in the *NAT2*6* cluster possesses a G590A SNP, and so on. To study the functional effect of each SNP separately, human *NAT2*4* and 12 variant *NAT2* alleles possessing SNPs in the coding region were expressed in yeast *(51,52)*. The effects of each SNP on *N*-acetylation and *O*-acetylation were highly correlated for human NAT1 and NAT2 *(55)*. Differences in functional effects among the various SNPs were noted (Table 4), suggesting multiple mechanisms for human slow *NAT2* acetylator phenotype. Similarly, *NAT2*4* and fourteen variant *NAT2* alleles were recombinantly expressed in *Escherichia coli (25,54)*. The *NAT2*5* cluster (all possessing the T341C SNP) showed the greatest reduction in *N*-, *O*-, and *N,O*-acetylation activities, followed by the *NAT2*14* cluster (all possessing the G191A SNP), followed by the *NAT2*6* cluster (all possessing the G590A SNP) followed by the *NAT2*7* cluster (all possessing the G857A SNP). These results suggest that human slow acetylator phenotype is not homogeneous but rather consists of multiple phenotypes dependent on the inheritance of specific SNPs and alleles.

3. METHODS FOR DETERMINATION OF THE *N*-ACETYLATION PHENOTYPE

3.1. Determination of the NAT2 Phenotype

Accurate determination of acetylator phenotype is critical in testing a number of important hypotheses, including the link between disease risk and acetylator phenotype. Theoretically, any agent that is metabolized via NAT2 could serve as a substrate probe for determination of NAT2 acetylator phenotype. However, the ideal method would be accurate, reproducible, rapid, simple, and pose little risk to subjects in whom phenotype is to be determined. Methods for phenotype determination have evolved to better achieve these criteria.

As isoniazid was the first agent characterized as displaying polymorphic acetylation, it served as the prototype marker compound for characterizing the acetylator phenotype. Initially, studies were conducted by taking multiple blood samples after administration of an oral dose and determination of the half-life of isoniazid. While this provided an accurate method for discriminating phenotypes, it was labor and cost intensive. A simplified approach was necessary for use in characterizing larger populations of subjects. To this end, Evans et al. *(5)* examined the frequency distribution of the plasma isoniazid concentration 6 h after an oral dose. While being a useful and reasonably accurate method for distinguishing phenotypes, chemical analysis of isoniazid did not possess the desired specificity and simplicity for widespread use. This led to the development of sulfamethazine as an alternative probe for determining the acetylator phenotype *(57)*. Particularly strong discrimination between phenotypes was demonstrated with use of both urine and plasma measurements of sulfamethazine and acetylated sulfamethazine. However, the relative unavailability of sulfamethazine in the United States limited the utility of this probe.

In 1984, Grant et al. *(58)* reported the use of caffeine as a safe probe for determination of the NAT2 phenotype. While caffeine itself does not undergo *N*-acetylation, the detection of 5-acetylamino-6-formylamino-3-uracil (AFMU) in urine of subjects administered caffeine indicated that a demethylated metabolite of caffeine was subject to acetylation *(59)*. The scheme in Fig. 2 illustrates the metabolic fate of caffeine in humans. These investigators demonstrated that measuring AFMU and 1-methylxanthine in urine provided the means to segregate a sample of 146 subjects into three acetylator phenotypes. In a limited number of subjects, there was cosegregation of subjects when either caffeine or

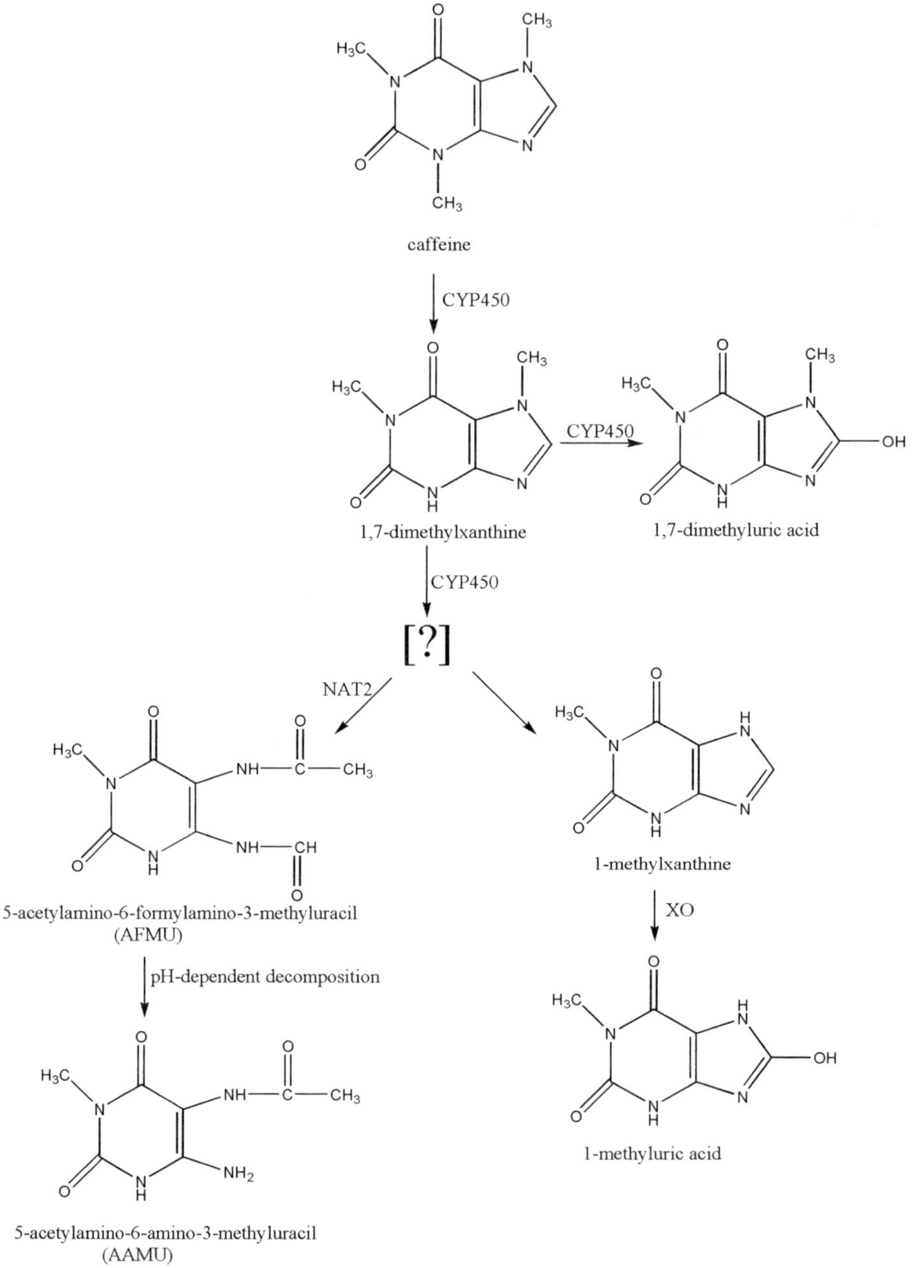

Fig. 2. Metabolic fate of caffeine. CYP450, Cytochromes P450; NAT2, *N*-acetyltransferase 2; XO, xanthine oxidase.

sulfamethazine were used to determine the NAT2 acetylator phenotype. Subsequent studies in larger populations confirmed the utility of caffeine as a probe for NAT2 acetylator phenotype determination *(60,61)*. Additional studies demonstrated that the acetylator phenotype assignment via caffeine is reproducible over time and independent of gender *(62,63)*.

There are, however, two potential sources of error with the method as described by Grant et al. The first arises from the instability of AFMU, which undergoes pH-dependent deformylation to 5-acetylamino-6-amino-3-methyluracil (AAMU). As urine pH varies widely, the degree of deformylation may vary from subject to subject—potentially confounding the measurement of AFMU and subsequent phenotype assignment. To overcome this potential source of variation, Tang et al. *(61)* published a modified method wherein AFMU in urine samples is converted to AAMU by the addition of base, followed by measurement of AAMU and 1-methylxanthine. A shortcoming of this approach is that it does not account for the variable basal level of AAMU in subjects not administered caffeine *(64)*. We found that some subjects excreted measurable concentrations of AAMU in urine despite a 2-wk caffeine-free diet (unpublished results), which is consistent with early reports *(64)*. Failure to account for this basal level of AAMU may result in erroneous phenotype assignment.

A second potential source of error with this method is the potential for variation in xanthine oxidase activity. With determination of the ratio of AFMU : 1-methylxanthine, alterations in xanthine oxidase may influence the ratio and therefore the assigned phenotype. To overcome this potentially confounding factor, Tang et al. *(61)* determined 1-methylxanthine (1X) and its product via xanthine oxidase, 1-methyluric acid (*see* Fig. 1). The ratio of these combined products correlated well with acetylator phenotype assigned in a group of 20 subjects via sulfamethazine. Table 5 summarizes the various urinary caffeine metabolite ratios that have been used for determination of NAT2 acetylator phenotype. Although theoretical considerations suggest that the AFMU/1X or AAMU/1X ratios to be most sensitive to changes in xanthine oxidase as a confounding factor *(65)*, the concordance of this ratio with more direct measures of acetylation (using dapsone or sulfamethazine) is not significantly different from that seen with the more complex metabolite ratios in the limited number of subjects in which comparison has been made *(58,60)*. Indeed, although Fuchs et al. *(66)* demonstrated that coadministration of allopurinol (an inhibitor of xanthine oxidase) reduces the AFMU/1X ratio, no subject changed assigned phenotype as a result of this coadministration. Thus, the magnitude of impact on the metabolite ratio appears to be relatively insignificant. As this observation is based on limited data, it is prudent to use the more extensive metabolite analysis in those situations where xanthine oxidase activity may be altered by disease or concomitant drug therapy.

Table 5
Caffeine Metabolite Urinary Ratios Used for Determination of NAT2 Phenotype

Metabolite ratio	References
$\dfrac{\text{AFMU}}{1\text{X}}$	58,68
$\dfrac{\text{AAMU}}{1\text{X}}$	60,61,69
$\dfrac{\text{AFMU}}{1\text{X} + 1\text{U}}$	70
$\dfrac{\text{AFMU}}{\text{AFMU} + 1\text{X} + 1\text{U}}$	70
$\dfrac{\text{AAMU}}{\text{AAMU} + 1\text{X} + 1\text{U}}$	60,61,69
$\dfrac{\text{AFMU}}{\text{AFMU} + 1\text{X} + 1\text{U} + 17\text{X} + 17\text{U}}$	58

AAMU, 5-Acetylamino-6-amino-3-uracil; AFMU, 5-acetylamino-6-formylamino-3-uracil; 1U, 1-methylurate; 1X, 1-methylxanthine; 17U, 1,7-dimethyluric acid; 17X, 1,7-dimethylxanthine (paraxanthine).

Although caffeine has been widely used as a probe to phenotype NAT2 activity, accurately quantifying low concentrations of an unstable metabolite in urine presents a significant analytical challenge, especially when used in populations that are receiving other medicines, herbal products, and/or nutritional supplements. Our experience in AIDS patients, who are often receiving many medications (in addition to self-treatment with herbal preparations), indicates that special care is needed for peak identification in urine samples. For this reason, we have developed a three-step method for assuring accurate peak identification that involves three serial analyses of each sample (67). Specifically, each urine sample is analyzed via standard liquid–liquid extraction followed by separation and quantification via high-performance liquid chromatography. Each sample is then analyzed after basic hydrolysis to ensure that the peak identified as AFMU in the normally processed sample disappears. Finally, each sample is assayed after the addition of pure AFMU, with verification that the peak previously identified as AFMU increases symmetrically after external addition of metabolite. This three-step process of analysis gives added confidence to peak identification in urine samples and removes the ambiguities that may arise due to intraday fluctuations in compound elution time during chromatographic analysis.

3.2. Determination of the NAT1 Phenotype

The identification of allelic variants of *NAT1* led to a reconsideration of the widespread view that compounds metabolized by this enzyme displayed a monomorphic frequency distribution pattern. Weber and Vatsis *(71)* provided evidence that a frequency distribution plot of *p*-aminobenzoic acid *N*-acetylation activity in human whole blood is not normally distributed. However, no clear polymorphic pattern was evident. Subsequently, Hughes et al. *(35)* examined the in vivo metabolism of *p*-aminosalicylate (PAS), an NAT1 selective probe, in 148 healthy subjects. Although a 65-fold variation in the urinary acetyl-PAS/PAS ratio was observed, no clear polymorphic pattern was evident. These investigators did, however, identify a subject with 10-fold lower urinary acetyl-PAS/PAS ratio who also possessed two novel NAT allelic variants (*NAT1*14* and *NAT1*15*). The expressed *NAT1*14* variant was found to exhibit decreased activity, while the *NAT1*15* was completely inactive. Although the low frequency of these variant alleles results in the lack of a clear polymorphic pattern for the NAT1 phenotype, substrates for this enzyme may be useful in identifying subjects possessing these allelic variants. Indeed, Hughes et al. *(35)* demonstrated that the metabolism of PAS in whole blood lysates from a subject with the *NAT1*14/NAT1*15* genotype was substantially less than that seen in subjects of other genotypes. Thus, in vitro screening may allow for large-scale population studies to identify variant phenotypes.

4. METHODS FOR DETERMINATION OF *N*-ACETYLATION GENOTYPE

Original *NAT1* and *NAT2* genotyping methods were designed to detect the most frequent SNPs (usually three or four) by restriction fragment length polymorphism (RFLP) analysis. Because of the limited number of SNPs screened, these assays had potential for genotype misclassifications (reviewed by Hein et al. *[72]*). *NAT1* genotyping assays developed subsequently include RFLP *(67,73–75)*, single-strand conformation polymorphism *(76)*, automated DNA sequencing *(77)*, allele discrimination *(78,79)*, and a READIT assay *(80)*. Similarly, *NAT2* genotyping methods include RFLP analysis *(81–86)*, allele-specific assays *(87,88)* and allele discrimination assays *(89,90)*. A method for simultaneous determination of *NAT1* and *NAT2* genotypes by reverse line blot hybridization also has been reported *(91)*. The impact of genotype misclassification in genotype–exposure interaction studies was recently documented for the *NAT2* genotype, smoking, and urinary bladder cancer risk *(92)*, and is a factor to consider in molecular epidemiology studies and genotype/phenotype discrepancies.

Table 6
Frequency of Genotype–Phenotype Discordance for NAT2

Frequency (%)	Probe	Population type	Reference
0/49 (0%)	Caffeine	Leprosy patients	Ilett et al. *(93)*
9/80 (11%)[a]	Dapsone	Bladder cancer and controls	Hayes et al. *(94)*
10/84 (12%)	Dapsone	Healthy	Rothman et al. *(95)*
5/120 (4%)	SMZ	Children; IDDM and controls	Mrozikiewicz et al. *(96)*
5/67 (8%)	SMZ	Children	Mrozikiewicz et al. *(85)*
38/563 (7%)	Caffeine	Mixed	Cascorbi et al. *(83)*
2/50 (4%)	Caffeine	HIV+ patients	Kaufmann et al. *(97)*
3/26 (12%)	SMZ	Healthy	Meisel et al. *(98)*
18/50 (36%)	Caffeine	HIV+ patients	O'Neil et al. *(99)*
20/90 (33%)	Caffeine	AIDS and healthy	O'Neil et al. *(67)*
9/60 (15%)	Dapsone	AIDS patients	O'Neil et al. *(67)*
26/74 (35%)[b]	Caffeine	AIDS patients	Wolkenstein et al. *(100)*
5/28 (18%)	Dapsone	AIDS patients	O'Neil et al. *(101)*
8/66 (12%)[c]	Dapsone	HIV+ and healthy	Alfirevic et al. *(102)*

[a]Reanalysis of genotype and phenotype resolved discordance in seven subjects.
[b]Full-length sequencing failed to resolve any discordant assignments.
[c]Discordance was resolved in four subjects by sequencing the entire *NAT2* exon.
HIV+, Patients infected with the human immunodeficiency virus; IDDM, insulin dependent diabetes mellitus; SMZ, sulfamethazine.

5. CONCORDANCE BETWEEN DEDUCED AND MEASURED *N*-ACETYLATION PHENOTYPE

Development of rapid, specific and economical methods for determination of *NAT2* genotype has led to many studies examining the relationship between variant alleles and disease incidence. Increasingly, these studies rely solely on the measurement of genotype, with the assumption that phenotype may be accurately deduced from genotype. As shown in Table 6, however, there is a fairly wide degree of variability in the frequency of discordance between genotype and phenotype, especially when caffeine is used as a probe for phenotype determination. Some of the early studies may have resulted in discordance owing to a failure to detect infrequently occurring variants of *NAT2*. However, in subsequent studies full-length sequencing has not always resolved the discordant assignments. The frequency of discordance is greatest in patients infected with the human immunodeficiency virus in whom caffeine is used as a substrate. These data suggest that disease-induced alterations in the disposition of caffeine may confound the analysis of NAT2 acetylator phenotype in this population and other probes are preferred. However, there is also significant discordance with other probe substrates (i.e., dapsone, sulfamethazine). Recognizing the potential for discordance between deduced and actual phenotype, investigators must be cautious in the conclusions drawn from studies that rely solely on deduced phenotype. On the other hand, when the hypothesis being tested relates to the association of a phenomenon with the occurrence variant alleles (as opposed to association with deduced phenotype), genotypic analysis alone is valid.

REFERENCES

1. Weber WW. Human variation in acetylation. In: Weber WW, ed. The Acetylator Genes and Drug Response. New York: Oxford University Press, 1987:19–31.
2. Selikoff IJ, Robitzek EH, Ornstein GG. Treatment of pulmonary tuberculosis with hydrazine derivatives of isonicotinic acid. JAMA 1952;150:973–980.
3. Hughes HB, Biehl JP, Jones AP, Schmidt LH. Metabolism of isoniazid in man as related to the occurrence of peripheral neuritis. Am Rev Tuberc 1954;70:266–273.
4. Weber WW. The genetics of acetylation. In: Weber WW, ed. The Acetylator Genes and Drug Response. New York: Oxford University Press; 1987:32–49.
5. Evans DJP, Manley KA, McKusick VA. Genetic control of isoniazid metabolism in man. Br Med J 1960;2:485–491.
6. Sunahara S, Urano M, Agawa M. Genetical and geographic studies on isoniazid inactivation. Science 1961;134:1530–1531.
7. Dufour AP, Knight RA, Harris HW. Genetics of isoniazid metabolism in caucasian, negro, and japanese populations. Science 1964;145:391.
8. Parkin DP, Vandenplas S, Botha FJH, et al. Trimodality of isoniazid elimination. Phenotype and genotype in patients with tuberculosis. Am J Respir Crit Care Med 1997;155:1717–1722.
9. Evans DJP, White TA. Human acetylation polymorphism. J Lab Clin Med 1964;63: 394–403.
10. Evans DJP, Davison K, Pratt RTC. The influence of acetylator phenotype on the effects of depression with phenelzine. Clin Pharmacol Ther 1965;6:430–435.
11. Gelber R, Peters J, Gordon G, Glazko A, Levy L. The polymorphic acetylation of dapsone in man. Clin Pharmacol Ther 1971;12:225–238.
12. Jenne JW. Partial purification and properties of the isoniazid transacetylase in human liver: its relationship to the acetylation of *p*-aminosalicylic acid. J Clin Invest 1965;44:1992–2002.
13. Grant DM, Blum M, Beer M, Meyer UA. Monomorphic and polymorphic human arylamine *N*-acetyltransferases: a comparison of liver isozymes and expressed products of two cloned genes. Mol Pharmacol 1991;39:184–191.
14. Hein DW, Doll MA, Fretland AJ, et al. Rodent models of the human acetylation polymorphism: comparisons of recombinant acetyltransferases. Mutat Res 1997; 376:101–106.
15. Hein DW. Acetylator genotype and arylamine-induced carcinogenesis. Biochim Biophys Acta 1988;948:37–66.

16. Vatsis KP, Martell KJ, Weber WW. Diverse point mutations in the human gene for polymorphic N-acetyltransferase. Proc Natl Acad Sci USA 1991;88:6333–6337.
17. Blum M, Demierre A, Grant DM, Heim M, Meyer UA. Molecular mechanism of slow acetylation of drugs and carcinogens in humans. Proc Natl Acad Sci USA 1991;88:5237–5241.
18. Hickman D, Risch A, Buckle V, et al. Chromosomal localization of human genes for arylamine N-acetyltransferase. Biochem J 1994;297:441–444.
19. Blum M, Grant DM, McBride W, Heim M, Meyer UA. Human arylamine N-acetyltransferase genes: isolation, chromosomal localization, and functional expression. DNA Cell Biol 1990;9:193–203.
20. Pompeo F, Brooke E, Kawamura A, Mushtaq A, Sim E. The pharmacogenetics of NAT: structural aspects. Pharmacogenomics 2002;3:19–30.
21. Dupret JM, Grant DM. Site-directed mutagenesis of recombinant human arylamine N-acetyltransferase expressed in Escherichia coli. Evidence for direct involvement of Cys68 in the catalytic mechanism of polymorphic human NAT2. J Biol Chem 1992;267:7381–7385.
22. Goodfellow GH, Dupret MM, Grant DM. Identification of amino acids imparting acceptor substrate selectivity to human arylamine acetyltransferases NAT1 and NAT2. Biochem J 2000;348:159–166.
23. Lima-Rodrigues F, Delomenie C, Goodfellow GH, Grant DM, Dupret J-M. Homology modelling and structural analysis of human arylamine N-acetyltransferase NAT1: evidence for the conservation of a cysteine protease catalytic domain and an active-site loop. Biochem J 2001;356:327–334.
24. Lima-Rodrigues F, Dupret J-M. 3D model of human arylamine N-acetyltransferase 2: structural basis of the slow acetylator phenotype of the R64Q variant and analysis of the active-site loop. Biochem Biophys Res Commun 2002;291:116–123.
25. Hein DW, Doll MA, Rustan TD, Ferguson RJ. Metabolic activation of N-hydroxyarylamines and N-hydroxyarylamides by 16 recombinant human NAT2 allozymes: effects of 7 specific NAT2 nucleic acid substitutions. Cancer Res 1995;55:3531–3536.
26. Hein DW, Rustan TD, Bucher KD, Miller LS. Polymorphic and monomorphic expression of arylamine carcinogen N-acetyltransferase isozymes in tumor target organ cytosols of Syrian hamsters congenic at the polymorphic acetyltransferase locus. J Pharmacol Exp Ther 1991;259:699–704.
27. Fretland AJ, Devanaboyina US, Doll MA, Zhao S, Xiao GH, Hein DW. Metabolic activation of 2-hydroxyamino-1-methyl-6-phenylimidazo[4,5-b]pyridine in Syrian hamsters congenic at the N-acetyltransferase 2 (NAT2) locus. Toxicol Sci 2003;74:253–259.
28. Minchin RF, Reeves PT, Teitel CH, et al. N- and O-acetylation of aromatic and heterocyclic amine carcinogens by human monomorphic and polymorphic acetyltransferases expressed in COS-1 cells. Biochem Biophys Res Commun 1992;185:839–844.
29. Hein DW, Doll MA, Rustan TD, et al. Metabolic activation and deactivation of arylamine carcinogens by recombinant human NAT1 and polymorphic NAT2 acetyltransferases. Carcinogenesis 1993;14:1633–1638.

30. Hein DW, Rustan TD, Ferguson RJ, Doll MA, Gray KR. Metabolic activation of aromatic and heterocyclic N-hydroxyarylamines by wild-type and mutant recombinant human NAT1 and NAT2 acetyltransferases. Arch Toxicol 1994;68:129–133.
31. Vatsis K, Weber W, Bell D, et al. Nomenclature for N-acetyltransferases. Pharmacogenetics 1995;5:1–17.
32. Hein DW, Grant DM, Sim E. Update on consensus N-acetyltransferase gene nomenclature. Pharmacogenetics 2000;10:291–292.
33. Doll MA, Jiang W, Deitz AC, Rustan TD, Hein DW. Identification of a novel allele at the human NAT1 acetyltransferase locus. Biochem Biophys Res Commun 1997; 233:584–591.
34. Butcher NJ, Ilett KF, Minchin RF. Functional polymorphism of the human arylamine N-acetyltransferase type 1 gene caused by C190T and G560A mutations. Pharmacogenetics 1998;8:67–72.
35. Hughes N, Janezic S, McQueen K, et al. Identification and characterization of variant alleles of human acetyltransferase NAT1 with defective function using p-aminosalicylate as an in-vivo and in-vitro probe. Pharmacogenetics 1998;8:55–66.
36. Lin HJ, Probst-Hensch NM, Hughes NC, et al. Variants of N-acetyltransferase NAT1 and a case-control study of colorectal adenomas. Pharmacogenetics 1998; 8:269–281.
37. Payton MA, Sim E. Genotyping human arylamine N-acetyltransferase Type 1 (NAT1): the identification of two novel allelic variants. Biochem Pharmacol 1998; 55:361–366.
38. de Leon JH, Vatsis KP, Weber WW. Characterization of naturally occurring and recombinant human N-acetyltransferase variants encoded by NAT1. Mol Pharmacol 2000;58:288–299.
39. Fretland AJ, Doll MA, Leff MA, Hein DW. Functional characterization of nucleotide polymorphisms in the coding region of human N-acetyltransferase 1. Pharmacogenetics 2001;11:511–520.
40. Bell DA, Badawi AF, Lang NP, Ilett KF, Kadlubar FF, Hirvonen A. Polymorphism in the NAT1 polyadenylation signal: association of NAT1*10 allele with higher N-acetylation activity in bladder and colon tissue samples. Cancer Res 1995;55: 5226–5229.
41. Badawi AF, Bell DA, Hirvonen A, Kadlubar FF. Role of aromatic amine acetyltransferases, NAT1 and NAT2, in carcinogen-DNA adduct formation in the human urinary bladder. Cancer Res 1995;55:5230–5237.
42. Butcher N, Ilett K, Minchin R. Substrate-dependent regulation of human arylamine N-acetyltransferase-1 in cultured cells. Mol Pharmacol 2000;57:468–473.
43. Upton A, Johnson N, Sandy J, Sim E. Arylamine N-acetyltransferases—of mice, men and microorganisms. Trends Pharmacol Sci 2001;22:140–146.
44. Delomenie C, Sica L, Grant DM, Krishnamoorthy R, Dupret J-M. Genotyping of the polymorphic N-acetyltransferase (NAT2*) gene locus in two native African populations. Pharmacogenetics 1996;6:177–185.
45. Weber WW, Hein DW. N-Acetylation pharmacogenetics. Pharmacol Rev 1985;37: 25–79.

46. Grant DM, Morike K, Eichelbaum M, Meyer UA. Acetylation pharmacogenetics. The slow acetylator phenotype is caused by decreased or absent arylamine N-acetyltransferase in human liver. J Clin Invest 1990;85:968–972.
47. Deguchi T. Sequences and expression of alleles of polymorphic arylamine N-acetyltransferase of human liver. J Biol Chem 1992;267:18140–18147.
48. Deguchi T, Mashimo M, Suzuki T. Correlation between acetylator phenotypes and genotypes of polymorphic arylamine N-acetyltransferase in human liver. J Biol Chem 1990;265:12757–12760.
49. Abe M, Deguchi T, Suzuki T. The structure and characteristics of a fourth allele of polymorphic N-acetyltransferase gene found in the Japanese population. Biochem Biophys Res Commun 1993;191:811–816.
50. Leff MA, Fretland AJ, Doll MA, Hein DW. Novel human N-acetyltransferase 2 alleles that differ in mechanism for slow acetylator phenotype. J Biol Chem 1999; 274:34519–34522.
51. Fretland AJ, Leff MA, Doll MA, Hein DW. Functional characterization of human N-acetyltransferase 2 (NAT2) single nucleotide polymorphisms. Pharmacogenetics 2001;11:207–215.
52. Zhu Y, Doll MA, Hein DW. Functional genomics of C190T single nucleotide polymorphism in human N-acetyltransferase 2. Biol Chem 2002;383:983–987.
53. Ferguson AJ, Doll MA, Rustan TD, Gray K, Hein DW. Cloning, expression, and functional characterization of two mutant (NAT2 191 and NAT2 341/803) and wild-type human polymorphic N-acetyltransferase (NAT2) alleles. Drug Metab Dispos 1994;22:371–376.
54. Hein DW, Ferguson AJ, Doll MA, Rustan TD, Gray K. Molecular genetics of human polymorphic N-acetyltransferase: enzymatic analysis of 15 recombinant human wild-type, mutant, and chimeric NAT2 allozymes. Hum Mol Genet 1994;3:729–734.
55. Hein DW. Molecular genetics and function of NAT1 and NAT2: role in aromatic amine metabolism and carcinogenesis. Mutat Res 2002;506–507:65–77.
56. Zang Y, Doll MA, Hein DW. Functional characterization of two newly found human N-acetyltransferase 2 alleles containing G364A(D122M) or A411T(L137F) single nucleotide polymorphisms (SNPs). Proceedings of the American Association for Cancer Research Conference on Molecular and Genetic Epidemiology of Cancer, 2003.
57. Evans DJP. An improved and simplified method of detecting the acetylator phenotype. J Med Genet 1969;21:243–253.
58. Grant D, Tang B, Kalow W. A simple test for acetylator phenotype using caffeine. Br J Clin Pharmacol 1984;17:459–464.
59. Tang BK, Grant DM, Kalow W. Isolation and identification of 5-acetylamino-6-formylamino-3-methyluracil as a major metabolite of caffeine in man. Drug Metab Dispos 1983;11:218–220.
60. Kilbane AJ, Silbart LK, Manis M, Beitins IZ, Weber WW. Human N-acetylation genotype determination with urinary caffeine metabolites. Clin Pharmacol Ther 1990;47:470–477.

61. Tang BK, Kadar D, Kalow W. An alternative test for acetylator phenotyping with caffeine. Clin Pharmacol Ther 1987;42:509–513.
62. McQuilkin SH, Nierenberg DW, Bresnick E. Analysis of within-subject variation of caffeine metabolism when used to determine cytochrome P4501A2 and N-acetyltransferase-2 activities. Cancer Epidemiol Biomark Prev 1995;4:139–146.
63. Kashuba A, Bertino J, Kearns G, et al. Quantitation of three-month intraindividual variability and influence of sex and menstrual cycle phase on CYP1A2, N-acetyltransferase-2, and xanthine oxidase activity determined with caffeine phenotyping. Clin Pharmacol Ther 1998;63:540–551.
64. Fink K, Adams ML, Pfleiderer W. A new pyrimidine, 5-acetylamino-6-amino-3-methyluracil. Its isolation, identification, and synthesis. J Biol Chem 1964;239: 4250–4256.
65. Rostami-Hodjegan A, Nurminen S, Jackson PR, Tucker GT. Caffeine urinary metabolite ratios as markers of enzyme activity: a theoretical assessment. Pharmacogenetics 1996;6:121–149.
66. Fuchs P, Haefeli W, Ledermann H, Wenk M. Xanthine oxidase inhibition by allopurinol affects the reliability of urinary caffeine metabolic ratios as markers for N-acetyltransferase 2 and CYP1A2 activities. Eur J Clin Pharmacol 1999;54: 869–876.
67. O'Neil WM, Drobitch RK, MacArthur RD, et al. Acetylator phenotype and genotype in patients infected with HIV: discordance between methods for phenotype determination and genotype. Pharmacogenetics 2000;10:171–182.
68. Butler MA, Lang NP, Young JF, et al. Determination of CYP1A2 and NAT2 phenotypes in human populations by analysis of caffeine urinary metabolites. Pharmacogenetics 1992;2:116–127.
69. Tang BK, Kadar D, Qian L, Iriah J, Yip J, Kalow W. Caffeine as a metabolic probe: validation of its use for acetylator phenotyping. Clin Pharmacol Ther 1991; 49:648–657.
70. Relling MV, Lin J-S, Ayers GD, Evans WE. Racial and gender differences in N-acetyltransferase, xanthine oxidase, and CYP1A2 activities. Clin Pharmacol Ther 1992;52:643–658.
71. Weber WW, Vatsis KP. Individual variability in p-aminobenzoic acid N-acetylation by human N-acetyltransferase (NAT1) in peripheral blood. Pharmacogenetics 1993; 3:209–212.
72. Hein DW, Doll MA, Fretland AJ, et al. Molecular genetics and epidemiology of the *NAT1* and *NAT2* acetylation polymorphisms. Cancer Epidemiol Biomark Prev 2000;9:29–42.
73. Deitz AC, Doll MA, Hein DW. A restriction fragment length polymorphism assay that differentiates human N-acetyltransferase-1 (NAT1) alleles. Anal Biochem 1997; 253:219–224.
74. Vaziri SAJ, Hughes NC, Sampson H, Darlington G, Jewett MAS, Grant DM. Variation in enzymes of arylamine procarcinogen biotransformation among bladder cancer patients and control subjects. Pharmacogenetics 2001;11:7–20.

75. Cascorbi I, Roots I, Brockmoller J. Association of NAT1 and NAT2 polymorphisms to urinary bladder cancer: significantly reduced risk in subjects with NAT1*10. Cancer Res 2001;61:5051–5056.
76. Lo-Guidice J-M, Allorge D, Chevalier D, et al. Molecular analysis of the N-acetyltransferase 1 gene (NAT1*) using polymerase chain reaction-restriction fragment-single strand conformation polymorphism assay. Pharmacogenetics 2000; 10:293–300.
77. Lan Q, Rothman N, Chow W-H, et al. No apparent association between NAT1 and NAT2 genotypes and risk of stomach cancer. Cancer Epidemiol Biomark Prev 2003;12:384–386.
78. Fronhoffs S, Bruning T, Ortiz-Pallardo E, et al. Real-time PCR analysis of the N-acetyltransferase NAT1 allele *3, *4, *10, *11, *14, and *17 polymorphisms in squamous cell cancer of the head and neck. Carcinogenesis 2001;22: 1405–1412.
79. Doll MA, Hein DW. Rapid genotype method to distinguish frequent and/or functional polymorphisms in human N-acetyltransferase-1 (NAT1). Anal Biochem 2002;301:328–332.
80. Iovannisci DM, Kupperman SO, Lloyd EW, Lammer EJ. The READIT assay as a method for genotyping NAT1*10 polymorphisms. Genet Test 2002;6:245–253.
81. Bell DA, Taylor JA, Butler MA, et al. Genotype/phenotype discordance for human arylamine N-acetyltransferase (NAT2) reveals a new slow-acetylator allele common in African Americans. Carcinogenesis 1993;14:1689–1692.
82. Lin HJ, Han C-Y, Link BK, Hardy S. Slow acetylator mutations in the human polymorphic N-acetyltransferase gene in 786 Asians, blacks, Hispanics, and whites: application to metabolic epidemiology. Am J Hum Genet 1993;52: 827–834.
83. Cascorbi I, Drakoulis N, Brockmoller J, Maurer A, Sperling K, Roots I. Arylamine N-acetyltransferase (NAT2) mutations and their allelic linkage in unrelated caucasian individuals: Correlation with phenotypic activity. Am J Hum Genet 1995;57: 581–592.
84. Doll M, Fretland A, Deitz AC, Hein D. Determination of human NAT2 acetylator genotype by restriction fragment-length polymorphism and allele specific amplification. Anal Biochem 1995;231:413–420.
85. Mrozikiewicz PM, Cascorbi I, Brockmoller J, Roots I. Determination and allelic allocation of seven nucleotide transitions within the arylamine N-acetyltransferase gene in the Polish population. Clin Pharmacol Ther 1996;59:376–382.
86. Deitz AC, Zheng W, Leff MA, et al. N-Acetyltransferase-2 genetic polymorphism, well-done meat intake, and breast cancer risk among postmenopausal women. Cancer Epidemiol Biomark Prev 2000;9:905–910.
87. Bigler J, Chen C, Potter JD. Determination of human NAT2 acetylator genotype by oligonucleotide ligation assay. Biotechniques 1997;22:682–690.
88. Labuda D, Krajinovic J, Richer C, et al. Rapid detection of CYP1A1, CYP2D6, and NAT variants by multiplex polymerase chain reaction and allele-specific oligonucleotide assay. Anal Biochem 1999;275:84–92.

89. Doll MA, Hein DW. Comprehensive human NAT2 genotype method using single nucleotide polymorphism-specific polymerase chain reaction primers and fluorogenic probes. Anal Biochem 2001;288:106–108.
90. Blomeke B, Sieben S, Spotter D, Landt O, Merk HF. Identification of *N*-acetyltransferase 2 genotypes by continuous monitoring of fluorogenic hybridization probes. Anal Biochem 1999;275:93–97.
91. Bunschoten A, Tiemersma E, Schouls L, Kampman E. Simultaneous determination of polymorphism in *N*-acetyltransferase 1 and 2 genes by reverse line blot hybridization. Anal Biochem 2000;285:156–162.
92. Deitz AC, Rothman N, Rebbeck TR, et al. Impact of misclassification in genotype-exposure interaction studies. Example of *N*-acetyltransferase 2 (NAT2), smoking, and bladder cancer. Cancer Epidemiol Biomark Prev 2004;13:in press.
93. Ilett KF, Chiswell GM, Spargo RM, Platt E, Minchin RF. Acetylation phenotype and genotype in Aboriginal leprosy patients from the north-west region of Western Australia. Pharmacogenetics 1993;3:264–269.
94. Hayes RB, Bi W, Rothman N, et al. *N*-Acetylation phenotype and genotype and risk of bladder cancer in benzidine-exposed workers. Carcinogenesis 1993;14:675–678.
95. Rothman N, Hayes RB, Bi W, et al. Correlation between *N*-acetyltransferase activity and NAT2 genotype in Chinese males. Pharmacogenetics 1993;3:250–255.
96. Mrozikiewicz PM, Drakoulis N, Roots I. Polymorphic arylamine *N*-acetyltransferase *(NAT2)* genes in children with insulin dependent diabetes mellitus. Clin Pharmacol Ther 1994;56:626–634.
97. Kaufmann G, Wenk M, Taeschner W, et al. *N*-Acetyltransferase 2 polymorphism in patients infected with human immunodeficiency virus. Clin Pharmacol Ther 1996;60:62–67.
98. Meisel P, Schroeder C, Wulff K, Siegmund W. Relationship between human genotype and phenotype of *N*-acetyltransferase (NAT2) as estimated by discriminant analysis and multiple linear regression: 1. Genotype and *N*-acetylation *in vivo*. Pharmacogenetics 1997;7:241–246.
99. O'Neil WM, Gilfix BM, DiGirolamo A, Tsoukas CM, Wainer IW. *N*-Acetylation among HIV-positive patients and patients with AIDS: when is fast, fast and slow, slow? Clin Pharmacol Ther 1997;62:261–271.
100. Wolkenstein P, Loriot M-A, Aractingi S, Cabelguenne A, Beaune P, Chosidow O. Prospective evaluation of detoxification pathways as markers of cutaneous adverse reactions to sulphonamides in AIDS. Pharmacogenetics 2000;10:821–828.
101. O'Neil WM, MacArthur RD, Farrough MJ, et al. Acetylator phenotype and genotype in HIV-infected patients with and without sulfonamide hypersensitivity. J Clin Pharmacol 2002;42:613–619.
102. Alfirevic A, Stalford AC, Vilar FJ, Wilkins EGL, Park BK, Pirmohamed M. Slow acetylator phenotype and genotype in HIV-positive patients with sulphamethoxazole hypersensitivity. Br J Clin Pharmacol 2003;55:158–165.

8

Methods and Approaches to Study Metabolism and Toxicity of Acetaminophen

Sam A. Bruschi

Summary

Although acetaminophen (also known as paracetamol) is a relatively safe and freely available analgesic, frequent organ toxicity (primarily in the liver) and admissions to emergency rooms occur. The aim of this chapter is to indicate selectively the most promising areas of research into the mechanisms of action of this drug and to highlight briefly new methodologies that are likely to maximize chances of filling gaps in our knowledge. As many other therapeutic and environmental chemicals mediate cell death and tissue damage by similar mechanisms as acetaminophen (i.e., via "reactive metabolites"), it is likely that any new information with respect to the toxicological mechanisms of acetaminophen will be generally applicable. The chapter highlights the metabolic scheme for both activation and detoxification of acetaminophen; summarizes current knowledge on the intracellular sequelae after exposure; assesses the relative importance of protein modification, oxidative stress, and mitochondrial injury in the mechanism of action; discusses evidence for the role of chemokines and cytokines in the "extrinsic" phase of acetaminophen-induced liver injury; assesses the role of nitric oxide and other reactive nitrogen species in injury; and discusses new approaches to studying liver injury, including the use of transgenic animals, RNA interference, DNA microarrays, and proteomic approaches.

Key Words

Acetaminophen; acute liver failure; acute tubular necrosis; *p*-aminophenol; apoptosis; centrilobular necrosis; chemokines; cyclooxygenases; cytochrome P450; CYP2E1; DNA microarrays; glucuronidation; mitochondria; *N*-acetyl-*p*-benzoquinone imine; *N*-acetylcysteine; nitric oxide; oxidative stress; protein modifications; small interfering RNA; stress genes; sulfation; transgenic/knockout mice.

1. INTRODUCTION

Acetaminophen or paracetamol (4′-hydroxyacetanilide, acetyl-*p*-aminophenol) is a freely available nonnarcotic analgesic/antipyretic medication *(1)*. It should

From: *Methods in Pharmacology and Toxicology,
Drug Metabolism and Transport: Molecular Methods and Mechanisms*
Edited by: L. Lash © Humana Press Inc., Totowa, NJ

be emphasized from the outset that acetaminophen is a relatively safe drug, especially when administered appropriately, being preferred to aspirin and other nonsteroidal anti-inflammatory drugs because of a lower incidence of gastrointestinal bleeding and no known association with Reye's syndrome *(1,2)*. The latter benefit effectively makes acetaminophen a preferable choice in the home for pediatric analgesic or antipyretic use. Nonetheless, its increased general availability and use—either alone or in combination with other medications—results in frequent inadvertent or deliberate overdose. As a result, acetaminophen misuse constitutes a public health problem in many Western countries and is commonly considered to be the most clinically important of toxicants implicated in acute liver failure (ALF).

In the United Kingdom, acetaminophen represents approx 50% of all hospital admissions with respect to therapeutic accidents or misuse and is the leading cause of ALF *(3)*. This is despite the fact that there are generally excellent chances of recovery if appropriate treatment is begun early (approx 0.6% of the total number of cases progressing to ALF *[3]*). Similarly, acetaminophen is estimated to be a major contributor to the incidence of ALF in the United States (39% *[4,5]*) and other countries *(6)*. Acute acetaminophen toxicity is usually observed as a zone 3 (centrilobular) necrosis of the hepatic lobule in humans and experimental animals *(1,2)*. A lower incidence of nephrotoxicity, observed as an acute tubular necrosis, is also evident (<2% in all acetaminophen poisonings *[7]*) and is usually associated with fulminant hepatic failure *(8)*. Other complications, such as major idiosyncratic immune responses, are rare.

From an early biochemical perspective and its relationship to subsequent target organ toxicity, we *(9)* and others *(2)* have classified the toxicity of acetaminophen into an "intrinsic" (stage 1) phase of hepatocyte death followed by a later "extrinsic" phase (stage 2), corresponding to activation of the acute-phase response and recruitment of immune surveillance. For our purposes, this should correlate with a period before (intrinsic) and after (extrinsic) the loss of hepatocyte integrity within and surrounding the region of liver injury. Such a reductionist classification enables a view of the toxicological actions of acetaminophen with respect to time and is not incompatible with traditional models of centrilobular necrosis. From this perspective, future studies may more accurately define cause–effect relationships important for the development of acetaminophen-induced hepatotoxicity. This classification is, however, distinct from the clinical phases of acetaminophen toxicity as previously outlined (e.g., ref. *8*). Clinical signs are known to include anorexia, malaise, pallor, diaphoresis, nausea, and vomiting in the first 24 h followed by upper-quadrant pain and abnormalities of liver function from between 24 and 48 h if left untreated. With further progression, more common signs of severe, late-stage hepatotoxicity become evident from 48 to 96 h postingestion, including peak serum alanine and aspartate aminotransferase levels, increased prothrombin time, encephalopathy, and coagulopathy.

N-Acetylcysteine has been effectively used for over 20 yr and represents one of several therapy options (see Subheading 2.2.; also refs 8,10–12). N-Acetylcysteine is optimally administered before 8–10 h after acetaminophen ingestion and 100% recovery is generally observed under these circumstances. Effectiveness becomes limited, however, if N-acetylcysteine treatment is begun later (12–24 h), and for this reason more detailed studies into the cellular effects of acetaminophen will undoubtedly result in new treatment alternatives and further improvements in outcome for late-presenters.

A comprehensive summary of the considerable literature regarding acetaminophen-induced hepatotoxicity is not the aim of this chapter, rather, the aim is to indicate selectively the most promising areas of research into the mechanisms of action of this drug and to highlight briefly new methodologies that are likely to maximize chances of filling gaps in our knowledge. As many other therapeutic and environmental chemicals mediate cell death and tissue damage by similar mechanisms as acetaminophen (i.e., via "reactive metabolites") it is likely that any new information with respect to the toxicological mechanisms of acetaminophen will be generally applicable.

2. ACETAMINOPHEN METABOLISM, BIOACTIVATION, AND TOXICOLOGY

2.1. General Metabolic Scheme

The physiochemical properties of a drug will determine the relative rate of absorption, uptake, distribution, and peak plasma levels from which therapeutic benefit or toxicological effect is derived. Additionally, other factors such as metabolism and excretion are contributory factors to the duration of action for a given drug (i.e., the fields of "pharmacokinetics" and "toxicokinetics"). These general concepts are well established for acetaminophen and many other compounds, and the reader is referred to established texts for further details (e.g., refs. 1,13,14). Of relevance is a comprehensive review of the chemical and physical properties of acetaminophen that has been previously published (15). Many well-controlled studies have exhaustively characterized acetaminophen pharmacokinetics and established predictable and reproducible responses over a wide range of doses (e.g., refs. 1,14 and references therein).

The hepatic metabolism of acetaminophen quantitatively predominates and proceeds via structurally modifying phase I reactions and/or via phase II conjugation reactions. A simplified scheme for the metabolism of acetaminophen is shown in Fig. 1 and represents the work of several laboratories over

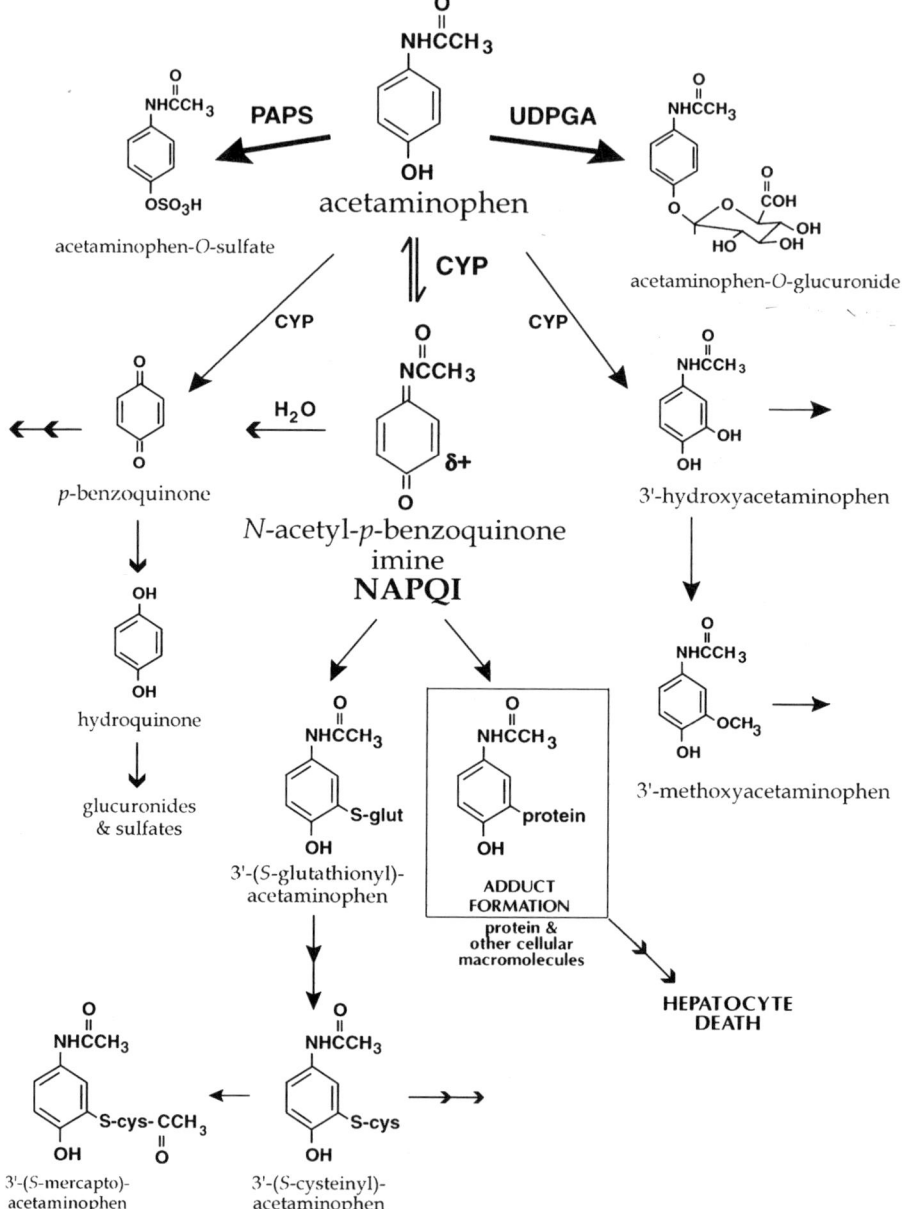

Fig. 1. Pathways of acetaminophen metabolism as adapted from ref. 60. Note: not all of these pathways have been detected in humans.

many years *(1,2,9,16–19)*. Glucuronidation (UDP-glucuronosyltransferases, UDPGA, primarily UGT1A6 *[20]*) and sulfation (sulfotransferases, PAPS *[21]*) represent approx 45–60% and 25–30% of a therapeutic dose, respectively, whereas approx 5% is excreted unchanged in the urine (Fig. 1). The resultant conjugates are inactive, nontoxic, more hydrophilic, and therefore suitable for excretion. Not shown in this scheme is the reversible conversion of acetaminophen to *p*-aminophenol *(9)*. It is generally assumed that acetaminophen crosses into the bloodstream from the mucosa by passive diffusion alone, although transporters for the glucuronide and glutathione conjugates of acetaminophen have been recently reported *(22–24)*. Variabilities in human plasma concentrations of acetaminophen at a given dose can be accounted for by such factors as interindividual differences in CYP (cytochrome P450) isoforms, body size, age, physiology and alcohol consumption (reviewed in ref. *9, see also* refs. *25–27*). Experimental approaches have also confirmed that the severity of acetaminophen hepatotoxicity in experimental animals can be altered considerably by changes in the metabolism pathways shown in Fig. 1. These are discussed further in Subheading 3.

2.2. Bioactivation of Acetaminophen and Important Intracellular Sequelae

Of central importance to acetaminophen toxicology is the CYP-mediated conversion of acetaminophen to a highly reactive quinone imine, *N*-acetyl-*p*-benzoquinone imine (NAPQI; Fig. 1). First proposed in 1973 by Mitchell and colleagues in a series of elegant studies *(28–31)*, the pivotal role for NAPQI in the toxicity of acetaminophen has been supported by many subsequent studies *(32–36)*. The electrophilic properties of NAPQI, which for the most part is generated by CYP2E1 oxidation in a minor pathway accounting for approx 5% of the total dose, generally results in an instantaneous conjugation with glutathione, the predominant protective nucleophile in the cell. Indeed, it is this mechanistic determination of protective role of glutathione that led directly to the development of *N*-acetylcysteine as an effective antidote and still represents the preferred treatment for acetaminophen toxicity today *(3,12,31)*.

In overdose situations, however, glutathione levels are exhausted and NAPQI can directly modify susceptible protein residues in what is widely believed to be the *first* step in a cascade of biochemical events leading to hepatocyte death *(2,9,18,19,28,30,36–44)*. The available evidence indicates that cysteine residues are the primary residues modified *(36,45)* and 3-(cysteinyl-*S*-yl) acetaminophen protein adducts have been observed in human acetaminophen overdose cases *(46)*. A comprehensive summary of the identities of all the proteins known to be modified by acetaminophen in experimental systems and their subcellular

2.3. Acetaminophen-Induced "Intrinsic" Hepatocyte Death: The Relative Importance of Protein Modification, Oxidative Stress, and Mitochondria

Such pathological changes in cellular biochemistry initiated by NAPQI are expected to follow the "reactive-metabolite hypothesis" of cell death and tissue injury, whereby the covalent modification and inhibition of critical cellular proteins results in functional deficits and the loss of cellular viability *(9,17,19,41)*. Acetaminophen is distinctive in this regard, as cellular perturbations following excessive doses appear to result from a combination of protein modification events *and* oxidative stress. Indeed, these may not be mutually exclusive phenomena, inasmuch as NAPQI, as a quinone imine, is both a strong oxidant per se and an electrophile capable of modifying proteins that function in a redox capacity within the cell (e.g., thioredoxin reductase and glutathione peroxidase) *(38,47,48)*. Despite considerable attention, the relative importance of protein covalent modifications to cellular redox alterations has not yet been well defined for acetaminophen-induced cytotoxicity/hepatotoxicity and this remains as a challenge for future studies and new technologies. By comparison, other compounds are known to initiate cell death primarily by covalently modifying proteins (e.g., chloramphenicol, tetrafluoroethyl-L-cysteine (TFEC), thioacetamide,) or by altering the cellular redox state exclusively (i.e., "oxidative stress" due to adriamycin, paraquat, or *tert*-butyl hydroperoxide) *(49–51)*.

What is known with increasing assurance, however, is that alterations to parenchymal cell mitochondria are important in the critical steps leading to acetaminophen-induced hepatocyte death. That mitochondria appear as critical "targets" is of interest as these observations have parallels to research in the broader area of apoptosis. Early studies defined the locus of acetaminophen action by indicating a preferential depletion of intramitochondrial glutathione levels, adenine nucleotide pools and redistributions of organellar calcium (e.g., refs. *47,52–57*). Very early changes in mitochondrial fatty-acyl-chain resonances have just been demonstrated, supporting these earlier studies *(58)*. Recently, our laboratory has also shown redistributions of the proapoptotic Bcl-2 family member Bax from the cytosol to mitochondria as an early event in acetaminophen-induced hepatotoxicity *(43)*. It is interesting to note, therefore, that Bax is generally accepted to function at the level of the mitochondrion and a recently proposed action links it to mitochondrial and endoplasmic reticulum organellar calcium ion sequestration in the direct control of apoptosis *(59)*.

Given the proteotoxic potential of NAPQI following intracellular glutathione depletion, it would seem compulsory to identify the primary protein "targets" for NAPQI modification. This has been accomplished with proteomic studies identifying proteins arylated by the reactive metabolite of acetaminophen by comparison to its nonhepatotoxic positional isomer 3′-hydroxyacetanilide (the *meta* isomer of acetaminophen) *(37,38)*. These studies complement numerous previous reports, using more classical procedures, that have identified the most prominent of acetaminophen-modified proteins (for an extensive review *see* ref. 60). Furthermore, it had already been shown that 3′-hydroxyacetanilide covalently binds to cellular proteins at least as well as, and probably more than, equivalent doses of acetaminophen but does not deplete cellular glutathione *(57,61)*. Consequently, the rationale for these proteomic studies was that a subset of modified cellular proteins should become evident that can only be observed with acetaminophen treatment and that these likely represent important "target proteins" for the eventual expression of hepatocyte death and hepatotoxicity. This was shown to be the case by the observation that acetaminophen modifies mitochondrial proteins (amongst others) whereas 3′-hydroxyacetanilide does not *(37,38)*. Some of the significant proteins identified included the ATP synthetase α-subunit, glutathione peroxidase, and the proteasome C8 subunit.

From a cell biology perspective, how do these proteomic studies relate to acetaminophen toxicity? We previously reported characterizations of a well-differentiated hepatocyte line (the TAMH line) that closely resembled acetaminophen-induced hepatotoxicity in vivo *(44)*. This cell culture model maintains CYP and other differentiation markers, activates acetaminophen to NAPQI and results in cell killing at relatively low concentrations (0.5–1.0 mM), which are comparable to the plasma levels observed during acetaminophen poisoning in humans *(1)*. As a result, the TAMH line obviates the concerns of spontaneous apoptosis following isolation of primary hepatocytes ex vivo *(62,63)*. An observation made by us at the time was of markedly increased mitochondrial number in TAMH cells following acetaminophen exposure (0.5–5.0 mM; ≥12 h). Accumulating evidence from the literature now suggests that mitochondrial fission events are mechanistically linked to apoptosis *(64–67)* and compatible with acetaminophen-induced Bax translocation in vivo (*see* earlier). Consequently, we chose to examine the functional state of TAMH mitochondria by flow cytometry, using a normalized function of mitochondrial membrane potential to absolute mitochondrial mass to account for mitochondrial fission (Fig. 2).

TAMH cells in culture were treated with 0.5 mM acetaminophen for 24 h and compared to a control vehicle. The upper set of plots of Fig. 2 represent selective fluorescent dye staining of control and acetaminophen-treated cultures

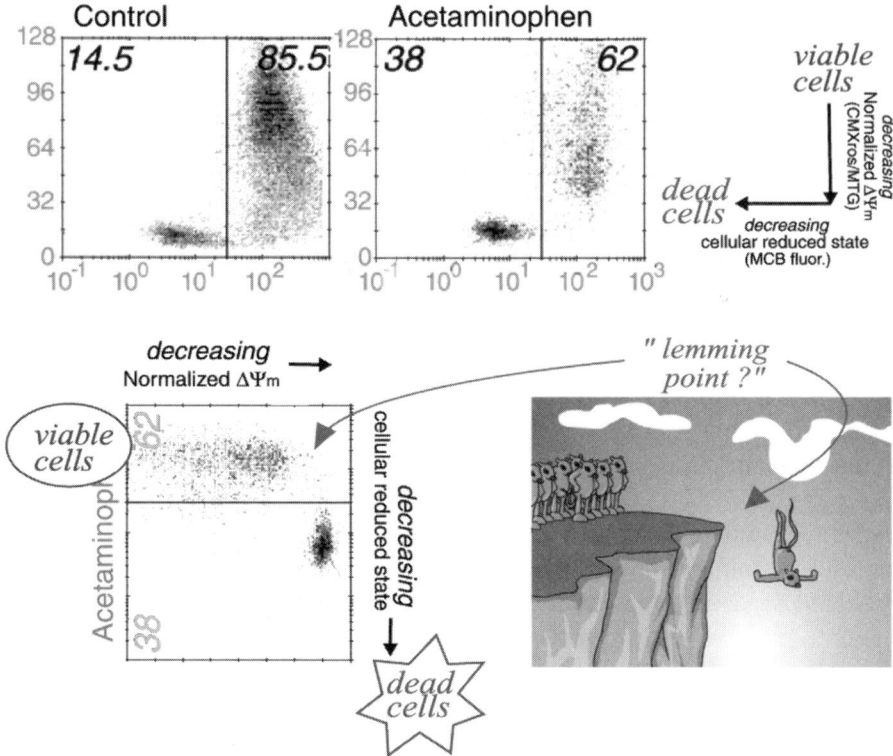

Fig. 2. Flow cytometric analyses of mitochondria following acetaminophen treatment of TAMH cells in culture. **(Upper panels)** Using selective fluorescent dyes, acetaminophen was first observed to decrease mitochondrial inner membrane potential (expressed as a normalized function) and then decrease cellular redox state (*see* text for details). **(Lower panels)** A whimsical analogy is made to another biological phenomenon to explain the biochemical events associated with acetaminophen-induced TAMH cell death.

for mitochondrial membrane potential ($\Delta\psi_m$; using the noncytotoxic dye CMX-rosamine), normalized to the total number of mitochondria (y-axis; using Mitotracker Green® [MTG]) and plotted against the total reduced cellular thiols on the x-axis (monochlorobimane [MCB] dye staining). The data indicate that cells first lose their normalized membrane potential ($\Delta\psi_m$/MTG) prior to changes in cellular redox state (MCB fluorescence) and this is represented by the percentages of cells shown in the top left of each divided panel. In the two lower panels of Fig. 2, we have rotated the upper plot 90° clockwise to provide an analogy with a well known phenomenon and to indicate that a cell death "decision" point (the "lemming point") precedes oxidative stress and cell death. The biochemical and cell biological characteristics of the "lemming point" still remain to be defined but may be related to mitochondrial fission and be Bcl-xL inhibitable (*see also* Fig. 4). Related to these findings is the recent report that the mitochondrial permeability transition appears to contribute to acetaminophen-induced hepatotoxicity and death in vivo with an elegant demonstration of increased survival following systemic cyclosporin A treatment *(68)*.

Changes in the ultrastructural morphology of mitochondria could also be observed in both our in vitro studies *(44)* and in livers of mice treated with 500 mg/kg (ip) acetaminophen (Fig. 3). First, in comparison to control animals, electron microscopy of hepatic tissue from animals treated for 6 h confirmed mitochondrial proliferation as a response to acetaminophen (Fig. 3 *[43]*) with closely packed mitochondria (m) in the cytoplasm and often tightly enclosed in a double-membrane structure of endoplasmic reticulum (er) origin (Fig. 3A,B). Vehicle-treated control animals showed unremarkable mitochondria (m) in a loose association with rough endoplasmic reticulum (er) (Fig. 3, upper panels). On closer examination, acetaminophen-treated hepatic mitochondria in the same field could be subdivided into two classes, namely (1) those with clearly defined double membrane enclosures, and (2) mitochondria with a diffuse "halo" of granularity (Fig. 3B, er vs er*). We have interpreted the latter as mitochondria enclosed by endoplasmic reticulum undergoing remodeling or disintegration.

These observations are consistent with our previous work indicating an induction of the stress genes *gadd153* and *atf3* as part of an upregulation of the endoplasmic reticulum-directed, unfolded protein response by acetaminophen *(44,69,70)*. At later time points (e.g., 24 h), acetaminophen-treated animals showed evidence of structurally abnormal, ring-shaped and elongated mitochondria (m*) with or without evidence of matrix swelling (Fig. 3c). At least one other group has also reported the presence of elongated mitochondria following acetaminophen treatment *(48)*. In cases of apparent advanced cellular decay, mitochondrial–endoplasmic reticulum associations had progressed to multilaminated structures with altered mitochondria (m*) at the center. These structures are suggestive of highly developed autophagy *(71)*. In summary, these observations provide further support for mitochondria as crucial to the initiation and progression of acetaminophen-induced liver injury. But, more importantly, these findings indicate that mitochondrial alterations are intimately associated with endoplasmic reticulum remodeling and provide an extended framework for the interpretation of forthcoming microarray, proteomic, and transgenic animal studies with acetaminophen. Likewise, recent reports increase our understanding of the biological events occurring during the "extrinsic" phase of acetaminophen injury (*see* Subheading 2.4.).

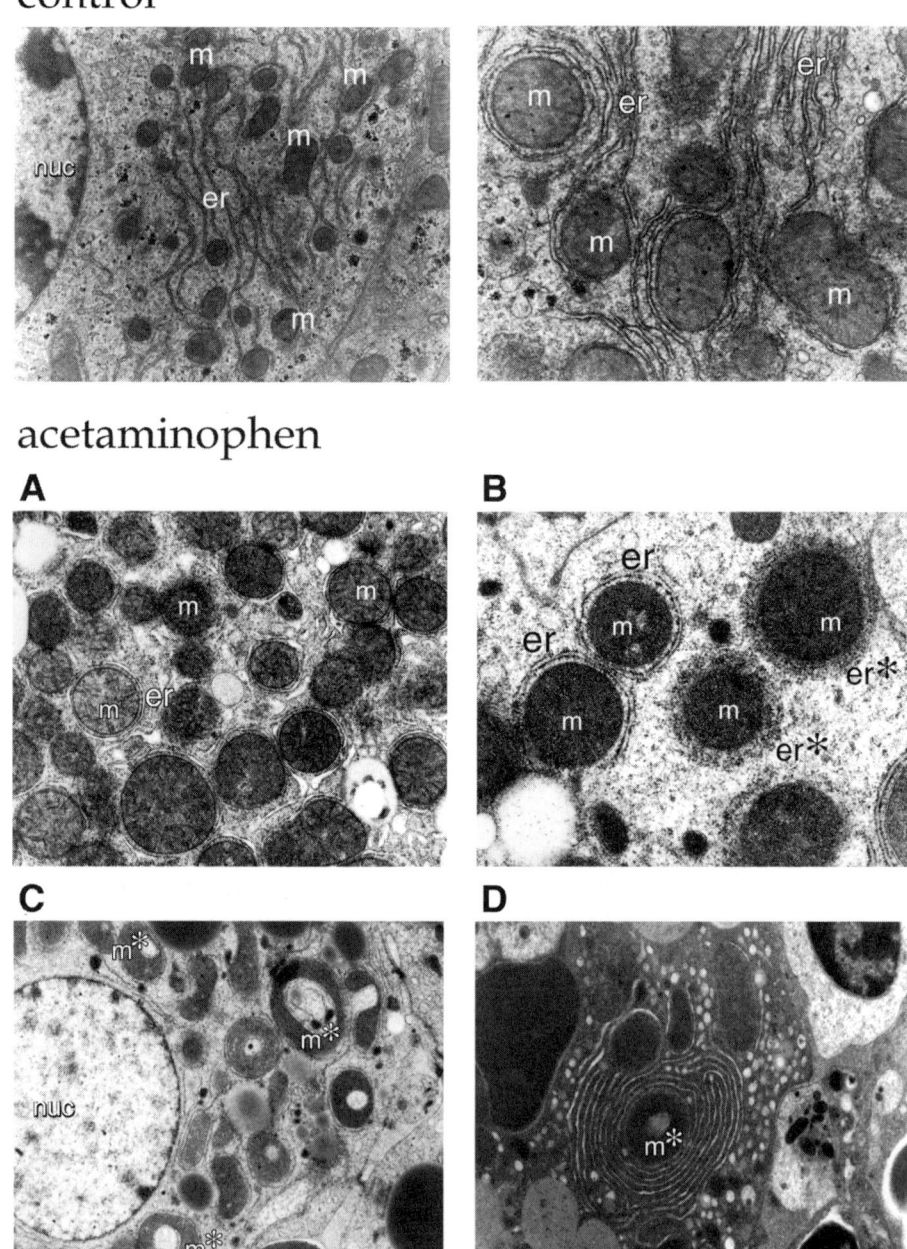

Mitochondrial matrix swelling (Fig. 3) and membrane potential loss (Fig. 2) are diagnostic features of a form of apoptotic cell death requiring the formation of a nonspecific pore on the outer mitochondrial membrane—the permeability transition pore *(68,72–74)*. The Bcl-2 family of proteins are recognized as important factors in the control of pore formation and downstream events in apoptosis *(75–77)*. Despite a lack of evidence for caspase activation during acetaminophen-induced damage by us *(43,44)* and others *(78)*, we examined whether acetaminophen-induced cell killing in the TAMH line might be modulated by a liver-specific and antiapoptotic member of the Bcl-2 family, that is, Bcl-xL (Fig. 4). Bcl-xL was observed to potently inhibit cell killing in this stably transfected cell culture system, even to *supratoxicological* concentrations of acetaminophen, in comparison to cells expressing an empty vector control (TAMH-Vc) or the parental cell line (TAMH; Fig. 4). These preliminary findings may eventually lead to exciting and novel therapeutic strategies if confirmed first in an in vivo animal system (e.g., acetaminophen hepatotoxicity in Bax-null mice) and, ultimately, in a system of greater relevance to humans (e.g., human liver slices). As Bcl-xL functions, at least in part, by heterodimerizing and inactivating proapoptotic Bax, it is conceivable that an effective and nontoxic Bax inhibitor could be incorporated into acetaminophen formulations to prevent overdose scenarios at the very earliest of stages, that is, initial ingestion. The feasibility of such an inhibitor has been boosted recently by observations of specific suppression of Bax function by a small peptide ubiquitously encoded by mammalian genomes *(79)*.

Fig. 3. *(see opposite page)* Ultrastructural examinations of hepatic parenchymal cell morphology from mice treated with acetaminophen or a vehicle control. (**Upper panels**) In control animals there was an unremarkable association of typical mitochondria *(m)* with rough endoplasmic reticulum *(er)*. Representative fields are shown at ×6000 (left) and ×12,000 (right) magnification. (**Lower panels**) (**A**) Acetaminophen treatment for 6 h was observed to alter both the morphology and density of mitochondria *(m)* in the cytoplasm. Closely packed mitochondria were often surrounded by a double-membrane structure of endoplasmic reticulum *(er)* origin (**B**). At higher magnification, surrounding membranes can be observed as either well-formed double membranes *(er)* or diffuse, granular structures *(er*)*. (**C,D**) Later time points (12–24 h) revealed the presence of numerous ring-shaped and elongated abnormal mitochondria *(m*)* possibly with matrix swelling. Mitochondrial autophagy and end-stage tissue decay was suggested by the presence of multilaminated structures with altered mitochondria *(m*)* at the center (**D**). Original magnification: ×6000 (**A,C**) and ×12,000 (**B,D**).

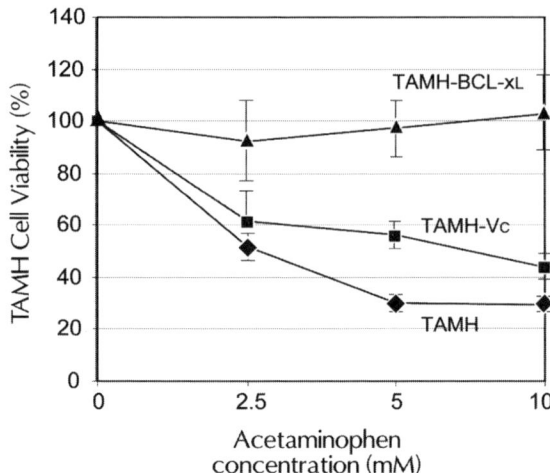

Fig. 4. Inhibition of acetaminophen-induced hepatocyte death in stable transfectants of TAMH cultures by overexpression of the anti-apoptotic protein Bcl-xL (TAMH-BCL-xL) in comparison to either the parental cell line (TAMH) or a stable transfectant of the parental cell line containing an empty vector control (TAMH-Vc).

2.4. Recent Developments in the "Extrinsic Phase" of Acetaminophen-Induced Liver Damage

2.4.1. A Role for Chemokines and Cytokines?

The therapeutic actions of acetaminophen now appear to be mediated by preferential inhibition of the cyclooxygenase isoform termed COX-3, a splice variant of the *cox-1* gene *(80)*. Consequently, prostaglandins generated by cyclooxygenases are increasingly recognized as the important proinflammatory targets of acetaminophen. Disruptions to hepatic cytokine and chemokine levels are also favored to play a role in the "extrinsic" phase of acetaminophen-induced injury. For example, the remarkable increases in mortality following acetaminophen treatment of *cox-2* null or heterozygous mice in comparison to either wild-type or *cox-1* null animals argues for a protective role during hepatotoxicity for the inflammatory mediators PGD2 and PGE2 *(81)*. Only further studies will more clearly define the contribution(s) of COX-3 and, as yet undetected but hypothesized, *cox-2* derived splice variants, in injury *(80,81)*. Likewise, comparable studies have shown that interleukin-6 (IL-6) null mice are more sensitive to toxic effects of acetaminophen *(82)*. Other related reports now implicate various cytokines (e.g., IL-6, IL-1, leukemia inhibitory factor, oncostatin M, and macrophage migration inhibitory factor) in poorly defined but interrelated functions during progression and/or recovery from hepatic injury (Table 1; *see* pp. 212–214). As reviewed earlier by us, there still appears to be considerable disagreement on the relative role of the cytokine tumor necrosis factor-α (TNF) during the extrinsic phase of acetaminophen-induced liver injury *(60)*. Collectively, more recent reports have so far failed to clarify the contribution of TNF to this form of hepatotoxicity *(83–86)*. Similar conflicts also arise for the role of the C-C chemokine receptor (CCR2) during acetaminophen-induced injury in *ccr2* null mice *(87,88)*.

2.4.2. What Role for NO and Other Reactive Nitrogen Species?

Finally, reactive nitrogen species have been hypothesized to contribute to the hepatotoxicity of acetaminophen as part of a systemic acute-phase and inflammatory response to organ damage *(85,89–93)*. Although the available evidence indicates formation of nitrotyrosine in areas of centrilobular damage *(84,90,92–94)* and partial protection from acetaminophen hepatic injury in *nos2* null mice (~50% *[84,89]*), many reports still appear to be in direct conflict. These include studies examining the role of hepatic nonparenchymal cells in the generation of reactive nitrogen species *(86,95–98)* and the relative beneficial effects of iNOS/NOS2 inhibitors *(84,92,98)* and nitric oxide donor molecules *(91,99–101)*. Some dispute also remains as to induction of the inducible form of nitric oxide synthase (iNOS/NOS2) following acetaminophen treatment in vivo *(84,90,102,103)*.

Studies with iNOS "selective" inhibitors are especially contentious with, for example, aminoguanine shown to increase or have little effect *(89,92)* or decrease *(84)* acetaminophen-induced liver injury. An implicit rationale for these studies has been that reactive nitrogen and related species are obligatory determinants of acetaminophen injury progression *(102,104)*. At present, these disparities do not appear to be easily attributable to methodological differences. Importantly, many of these studies have not detailed dose-dependent inhibitor effects on acetaminophen-mediated liver injury with only a single-dose observation usually reported. In direct contrast, clear dose-related inhibition of acetaminophen-induced hepatotoxicity was shown with a liver-selective, CYP-generated, nitric oxide *donor* prodrug (O[2]-vinyl 1-[pyrrolidin-1-yl]diazen-1-ium-1,2-diolate; V-PYRRO/NO) *(85,105)*. The hepatoprotective effects of V-PYRRO/NO were attributed to the prevention of late-stage sequelae in acetaminophen injury and this would seem to be consistent with a hepatoprotective role for reactive nitrogen species during the late extrinsic phase *(85)*.

Findings with the donor prodrug V-PYRRO/NO are supported by reports of hepatoprotection with a novel, nitric oxide-releasing, nitroxybutyl ester derivative of acetaminophen ("nitroparacetamol" or NCX-701 *[91,99–101]*). In comparison to acetaminophen, which is only a weak anti-inflammatory agent, animal studies have observed that nitroparacetamol is an effective anti-inflammatory *(101)*, is up to 20 times more potent as an analgesic in some models of nociception *(101)*, and does not appear to cause liver damage on an equimolar basis *(91,99)*. Interestingly, lack of nitroparacetamol hepatotoxicity is evident despite comparable glutathione depletion following equimolar doses of either acetaminophen or the "nitro" derivative *(91)*.

Although the precise mechanisms have not yet been determined, it does appear that the nitroxybutyl functionality is important for nitric oxide release and hepatoprotection for several reasons. For example, nitroparacetamol coadministration protects against either acetaminophen-induced or Fas ligand/HBV transgenic models of liver injury. Furthermore, a similar aspirin derivative ("nitroaspirin") protects against concanavalin A-induced liver injury *(91)*. The levels of nitrate/nitrite were also seen to rise only with the "nitro" derivative, providing solid evidence for a nitric oxide-mediated hepatoprotection *(91)*. From these and other studies, it has been argued that acetaminophen acts to kill hepatocytes by either upregulating *(85,91,106)* or antagonizing *(107,108)* liver Fas/FasL apoptotic pathways. These conflicting conclusions remain unresolved at present. Nonetheless, from a clinical standpoint, these findings with NO-releasing derivatives of acetaminophen are exciting, especially when considered alongside apparently successful phase II trials with this drug.

Despite the unresolved nature of many aspects of the extrinsic phase of acetaminophen-induced injury, it is clear that an activation of immune surveillance and acute phase responses is an integral part of the biology—for better or worse. The cytokine responsive transcription factor nuclear factor κB (NF-κB) is an essential and major component of the innate and adaptive immune response through its central role in regulating numerous genes controlling, for example, cell proliferation and apoptosis *(109,110)*. In a simplified model for activation, NF-κB is usually kept inactive in the cytoplasm by way of binding to inhibitory proteins known as I-κB. Activation occurs by removal of these inhibitory proteins via specific I-κB-directed kinases, which phosphorylate known I-κB serine residues, thereby resulting in ubiquitination and degradation by the proteasome *(111)*. I-κB degradation unmasks nuclear localization signals on NF-κB, resulting in translocation into the nucleus, DNA binding and gene activation. Some of the more important gene products upregulated by NF-κB that are relevant to intrinsic or extrinsic acetaminophen toxicity, include regulators of apoptosis and cell division, such as cIAPs (cellular inhibitors of apoptosis proteins that directly inhibit caspase activities), Bcl-xL, Bax (perhaps indirectly), Fas ligand, IL-2/6/8, TNF, COX-2, cyclin D1, and the protooncogene c-*myc*. Essentially, it appears that NF-κB activates multiple target genes whose products function to block mitochondrially mediated apoptosis and it is this antiapoptotic function that serves to stimulate the immune system and inflammation. Consequently, nuclear localization of NF-κB is an important indicator of NF-κB activation. We chose to examine NF-κB subcellular localization following acetaminophen administration in mice to determine the extent of NF-κB activation with damage (Fig. 5).

Tissue sections (5 μm) from formalin-fixed, paraffin-embedded, liver tissue of mice treated with acetaminophen (500 mg/kg, ip; 24 h) were subjected to heat-induced antigen retrieval using DAKO TRS™ solution (DAKO, Carpinteria, CA). Immunohistochemical localization of the p65/RelA subunit, as representative of the most abundant form of heterodimeric NF-κB (Santa Cruz, SC-372; 1:200), was conducted after inactivation of endogenous peroxidase activity for 5 min with 3% (v/v) hydrogen peroxide solution. Biotinylated goat antirabbit antibody (DAKO) was used as a secondary antibody followed by incubation with horseradish peroxidase-conjugated strepavidin (DAKO). Slides were developed with diaminobenzidine (DAKO), thereby forming a colored precipitate on the slide at the location of the antigen. Slides were finally counterstained with hematoxylin. Analysis by standard light microscopy indicated little p65/RelA specific staining in either the undamaged areas or areas of overt centrilobular necrotic damage surrounding the central vein (Fig. 5A [×100] and Fig. 5B [×200]). On the periphery of damaged areas, however, p65/RelA specific staining was observed with hepatocytes showing either cytoplasmic staining (open arrowheads) or nuclear staining of p65/RelA (solid arrowheads). Moreover, closer examination indicated that immunostained cells adjoining areas of necrotic damage also had evidence of microvesicular steatosis (associated with acetaminophen damage in vivo *[43]*). In addition, nuclear translocation of p65/RelA was evident in sinusoidal lining cells, both within the area of centrilobular necrosis and at the junction between the necrotic and viable zones.

An inhibition of gel-shift DNA binding of NF-κB has been previously reported using both in vitro *(112)* and in vivo systems *(113,114)*. In vitro studies have used very high doses of acetaminophen only (~10 mM) and so are unlikely to be relevant to clinical overdose situations. In vivo studies remain to be consolidated with evidence for either activation *(83)* or inactivation of NF-κB DNA binding *(113,114)*. We argue from our own data with p65/RelA immunohistochemistry and other reports in the literature *(83)*, that NF-κB activation represents a bona fide response to acetaminophen exposure in the liver. It is interesting to note here that other proteins have also been observed to translocate into the nucleus following acetaminophen treatment in experimental animals in what appears to be a coordinated cellular stress response to this drug *(44,60,78)*.

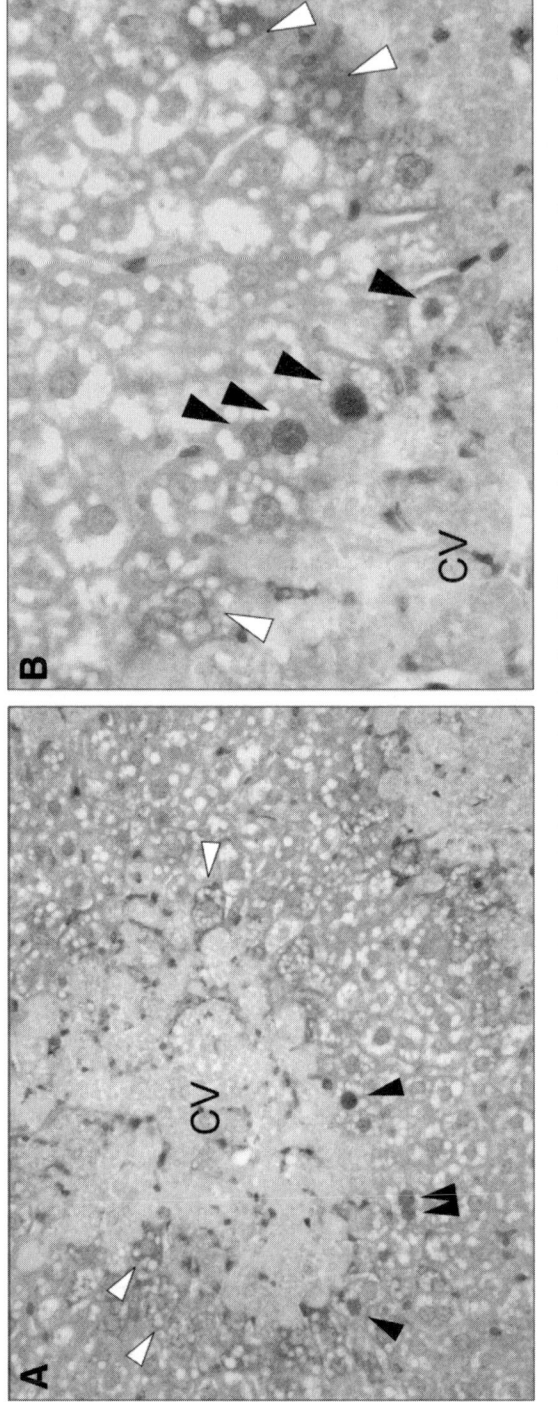

Fig. 5. Immunohistochemical localization of p65/RelA subunit of NF-κB transcription factor in sections from acetaminophen treated liver tissue. Cytoplasmic staining of activated p65/RelA antigen was observed on the periphery of centrilobular damage around the central vein (CV) in parenchymal cells with or without evidence of microvesicular steatosis (*open arrowhead*). Exclusive nuclear localization of activated p65/RelA subunit was observed in some cells on the margin of necrotic injury (*closed arrowheads*). Original magnification: ×100 (**A**) and ×200 (**B**). (A color version of this figure is available from the author on request.)

3. NEW APPROACHES TO THE STUDY OF ACETAMINOPHEN-INDUCED HEPATOCYTE KILLING AND LIVER TOXICITY

3.1. Transgenic Animal Models

Standard genetic analyses use selective inactivation or removal of a gene in vivo or in vitro as a key methodology to elucidate the function of that gene and its protein product. Such "loss-of-function" approaches have proven to be enormously powerful and can provide considerable detail on the biological function of a gene and its product(s). In conceptually related methodologies, the levels of a gene or protein of interest can be elevated by selective overexpression in either a constitutive or an inducible manner. More than 20 studies have now examined acetaminophen-induced liver injury and mortality in "knockout" and overexpressing transgenic mouse models, and these are briefly summarized in Table 1. Much of the promise of using transgenic animal models in the elucidation of acetaminophen toxicity has yet to be realized, with many studies providing unexpectedly contradictory or counterintuitive findings that are difficult to integrate into the accepted metabolic and toxicological paradigms. Nonetheless, transgenic animal studies are also likely to bring about a broader appreciation of the cell biological consequences of acetaminophen, as evidenced by studies that have confirmed preconceptions of acetaminophen-mediated toxicity as indicated in Fig. 1 (*see also* Table 1, pp. 214–216).

Confirmatory evidence for the central role of CYP (cytochrome P450) isoforms in acetaminophen bioactivation comes from several studies that either directly *(115–117)* or indirectly *(118)* modulate CYP enzyme levels in transgenic systems. Studies with mice deficient in both CYP2E1 and CYP1A2 (i.e., CYP2E1/1A2 "double null") indicated considerable resistance to hepatotoxicity, with protection appearing additive in comparison with either CYP2E1 or CYP1A2 single-knockout mice *(115–117)*. From these studies, a prominent role for CYP2E1 can be inferred with only a minor metabolic contribution from CYP1A2 to acetaminophen hepatotoxicity in the mouse *(116,117)*. The relative contribution of other CYP isoforms, notably CYP3A (CYP3A4 in human), CYP2A6 and CYP2D6, have not yet been reported using transgenic models and may be only of academic interest given the extent of protection observed with CYP2E1/1A2 double-null animals. An important cautionary note should be remembered when extrapolation of these studies to the human situation is attempted. As indicated in a recent review, there is considerable complexity and variability between mammalian species in the CYP superfamily *(119)*. Moreover, substantial interindividual polymorphic variability is observed in human metabolism, which contributes to idiosyncratic responses to drug, toxicant, and carcinogen exposure *(119)*.

Table 1
Summary of Transgenic Animal Studies Involving Acetaminophen Hepatotoxicity

Protein/gene	Experimental model	Hepatotoxicity compared to WT	Reference	Comments	Predictable?
Intrinsic Phase					
Bcl-2	Transgenic overexpression	Increase approx 300%	(43)	Acetaminophen increases proteolysis of BCL-2	No
Constitutive androstane receptor (CAR)	Knockout, humanized transgenic	Decrease approx 40%	(118)	CYP isoforms and GST Pi are CAR target genes	Yes
CYP1A2	Knockout	Marginal/minor	(116)		?
CYP2E1	Knockout	Decrease 100%	(117)	Approx 100% protection until 600 mg/kg	Yes
CYP1A2/2E1	Double knockout	Decrease approx 100%	(115)	Complete protection, absence of bioactivation	Yes (?)
Glutathione synthetase	Transgenic overexpression	Increase >200%	(139)		No
Glutathione transferase Pi1/Pi2 (GST Pi1/2)	Knockout	Decrease <20%	(130)	Major SeBP target downregulated (156)	No
Glutathione peroxidase (extracellular)	Transgenic overexpression	Decreased mortality	(131)	Expected function during "extrinsic" phase	Yes (?)
Glutathione peroxidase (intracellular)	Transgenic overexpression	Increased mortality	(131)	Expected function during "intrinsic" phase	No
Keratins 8, 18	Transgenic overexpression of mutant	45% increase in lethality	(160)	arg89 to cys mutant of human K18 providing extra Cys for adduction proposed relevance to nonimmunological idiosyncratic risk factor mechanism unknown/ phenomenological	?

Gene/Protein	Method	Effect	Reference	Comment	
Peroxisome proliferator-activated receptor α	Knockout	(See comment)	(113,129)	Failure of clofibrate to protect in PPAR-null animals cf. WT streptozotocin-induced diabetic mice are resistant to acetaminophen presumably via a PPARα-dependent mechanism	?
Metallothionein 1 and 2	Double knockout	Increase (3- to 13-fold)	(161,162)	Expected cytoprotective function broadly supported by microarray data	Yes (?)
Nuclear response factor 2 (NRF2)	Knockout	Large increase (approx 100-fold)	(163)	GST Pi2, SOD1, catalase, glutathione peroxidase are NRF2-dependent genes (164)	?
Cu/Zn superoxide dismutase (SOD1)	Transgenic overexpression	Decreased mortality	(131)	Expected function during "intrinsic" phase	Yes
Bax	Not yet reported	Unknown			
Selenium or acetaminophen binding protein (SeBP)	Not yet reported	Unknown		Closely related but little known of biological function(s) (133)	
Extrinsic phase					
C-C Chemokine Receptor 2	Knockout	Either no effect or apparent increase of up to 120-fold	(87,88)		?
Cyclooxygenase 1 (COX-1)	Knockout	No effect	(81)		?
COX-2	Knockout	Increase 75–200%	(81)		No (?)

(*continued*)

Table 1
Summary of Transgenic Animal Studies Involving Acetaminophen Hepatotoxicity *(continued)*

Protein/gene	Experimental model	Hepatotoxicity compared to WT	Reference	Comments	Predictable?
Interleukin 6 (IL-6)	Knockout	Increase 40–200%	(82)	Protective HSPs induced	No (?)
IL-10 and IL-10/iNOS double knock-out	Knockout, double knock-out	Variously increased	(103)	Extent of injury is less in IL-10/iNOS double-null cf. IL-10 knock-out alone	No (?)
Macrophage infiltration factor	Knockout	Survival 40% protected	(165)	Serum peak enzyme levels are same as controls	No (?)
Nitric oxide synthase 2 (iNOS)	Knockout	Decrease approx 50%	(84,89,103)	Marginal pathology; potentially cytokine-mediated	Yes (?)
Tumor necrosis factor receptor 1	Knockout	Typically 200% increase	(83,166)		?
Tumor necrosis factor/ lymphotoxin α	Double knockout	No effect	(166)		?

Acetaminophen target proteins identified from previous studies are indicated as underlined.

Recently, novel findings regarding a contribution to acetaminophen-induced hepatotoxicity from the "constitutive androstane receptor" (CAR) were reported *(118)*. CAR is a member of the nuclear orphan receptor family of important transcriptional regulators previously characterized in the expression of CYP2B10 *(120)*, CYP2C9 *(121)*, and other CYP isoforms *(122,123)*. Consequently, modulation of acetaminophen liver injury by CAR is consistent with the model shown in Fig. 1, as CAR regulates early steps in acetaminophen bioactivation. In this study, CAR null mice were protected from subtoxic doses of acetaminophen following CYP-induction under a CAR-specific regime using phenobarbital. In addition, acetaminophen-induced hepatotoxicity was similarly phenobarbital-dependent in transgenic animals constructed to express only the human CAR ortholog *(118)*. The relevance of these studies to humans remains to be established, however, as there are marked differences in pharmacology between mouse and human CAR and other related members of the nuclear orphan receptor family *(124,125)*. Nonetheless, observations of hepatoprotection in wild-type mice using CAR-specific antagonism with androstanol *(126)* following even high doses of acetaminophen *(118)* is of clinical interest as androstanol has been reported to act by similar mechanisms in both mice and humans *(124,125)*. Much more work will be required in this area to provide an alternative to *N*-acetylcysteine as androstanol, even though equipotent with *N*-acetylcysteine, was only effective at very early time points after acetaminophen administration *(118)*. Of related but tangential interest is the observation that activation of another orphan nuclear receptor superfamily member (the PPAR or "peroxisome proliferator-activated receptor") prevents acetaminophen-induced hepatotoxicity by incompletely defined mechanisms *(127–129)*.

As an example of transgenic/knockout models that have yielded unexpected findings are the studies which have altered the expression of proteins previously identified as arylated by NPPQI. These include studies with glutathione transferase (GST Pi1 and/or Pi2 *[130]*) and the intracellular form of glutathione peroxidase *(131)*. Transgenic studies have not yet been reported that modify expression of either selenium- or acetaminophen-binding proteins, which represent the predominant proteins arylated by NAPQI in the hepatocyte *(39,132)*. These are closely related proteins differing by only 18 residues (8 conservative substitutions) and, although the biological function(s) are mostly unknown, there is evidence for a role in protein transport within the Golgi *(133)*.

The unexpected alterations in acetaminophen-induced hepatotoxicity that have been observed in GST Pi1/Pi2 null animals and intracellular glutathione peroxidase overexpressing transgenics might either be attributable to a previously unrecognized protein function or to a more trivial explanation. In the case of GST Pi1/Pi2, a new function has been proposed that incorporates observations of increased activity of an important stress-signaling kinase, JNK (c-Jun

N-terminal kinase), in GST Pi null animals *(134,135)*. From these studies, it has been inferred that constitutive JNK signaling represents a cytoprotective mechanism in GST Pi1/Pi2 knockouts exposed to acetaminophen *(135)*. Although the JNK signal transduction pathway is known to be either prosurvival or proapoptotic, these observations are at present difficult to reconcile with the accumulating evidence for a Bax-mediated, mitochondrially directed, pro-death function for sustained JNK activity *(136–138)*. Pending confirmation of alternative biological functions for acetaminophen-targeted proteins, a simpler scheme can be envisaged that still adequately explains such unexpected variations to acetaminophen-induced hepatotoxicity *(60)*.

In this proposed scheme, transgenic modulation of acetaminophen-targeted proteins (located intracellularly) before dosing will result in a decrease or an increase in the available pool of proteins that can be arylated by NAPQI once it is formed (i.e., the reactive metabolite "sink" hypothesis). In situations of severely compromised ATP production, many of the cellular protein quality control mechanisms will become ineffectual and cytotoxic protein aggregates will accumulate. Only further studies will discriminate between this more trivial scheme and other schemes that propose new biological functions for acetaminophen target proteins.

Unpredictable findings using transgenic animals are not limited to proteins directly modified by NAPQI. Our own studies have shown that overexpression of the antiapoptotic Bcl-2 protein *increases* acetaminophen-induced hepatotoxicity, contrary to expectations *(43)*. Similarly, transgenic mice with elevated intracellular glutathione levels from overexpression of a major enzyme in glutathione biosynthesis were not protected from acetaminophen overdose *(139)*. In fact, glutathione synthetase transgenic animals were even more sensitive to acetaminophen-induced hepatotoxicity than wild-type animals. It is conceivable that both of these anomalous cases may also be explained by the reactive metabolite "sink" hypothesis in as much as both involve overexpression of cysteine-containing proteins. Further proteomic studies are necessary to determine if "nontarget" proteins can also provide an increased pool for acetaminophen-derived reactive metabolites, as mentioned earlier and detailed elsewhere *(60)*.

3.2. RNA Interference (siRNA)

That very small RNA species can serve important and fundamental regulatory functions in eukaryotic gene expression is a remarkable and unexpected discovery that is fully expected to revolutionize genetic analyses in the future. "RNA interference" (alternatively, siRNA or RNAi) can specifically repress the mRNA product of a gene, resulting in a null or hypomorphic phenotype ("knockdown" *[140,141]*). Unlike single-stranded antisense DNA techniques, siRNA is believed to act catalytically on homologous target mRNAs as hundreds of complementary mRNAs are destroyed before the siRNA loses its potency *(140–142)*.

There are immediate and obvious applications for this technology in toxicology (as indeed there have been for transgenic animal model systems). For example, with siRNA comes the capability to define the exact contribution each of the acetaminophen target proteins makes to the eventual expression of hepatocyte cell death. siRNA technology has recently progressed so rapidly that these studies can be carried out in either an appropriate mammalian cell culture system (*[141–144]*; e.g., ref. *44*) or in vivo with systemic portal or tail vein injection of siRNA's *(145)*. The application of siRNA technologies to dissecting out the relative contribution of each of the acetaminophen/NAPQI target proteins, or any other proteins presumed important to the eventual expression of hepatocyte death, is eagerly awaited. It is expected that findings using siRNA techniques will be complementary to those derived from knockout transgenic analyses (*see* Subheading 3.1.).

3.3. Microarray, Genome/Transcriptome, and Proteome Analyses

The complexity of acetaminophen-mediated organ damage has so far prevented the development of a holistic view for this type of injury. A global view of acetaminophen toxicity at both the cellular ("intrinsic") or organismal ("extrinsic") levels appears warranted given the number of studies published to date that have indicated a level of adaptive and coordinated complexity in the response to acetaminophen. Our understanding and appreciation of these adaptive responses are likely to ultimately increase with the application of new genome- and proteome-wide analysis technologies. For microarray analyses, this represents the ability to determine which of the many thousands of genes are newly expressed in response to a drug or chemical and can even be applied to the entire mammalian genome in a single experiment. Indeed, there is a general belief that microarray technologies alone can precisely define the biological effects of a drug or chemical *(146)*. This expectation may prove unrealistic for several reasons, including: (1) Some toxicological actions are not mediated at the level of *de novo* gene transcription (which is the basis for microarray analyses). Toxicological mechanisms involving apoptotic cell death and idiosyncratic immune reactions are two important and relevant examples (2) Genetic profiles obtained will vary considerably, depending on the choice of test systems (animal species/strain, in vivo or in vitro, and time/dose variations on gene expression). (3) Microarray analyses will require follow-up biochemical and proteomic studies as confirmation.

Several studies are now available and represent initial forays into the application of microarray techniques to acetaminophen-induced liver injury *(48,85,113,147–149)*. The findings to date are both heartening (with some surprising similarities) and sobering. As an indication of the varying model systems employed, studies have used the mouse (C57Bl/6x129/Ola *[147]*, 129SV *[113]*, and CD-1 *[48,85]*), rat (Sprague–Dawley *[149]*), isolated primary rat hepatocytes (Wistar *[148]*), and an immortalized hepatoblastoma-derived cell line (HepG2 *[150]*). In vivo studies have varied concentrations from nontoxic (150 mg/kg) to toxic (600 mg/kg) in the mouse (of which the Black 6 background is the most sensitive). In the far more resistant rat model, a single study has elevated the acetaminophen dose to 1000 mg/kg *(149)*.

Microarray studies using cell lines have similarly varied acetaminophen concentrations enormously from a toxicologically realistic 1 mM *(148)* to a supratoxicological 20 mM *(150)*. Unfortunately, in the former case 1 mM acetaminophen concentrations did not result in cytotoxicity for hepatocytes isolated from male rats (EC50 > 10 mM) and only marginal cytotoxicity in female hepatocytes (EC$_{50}$ > 8.1 mM) *(148)*. This represents a central concern for the field; namely, the choice of an in vitro system that is toxicologically relevant to the human (*see* Subheading 2.3. and later in this subheading).

As a source of reassurance, several genes are commonly upregulated in response to acetaminophen in most of these studies. These include metallothionein 1 and/or 2 *(48,85,147,150)*, heme oxygenase *(85,147)*, and other heat shock or stress proteins *(48,85,113,147)*. In contrast, whereas some studies observed upregulation of specific genes, e.g., *c-Jun/JunD (85,113,147)*, others did not *(48,148)*. Similarly, *gadd153* was upregulated in many studies *(85,113,147,148)* but one study failed to confirm co-upregulation of *gadd45* *(148)*. There was an apparent lack of agreement between all studies on the relative upregulation of CYP isoform genes (e.g., *cyp1a2, 2b1, 2e1, 3a1, 4a3/10/12*). In summary, the application of microarray technologies to the problem of acetaminophen-induced hepatotoxicity is still in its infancy. Many of the studies reviewed here provided only abridged lists of all the genes that were influenced by acetaminophen exposure in their chosen model systems. Clearly, a central repository of accumulated data, including complete gene lists that have been adequately annotated, will be necessary to provide a reasonable basis for direct comparison and to allow progress in the field.

It is self-evident that many of the variations listed above are attributable to differences in experimental design and the choice of model system. The use of whole animal systems will be necessary for the foreseeable future as only these can model the complexity of the extrinsic phase of injury However, there is considerable room for improvement in the choice of cell culture systems to investigate acetaminophen-induced intrinsic damage. For many, the use of primary cultured isolated hepatocytes represents the best test model due to maintenance of high metabolic activity. In the case of acetaminophen, however, intrinsic cytotoxic mechanisms are, at least in part, apoptotic *(43,44,91,151)*.

Consequently, the primary hepatocyte test system has well documented limitations associated with a spontaneous apoptotic capacity initiated on cell isolation *(62,63)*. Our own investigations have shown that a transforming growth factor-α (TGF-α) overexpressing transgenic mouse hepatocyte line obviates many of these concerns with both invariant maintenance of hepatocyte differentiation in vitro and high CYP-mediated metabolic capacity, including but not limited to acetaminophen bioactivation *(44)*. Moreover, many of the biological phenomena observed following toxicologically relevant dosing of acetaminophen in the TAMH cell line have clear in vivo correlates *(44)*, indicating that this cell line should provide an excellent mechanistic in vitro model to complement future in vivo microarray studies.

Finally, and all too briefly, several important issues still need to be addressed at the level of target proteins and proteomics. At present, the procedures by which NAPQI modification of protein cysteine residues results in altered and/or inhibited target protein function is not known. At best, only a relatively basic understanding exists *(152)*. Mass spectrometric analysis of hepatic proteins isolated under stable conditions to determine the number and location of arylated residues modified by NAPQI should provide additional valuable information regarding very early aspects of intrinsic cell death. Conceptually linked are a small number of proteomic studies that have attempted to define the changes in abundance for all cellular proteins following acetaminophen exposure *(38,48,153–156)*. Many of these were comparative studies whereby changes in protein levels were also noted for the nonhepatotoxic isomer 3′-hydroxyacetanilide. Only one study, however, has extended proteomic analysis to determine protein changes in a transgenic animal model of hepatoprotection to acetaminophen *(156)*. This represents an attractive area for future endeavor that could easily incorporate new advances in quantitative proteomics using stable isotope labeling procedures *(157)*. For application to the field of acetaminophen-induced liver injury, however, these quantitative labeling procedures must be adapted so as to modify residues other than free cysteine residues, as originally designed *(158,159)*. Quantitative proteomic analyses might also be expected to confirm or negate the reactive metabolite "sink" hypothesis for either acetaminophen "target" and "nontarget" proteins as described above and detailed elsewhere *(60)*.

4. CONCLUSIONS

Modern and powerful techniques now promise an ability to delineate the critical steps necessary for expression of acetaminophen liver injury—but certain precautions would seem to still apply. Careful management and interpretation will be necessary for the copious amount of microarray, siRNA and transgenic information that will be generated in the future. In addition, much of this information will amount to little if an understanding and appreciation of the biology of acetaminophen-induced hepatotoxicity is neglected. Careful choices regarding model systems, toxicologically relevant doses of acetaminophen and appropriate time points for observation should yield remarkable insights into the biology of the intrinsic and extrinsic phases of acetaminophen-initiated damage. For basic mechanistic research into both the intrinsic and extrinsic phases of acetaminophen injury, the ultimate "proof-of-concept" will come with the eventual application of successful clinical treatments that complement existing strategies.

ACKNOWLEDGMENTS

Many thanks go to my colleagues *par excellence* Rob Pierce, Zhong-Hua Hu, Han K. Ho, Michael Adams, Jean Campbell, Chris Franklin, Terry Kavanagh, Theo Bammler, Dave Hockenbery, Nelson Fausto, and Sid Nelson. This work was supported by NIH Grant GM51916 to S.B.

DEDICATION

This chapter is dedicated to the memory of my father and his love of knowledge.

REFERENCES

1. Prescott LF. Paracetamol (Acetaminophen): A Critical Bibliographic Review. London: Taylor and Francis; 1996.
2. Bessems JG, Vermeulen NP. Paracetamol (acetaminophen)-induced toxicity: molecular and biochemical mechanisms, analogues and protective approaches. Crit Rev Toxicol 2001;31:55–138.
3. Dargan PI, Jones AL. Management of paracetamol poisoning. Trends Pharmacol Sci 2003;24:154–157.
4. Ostapowicz G, Fontana RJ, Schiodt FV, et al. Results of a prospective study of acute liver failure at 17 tertiary care centers in the United States. Ann Intern Med 2002;137:947–954.
5. Lee WM. Drug-induced hepatotoxicity. N Engl J Med 2003;349:474–485.
6. Gow PJ, Smallwood RA, Angus PW. Paracetamol overdose in a liver transplantation centre: an 8-year experience. J Gastroenterol Hepatol 1999;14:817–821.
7. Blakely P, McDonald BR. Acute renal failure due to acetaminophen ingestion: a case report and review of the literature. J Am Soc Nephrol 1995;6:48–53.
8. Mokhlesi B, Leikin JB, Murray P, Corbridge TC. Adult toxicology in critical care: Part II: specific poisonings. Chest 2003;123:897–922.
9. Nelson SD, Bruschi SA. Mechanisms of acetaminophen-induced liver disease. In: Kaplowitz N, DeLeve LD, eds. Drug-Induced Liver Disease. New York and Basel: Marcel Dekker; 2002:287–325.
10. Lyons L, Studdiford JS, Sommaripa AM. Treatment of acetaminophen overdosage with N-acetylcysteine. N Engl J Med 1977;296:174–175.

11. Piperno E, Berssenbruegge DA. Reversal of experimental paracetamol toxicosis with N-acetylcysteine. Lancet 1976;2(7988):738–739.
12. James LP, Wells E, Beard RH, Farrar HC. Predictors of outcome after acetaminophen poisoning in children and adolescents. J Pediatr 2002;140: 522–526.
13. Parkinson A. Biotransformation of xenobiotics. In: Klaassen CD, ed. Toxicology—The Basic Science of Poisons, 5th edit. New York: McGraw-Hill; 1996:113–186.
14. Prescott LF. Kinetics and metabolism of paracetamol and phenacetin. Br J Clin Pharmacol 1980;10 (Suppl 2):291S–298S.
15. Fairbrother JE. Acetaminophen. New York and London: Academic Press; 1974.
16. Black M. Acetaminophen hepatotoxicity. Gastroenterology 1980;78:382–392.
17. Cohen SD, Khairallah EA. Selective protein arylation and acetaminophen-induced hepatotoxicity. Drug Metab Rev 1997;29:59–77.
18. Hinson JA, Pohl LR, Monks TJ, Gillette JR. Acetaminophen-induced hepatotoxicity. Life Sci 1981;29:107–116.
19. Nelson SD, Pearson PG. Covalent and noncovalent interactions in acute lethal cell injury caused by chemicals. Annu Rev Pharmacol Toxicol 1990;30:169–195.
20. Burchell B, Brierley CH, Rance D. Specificity of human UDP-glucuronosyltransferases and xenobiotic glucuronidation. Life Sci 1995;57:1819–1831.
21. Blackledge HM, O'Farrell J, Minton NA, McLean AE. The effect of therapeutic doses of paracetamol on sulphur metabolism in man. Hum Exp Toxicol 1991;10: 159–165.
22. Xiong H, Suzuki H, Sugiyama Y, Meier PJ, Pollack GM, Brouwer KL. Mechanisms of impaired biliary excretion of acetaminophen glucuronide after acute phenobarbital treatment or phenobarbital pretreatment. Drug Metab Dispos 2002; 30:962–969.
23. Xiong H, Turner KC, Ward ES, Jansen PL, Brouwer KL. Altered hepatobiliary disposition of acetaminophen glucuronide in isolated perfused livers from multidrug resistance-associated protein 2-deficient TR(–) rats. J Pharmacol Exp Ther 2000;295:512–518.
24. Silva VM, Chen C, Hennig GE, Whiteley HE, Manautou JE. Changes in susceptibility to acetaminophen-induced liver injury by the organic anion indocyanine green. Food Chem Toxicol 2001;39:271–278.
25. Zimmerman HJ, Maddrey WC. Acetaminophen (paracetamol) hepatotoxicity with regular intake of alcohol: analysis of instances of therapeutic misadventure. Hepatology 1995;22:767–773.
26. Thummel KE, Slattery JT, Ro H, Chien JY, Nelson SD, Lown KE, Watkins PB. Ethanol and production of the hepatotoxic metabolite of acetaminophen in healthy adults. Clin Pharmacol Ther 2000;67:591–599.
27. Novak D, Lewis JH. Drug-induced liver disease. Curr Opin Gastroenterol 2003;19:203–215.
28. Potter WZ, Davis DC, Mitchell JR, Jollow DJ, Gillette JR, Brodie BB. Acetaminophen-induced hepatic necrosis. 3. Cytochrome P-450-mediated covalent binding in vitro. J Pharmacol Exp Ther 1973;187:203–210.

29. Mitchell JR, Jollow DJ, Potter WZ, Davis DC, Gillette JR, Brodie BB. Acetaminophen-induced hepatic necrosis. I. Role of drug metabolism. J Pharmacol Exp Ther 1973;187:185–194.
30. Jollow DJ, Mitchell JR, Potter WZ, Davis DC, Gillette JR, Brodie BB. Acetaminophen-induced hepatic necrosis. II. Role of covalent binding in vivo. J Pharmacol Exp Ther 1973;187:195–202.
31. Mitchell JR, Jollow DJ, Potter WZ, Gillette JR, Brodie BB. Acetaminophen-induced hepatic necrosis. IV. Protective role of glutathione. J Pharmacol Exp Ther 1973;187:211–217.
32. Corcoran GB, Mitchell JR, Vaishnav YN, Horning EC. Evidence that acetaminophen and N-hydroxyacetaminophen form a common arylating intermediate, N-acetyl-p-benzoquinoneimine. Mol Pharmacol 1980;18:536–542.
33. Dahlin DC, Nelson SD. Synthesis, decomposition kinetics, and preliminary toxicological studies of pure N-acetyl-p-benzoquinone imine, a proposed toxic metabolite of acetaminophen. J Med Chem 1982;25:885–886.
34. Holme JA, Dahlin DC, Nelson SD, Dybing E. Cytotoxic effects of N-acetyl-p-benzoquinone imine, a common arylating intermediate of paracetamol and N-hydroxyparacetamol. Biochem Pharmacol 1984;33:401–406.
35. Dahlin DC, Miwa GT, Lu AY, Nelson SD. N-Acetyl-p-benzoquinone imine: a cytochrome P-450-mediated oxidation product of acetaminophen. Proc Natl Acad Sci USA 1984;81:1327–1331.
36. Streeter AJ, Dahlin DC, Nelson SD, Baillie TA. The covalent binding of acetaminophen to protein. Evidence for cysteine residues as major sites of arylation in vitro. Chem Biol Interact 1984;48:349–366.
37. Qiu Y, Benet LZ, Burlingame AL. Identification of hepatic protein targets of the reactive metabolites of the non-hepatotoxic regioisomer of acetaminophen, 3′-hydroxyacetanilide, in the mouse in vivo using two-dimensional gel electrophoresis and mass spectrometry. Adv Exp Med Biol 2001;500:663–673.
38. Qiu Y, Benet LZ, Burlingame AL. Identification of the hepatic protein targets of reactive metabolites of acetaminophen in vivo in mice using two-dimensional gel electrophoresis and mass spectrometry. J Biol Chem 1998;273:17940–17953.
39. Pumford NR, Martin BM, Hinson JA. A metabolite of acetaminophen covalently binds to the 56 kDa selenium binding protein. Biochem Biophys Res Commun 1992;182:1348–1355.
40. Hoivik DJ, Manautou JE, Tveit A, Mankowski DC, Khairallah EA, Cohen SD. Evidence suggesting the 58-kDa acetaminophen binding protein is a preferential target for acetaminophen electrophile. Fundam Appl Toxicol 1996;32:79–86.
41. Gibson JD, Pumford NR, Samokyszyn VM, Hinson JA. Mechanism of acetaminophen-induced hepatotoxicity: covalent binding versus oxidative stress. Chem Res Toxicol 1996;9:580–585.
42. Cohen SD, Pumford NR, Khairallah EA, et al. Selective protein covalent binding and target organ toxicity. Toxicol Appl Pharmacol 1997;143:1–12.
43. Adams ML, Pierce RH, Vail ME, et al. Enhanced acetaminophen hepatotoxicity in transgenic mice overexpressing bcl-2. Mol Pharmacol 2001;60:907–915.

44. Pierce RH, Franklin CC, Campbell JS, et al. Cell culture model for acetaminophen-induced hepatocyte death in vivo. Biochem Pharmacol 2002;64:413–424.
45. Hoffmann KJ, Streeter AJ, Axworthy DB, Baillie TA. Identification of the major covalent adduct formed in vitro and in vivo between acetaminophen and mouse liver proteins. Mol Pharmacol 1985;27:566–573.
46. Hinson JA, Roberts DW, Benson RW, Dalhoff K, Loft S, Poulsen HE. Mechanism of paracetamol toxicity. Lancet 1990;335(8691):732.
47. Tirmenstein MA, Nelson SD. Acetaminophen-induced oxidation of protein thiols. Contribution of impaired thiol-metabolizing enzymes and the breakdown of adenine nucleotides. J Biol Chem 1990;265:3059–3065.
48. Ruepp SU, Tonge RP, Shaw J, Wallis N, Pognan F. Genomics and proteomics analysis of acetaminophen toxicity in mouse liver. Toxicol Sci 2002;65:135–150.
49. Groves CE, Lock EA, Schnellmann RG. Role of lipid peroxidation in renal proximal tubule cell death induced by haloalkene cysteine conjugates. Toxicol Appl Pharmacol 1991;107:54–62.
50. James EA, Gygi SP, Adams ML, et al. Mitochondrial aconitase modification, functional inhibition, and evidence for a supramolecular complex of the TCA cycle by the renal toxicant S-(1,1,2,2-tetrafluoroethyl)-L-cysteine. Biochemistry 2002;41:6789–6797.
51. Suntres ZE. Role of antioxidants in paraquat toxicity. Toxicology 2002;180:65–77.
52. Schanne FA, Kane AB, Young EE, Farber JL. Calcium dependence of toxic cell death: a final common pathway. Science 1979;206:700–702.
53. Bruschi SA, Priestly B. Implications of alterations in intracellular calcium ion homeostasis in the advent of paracetamol-induced cytotoxicity in primary mouse hepatocyte cultures. Toxicol In Vitro 1990;4:743–749.
54. Burcham PC, Harman AW. Mitochondrial dysfunction in paracetamol hepatotoxicity: in vitro studies in isolated mouse hepatocytes. Toxicol Lett 1990;50:37–48.
55. Burcham PC, Harman AW. Acetaminophen toxicity results in site-specific mitochondrial damage in isolated mouse hepatocytes. J Biol Chem 1991;266:5049–5054.
56. Tirmenstein MA, Nelson SD. Subcellular binding and effects on calcium homeostasis produced by acetaminophen and a nonhepatotoxic regioisomer, 3'-hydroxyacetanilide, in mouse liver. J Biol Chem 1989;264:9814–9819.
57. Tirmenstein MA, Nelson SD. Hepatotoxicity after 3'-hydroxyacetanilide administration to buthionine sulfoximine pretreated mice. Chem Res Toxicol 1991;4:214–217.
58. Coen M, Lenz EM, Nicholson JK, Wilson ID, Pognan F, Lindon JC. An integrated metabonomic investigation of acetaminophen toxicity in the mouse using NMR spectroscopy. Chem Res Toxicol 2003;16:295–303.
59. Scorrano L, Oakes SA, Opferman JT, et al. BAX and BAK regulation of endoplasmic reticulum Ca^{2+}: a control point for apoptosis. Science 2003;300:135–139.
60. Nelson SD, Bruschi SA. Mechanisms of acetaminophen-induced liver disease. In: Kaplowitz N, DeLeve LD, eds. Drug-Induced Liver Disease. New York and Basel, Marcel Dekker, 2002.

61. Roberts SA, Price VF, Jollow DJ. Acetaminophen structure-toxicity studies: in vivo covalent binding of a nonhepatotoxic analog, 3-hydroxyacetanilide. Toxicol Appl Pharmacol 1990;105:195–208.
62. Bailly-Maitre B, de Sousa G, Zucchini N, Gugenheim J, Boulukos KE, Rahmani R. Spontaneous apoptosis in primary cultures of human and rat hepatocytes: molecular mechanisms and regulation by dexamethasone. Cell Death Differ 2002;9: 945–955.
63. Bailly-Maitre B, de Sousa G, Boulukos K, Gugenheim J, Rahmani R. Dexamethasone inhibits spontaneous apoptosis in primary cultures of human and rat hepatocytes via Bcl-2 and Bcl-xL induction. Cell Death Differ 2001;8:279–288.
64. Frank S, Gaume B, Bergmann-Leitner ES, et al. The role of dynamin-related protein 1, a mediator of mitochondrial fission, in apoptosis. Dev Cell 2001;1:515–525.
65. Karbowski M, Youle RJ. Dynamics of mitochondrial morphology in healthy cells and during apoptosis. Cell Death Differ 2003;10:870–880.
66. Karbowski M, Lee YJ, Gaume B, et al. Spatial and temporal association of Bax with mitochondrial fission sites, Drp1, and Mfn2 during apoptosis. J Cell Biol 2002;159:931–938.
67. Breckenridge DG, Stojanovic M, Marcellus RC, Shore GC. Caspase cleavage product of BAP31 induces mitochondrial fission through endoplasmic reticulum calcium signals, enhancing cytochrome c release to the cytosol. J Cell Biol 2003; 160:1115–1127.
68. Haouzi D, Cohen I, Vieira HL, et al. Mitochondrial permeability transition as a novel principle of hepatorenal toxicity in vivo. Apoptosis 2002;7:395–405.
69. Ma Y, Hendershot LM. The unfolding tale of the unfolded protein response. Cell 2001;107:827–830.
70. Kaufman RJ. Stress signaling from the lumen of the endoplasmic reticulum: coordination of gene transcriptional and translational controls. Genes Dev 1999;13:1211–1233.
71. Klionsky DJ, Emr SD. Autophagy as a regulated pathway of cellular degradation. Science 2000;290:1717–1721.
72. Newmeyer DD, Ferguson-Miller S. Mitochondria: releasing power for life and unleashing the machineries of death. Cell 2003;112:481–490.
73. Marchetti P, Castedo M, Susin SA, et al. Mitochondrial permeability transition is a central coordinating event of apoptosis. J Exp Med 1996;184:1155–1160.
74. Wei MC, Zong WX, Cheng EH, et al. Proapoptotic BAX and BAK: a requisite gateway to mitochondrial dysfunction and death. Science 2001;292:727–730.
75. Borner C. The Bcl-2 protein family: sensors and checkpoints for life-or-death decisions. Mol Immunol 2003;39:615–647.
76. Cory S, Adams JM. The Bcl2 family: regulators of the cellular life-or-death switch. Nat Rev Cancer 2002;2:647–656.
77. Gross A, McDonnell JM, Korsmeyer SJ. BCL-2 family members and the mitochondria in apoptosis. Genes Dev 1999;13:1899–1911.
78. El-Hassan H, Anwar K, Macanas-Pirard P, et al. Involvement of mitochondria in acetaminophen-induced apoptosis and hepatic injury: roles of cytochrome *c*, Bax, Bid. and caspases. Toxicol Appl Pharmacol 2003;191:118–129.

79. Guo B, Zhai D, Cabezas E, et al. Humanin peptide suppresses apoptosis by interfering with Bax activation. Nature 2003;423:456–461.
80. Chandrasekharan NV, Dai H, Roos KL, et al. COX-3, a cyclooxygenase-1 variant inhibited by acetaminophen and other analgesic/antipyretic drugs: cloning, structure, and expression. Proc Natl Acad Sci USA 2002;99:13926–13931.
81. Reilly TP, Brady JN, Marchick MR, et al. A protective role for cyclooxygenase-2 in drug-induced liver injury in mice. Chem Res Toxicol 2001;14:1620–1628.
82. Masubuchi Y, Bourdi M, Reilly TP, Graf ML, George JW, Pohl LR. Role of interleukin-6 in hepatic heat shock protein expression and protection against acetaminophen-induced liver disease. Biochem Biophys Res Commun 2003;304: 207–212.
83. Chiu H, Gardner CR, Dambach DM, et al. Role of p55 tumor necrosis factor receptor 1 in acetaminophen-induced antioxidant defense. Am J Physiol 2003;285: G959–G966.
84. Gardner CR, Laskin JD, Dambach DM, et al. Reduced hepatotoxicity of acetaminophen in mice lacking inducible nitric oxide synthase: potential role of tumor necrosis factor-alpha and interleukin-10. Toxicol Appl Pharmacol 2002;184:27–36.
85. Liu J, Li C, Waalkes MP, Myers P, Saavedra JE, Keefer LK. The nitric oxide donor, V-PYRRO/NO, protects against acetaminophen-induced hepatotoxicity in mice. Hepatology 2003;37:324–333.
86. Ju C, Reilly TP, Bourdi M, et al. Protective role of Kupffer cells in acetaminophen-induced hepatic injury in mice. Chem Res Toxicol 2002;15:1504–1513.
87. Dambach DM, Watson LM, Gray KR, Durham SK, Laskin DL. Role of CCR2 in macrophage migration into the liver during acetaminophen-induced hepatotoxicity in the mouse. Hepatology 2002;35:1093–1103.
88. Hogaboam CM, Bone-Larson CL, Steinhauser ML, et al. Exaggerated hepatic injury due to acetaminophen challenge in mice lacking C-C chemokine receptor 2. Am J Pathol 2000;156:1245–1252.
89. Michael SL, Mayeux PR, Bucci TJ, et al. Acetaminophen-induced hepatotoxicity in mice lacking inducible nitric oxide synthase activity. Nitric Oxide 2001;5:432–441.
90. Gardner CR, Heck DE, Yang CS, et al. Role of nitric oxide in acetaminophen-induced hepatotoxicity in the rat. Hepatology 1998;27:748–754.
91. Fiorucci S, Antonelli E, Mencarelli A, et al. A NO-releasing derivative of acetaminophen spares the liver by acting at several checkpoints in the Fas pathway. Br J Pharmacol 2002;135:589–599.
92. Hinson JA, Bucci TJ, Irwin LK, Michael SL, Mayeux PR. Effect of inhibitors of nitric oxide synthase on acetaminophen-induced hepatotoxicity in mice. Nitric Oxide 2002;6:160–167.
93. James LP, McCullough SS, Lamps LW, Hinson JA. Effect of N-acetylcysteine on acetaminophen toxicity in mice: relationship to reactive nitrogen and cytokine formation. Toxicol Sci 2003; 75:458–467.
94. Hinson JA, Michael SL, Ault SG, Pumford NR. Western blot analysis for nitrotyrosine protein adducts in livers of saline-treated and acetaminophen-treated mice. Toxicol Sci 2000;53:467–473.

95. Laskin DL, Laskin JD. Role of macrophages and inflammatory mediators in chemically induced toxicity. Toxicology 2001;160:111–118.
96. Laskin DL, Pendino KJ. Macrophages and inflammatory mediators in tissue injury. Annu Rev Pharmacol Toxicol 1995;35:655–677.
97. Goldin RD, Ratnayaka ID, Breach CS, Brown IN, Wickramasinghe SN. Role of macrophages in acetaminophen (paracetamol)-induced hepatotoxicity. J Pathol 1996;179:432–435.
98. Michael SL, Pumford NR, Mayeux PR, Niesman MR, Hinson JA. Pretreatment of mice with macrophage inactivators decreases acetaminophen hepatotoxicity and the formation of reactive oxygen and nitrogen species. Hepatology 1999;30:186–195.
99. Futter LE, al-Swayeh OA, Moore PK. A comparison of the effect of nitroparacetamol and paracetamol on liver injury. Br J Pharmacol 2001;132:10–12.
100. Keeble JE, Moore PK. Pharmacology and potential therapeutic applications of nitric oxide-releasing non-steroidal anti-inflammatory and related nitric oxide-donating drugs. Br J Pharmacol 2002;137:295–310.
101. al-Swayeh OA, Futter LE, Clifford RH, Moore PK. Nitroparacetamol exhibits anti-inflammatory and anti-nociceptive activity. Br J Pharmacol 2000;130:1453–1456.
102. Knight TR, Kurtz A, Bajt ML, Hinson JA, Jaeschke H. Vascular and hepatocellular peroxynitrite formation during acetaminophen toxicity: role of mitochondrial oxidant stress. Toxicol Sci 2001;62:212–220.
103. Bourdi M, Masubuchi Y, Reilly TP, et al. Protection against acetaminophen-induced liver injury and lethality by interleukin 10: role of inducible nitric oxide synthase. Hepatology 2002;35:289–298.
104. Knight TR, Ho Y-S, Farwood A, Jaeschke H. Peroxynitrite is a critical mediator of acetaminophen hepatotoxicity in murine livers: protection. J Pharmacol Exp Ther 2002;303:468–475.
105. Saavedra JE, Billiar TR, Williams DL, Kim YM, Watkins SC, Keefer LK. Targeting nitric oxide (NO) delivery in vivo. Design of a liver-selective NO donor prodrug that blocks tumor necrosis factor-α-induced apoptosis and toxicity in the liver. J Med Chem 1997;40:1947–1954.
106. Zhang H, Cook J, Nickel J, et al. Reduction of liver Fas expression by an antisense oligonucleotide protects mice from fulminant hepatitis. Nat Biotechnol 2000;18:862–867.
107. Jaeschke H, Knight TR, Bajt ML. The role of oxidant stress and reactive species in acetaminophen hepatotoxicity. Toxicol Lett 2003;144:279–288.
108. Lawson JA, Fisher MA, Simmons CA, Farhood A, Jaeschke H. Inhibition of Fas receptor (CD95)-induced hepatic caspase activation and apoptosis by acetaminophen in mice. Toxicol Appl Pharmacol 1999;156:179–186.
109. Karin M, Lin A. NF-κB at the crossroads of life and death. Nat Immunol 2002;3:221–227.
110. Taylor BS, Alarcon LH, Billiar TR. Inducible nitric oxide synthase in the liver: regulation and function. Biochemistry (Moscow) 1998;63:766–781.
111. Ghosh S, Karin M. Missing pieces in the NF-κB puzzle. Cell 2002;109(Suppl): S81–S96.

112. Boulares AH, Giardina C, Inan MS, Khairallah EA, Cohen SD. Acetaminophen inhibits NF-κB activation by interfering with the oxidant signal in murine Hepa 1-6 cells. Toxicol Sci 2000;55:370–375.
113. Shankar K, Vaidya VS, Corton JC, et al. Activation of PPAR-α in streptozotocin-induced diabetes is essential for resistance against acetaminophen toxicity. FASEB J 2003;17:1748–1750.
114. Blazka ME, Germolec DR, Simeonova P, Bruccoleri A, Pennypacker KR, Luster MI. Acetaminophen-induced hepatotoxicity is associated with early changes in NF-κB and NF-IL6 DNA binding activity. J Inflamm 1995;47:138–150.
115. Zaher H, Buters JT, Ward JM, et al. Protection against acetaminophen toxicity in CYP1A2 and CYP2E1 double-null mice. Toxicol Appl Pharmacol 1998;152:193–199.
116. Tonge RP, Kelly EJ, Bruschi SA, et al. Role of CYP1A2 in the hepatotoxicity of acetaminophen: investigations using Cyp1a2 null mice. Toxicol Appl Pharmacol 1998;153:102–108.
117. Lee SS, Buters JT, Pineau T, Fernandez-Salguero P, Gonzalez FJ. Role of CYP2E1 in the hepatotoxicity of acetaminophen. J Biol Chem 1996;271:12063–12067.
118. Zhang J, Huang W, Chua SS, Wei P, Moore DD. Modulation of acetaminophen-induced hepatotoxicity by the xenobiotic receptor CAR. Science 2002;298:422–424.
119. Gonzalez FJ, Kimura S. Study of P450 function using gene knockout and transgenic mice. Arch Biochem Biophys 2003;409:153–158.
120. Wei P, Zhang J, Egan-Hafley M, Liang S, Moore DD. The nuclear receptor CAR mediates specific xenobiotic induction of drug metabolism. Nature 2000;407:920–923.
121. Gerbal-Chaloin S, Daujat M, Pascussi JM, Pichard-Garcia L, Vilarem MJ, Maurel P. Transcriptional regulation of CYP2C9 gene. Role of glucocorticoid receptor and constitutive androstane receptor. J Biol Chem 2002;277:209–217.
122. Rosenfeld JM, Vargas R, Xie W, Evans RM. Genetic profiling defines the xenobiotic gene network controlled by the nuclear receptor pregnane X receptor. Mol Endocrinol 2003;17:1268–1282.
123. Maglich JM, Parks DJ, Moore LB, et al. Identification of a novel human constitutive androstane receptor (CAR) agonist and its use in the identification of CAR target genes. J Biol Chem 2003;278:17277–17283.
124. Moore LB, Parks DJ, Jones SA, et al. Orphan nuclear receptors constitutive androstane receptor and pregnane X receptor share xenobiotic and steroid ligands. J Biol Chem 2000;275:15122–15127.
125. Moore JT, Moore LB, Maglich JM, Kliewer SA. Functional and structural comparison of PXR and CAR. Biochim Biophys Acta 2003;1619:235–238.
126. Forman BM, Tzameli I, Choi H-S, et al. Androstane metabolites bind to and deactivate the nuclear receptor CAR-β. Nature 1998;395:612–615.
127. Nicholls-Grzemski FA, Calder IC, Priestly BG. Peroxisome proliferators protect against paracetamol hepatotoxicity in mice. Biochem Pharmacol 1992;43:1395–1396.

128. Manautou JE, Emeigh Hart SG, Khairallah EA, Cohen SD. Protection against acetaminophen hepatotoxicity by a single dose of clofibrate: effects on selective protein arylation and glutathione depletion. Fundam Appl Toxicol 1996;29:229–237.
129. Chen C, Hennig GE, Whiteley HE, Corton JC, Manautou JE. Peroxisome proliferator-activated receptor α-null mice lack resistance to acetaminophen hepatotoxicity following clofibrate exposure. Toxicol Sci 2000;57:338–344.
130. Henderson CJ, Wolf CR, Kitteringham N, Powell H, Otto D, Park BK. Increased resistance to acetaminophen hepatotoxicity in mice lacking glutathione S-transferase Pi. Proc Natl Acad Sci USA 2000;97:12741–12745.
131. Mirochnitchenko O, Weisbrot-Lefkowitz M, Reuhl K, Chen L, Yang C, Inouye M. Acetaminophen toxicity. Opposite effects of two forms of glutathione peroxidase. J Biol Chem 1999;274:10349–10355.
132. Bartolone JB, Birge RB, Bulera SJ, et al. Purification, antibody production, and partial amino acid sequence of the 58-kDa acetaminophen-binding liver proteins. Toxicol Appl Pharmacol 1992;113:19–29.
133. Porat A, Sagiv Y, Elazar Z. A 56-kDa selenium-binding protein participates in intra-Golgi protein transport. J Biol Chem 2000;275:14457–14465.
134. Elsby R, Kitteringham NR, Goldring CE, et al. Increased constitutive c-Jun N-terminal kinase signaling in mice lacking glutathione S-transferase Pi. J Biol Chem 2003;278:22243–22249.
135. Wolf CR. The Gerhard Zbinden memorial lecture: application of biochemical and genetic approaches to understanding pathways of chemical toxicity. Toxicol Lett 2002;127:3–17.
136. Chen YR, Wang X, Templeton D, Davis RJ, Tan TH. The role of c-Jun N-terminal kinase (JNK) in apoptosis induced by ultraviolet C and gamma radiation. Duration of JNK activation may determine cell death and proliferation. J Biol Chem 1996;271:31929–31936.
137. Tournier C, Hess P, Yang DD, et al. Requirement of JNK for stress-induced activation of the cytochrome c-mediated death pathway. Science 2000;288:870–874.
138. Huang S, Shu L, Dilling MB, Easton J, Harwood FC, Ichijo H, Houghton PJ. Sustained activation of the JNK cascade and rapamycin-induced apoptosis are suppressed by p53/p21(Cip1). Mol Cell 2003;11:1491–1501.
139. Rzucidlo SJ, Bounous DI, Jones DP, Brackett BG. Acute acetaminophen toxicity in transgenic mice with elevated hepatic glutathione. Vet Hum Toxicol 2000;42:146–150.
140. Tuschl T. Expanding small RNA interference. Nat Biotechnol 2002;20:446–448.
141. Elbashir SM, Harborth J, Lendeckel W, Yalcin A, Weber K, Tuschl T. Duplexes of 21-nucleotide RNAs mediate RNA interference in cultured mammalian cells. Nature 2001;411:494–498.
142. Caplen NJ, Parrish S, Imani F, Fire A, Morgan RA. Specific inhibition of gene expression by small double-stranded RNAs in invertebrate and vertebrate systems. Proc Natl Acad Sci USA 2001;98:9742–9747.
143. Brummelkamp TR, Bernards R, Agami R. A system for stable expression of short interfering RNAs in mammalian cells. Science 2002;296:550–553.

144. Yu JY, DeRuiter SL, Turner DL. RNA interference by expression of short-interfering RNAs and hairpin RNAs in mammalian cells. Proc Natl Acad Sci USA 2002;99:6047–6052.
145. Zender L, Hutker S, Liedtke C, et al. Caspase 8 small interfering RNA prevents acute liver failure in mice. Proc Natl Acad Sci USA 2003;100:7797–7802.
146. Ulrich R, Friend SH. Toxicogenomics and drug discovery: will new technologies help us produce better drugs? Nat Rev Drug Disc 2002;1:84–88.
147. Reilly TP, Bourdi M, Brady JN, et al. Expression profiling of acetaminophen liver toxicity in mice using microarray technology. Biochem Biophys Res Commun 2001;282:321–328.
148. De Longueville F, Atienzar FA, Marcq L, et al. Use of a low-density microarray for studying gene expression patterns induced by hepatotoxicants on primary cultures of rat hepatocytes. Toxicol Sci 2003;75:378–392.
149. Cunningham MJ, Liang S, Fuhrman S, Seilhamer JJ, Somogyi R. Gene expression microarray data analysis for toxicology profiling. Ann NY Acad Sci 2000;919:52–67.
150. Gore MA, Morshedi MM, Reidhaar-Olson JF. Gene expression changes associated with cytotoxicity identified using cDNA arrays. Funct Integr Genomics 2000;1:114–126.
151. El-Hassan H, Anwar K, Macanas-Pirard P, et al. Involvement of mitochondria in acetaminophen-induced apoptosis and hepatic injury. Roles of cytochrome c, Bax, Bid, and caspases. Toxicol Appl Pharmacol 2003;191:118–129.
152. Dietze EC, Schafer A, Omichinski JG, Nelson SD. Inactivation of glyceraldehyde-3-phosphate dehydrogenase by a reactive metabolite of acetaminophen and mass spectral characterization of an arylated active site peptide. Chem Res Toxicol 1997;10:1097–1103.
153. Myers TG, Dietz EC, Anderson NL, Khairallah EA, Cohen SD, Nelson SD. A comparative study of mouse liver proteins arylated by reactive metabolites of acetaminophen and its nonhepatotoxic regioisomer, 3'-hydroxyacetanilide. Chem Res Toxicol 1995;8:403–413.
154. Fountoulakis M, Berndt P, Boelsterli UA, et al. Two-dimensional database of mouse liver proteins: changes in hepatic protein levels following treatment with acetaminophen or its nontoxic regioisomer 3-acetamidophenol. Electrophoresis 2000;21:2148–2161.
155. Qiu Y, Benet LZ, Burlingame AL. Identification of hepatic protein targets of the reactive metabolites of the non-hepatotoxic regioisomer of acetaminophen, 3'-hydroxyacetanilide, in the mouse in vivo using two-dimensional gel electrophoresis and mass spectrometry. Adv Exp Med Biol 2001;500:663–673.
156. Kitteringham NR, Powell H, Jenkins RE, et al. Protein expression profiling of glutathione S-transferase pi null mice as a strategy to identify potential markers of resistance to paracetamol-induced toxicity in the liver. Proteomics 2003;3:191–207.
157. Patterson SD, Aebersold RH. Proteomics: the first decade and beyond. Nat Genet 2003;33(Suppl):311–323.

158. Smolka MB, Zhou H, Purkayastha S, Aebersold R. Optimization of the isotope-coded affinity tag-labeling procedure for quantitative proteome analysis. Anal Biochem 2001;297:25–31.
159. Gygi SP, Rist B, Gerber SA, Turecek F, Gelb MH, Aebersold R. Quantitative analysis of complex protein mixtures using isotope-coded affinity tags. Nat Biotechnol 1999;17:994–999.
160. Ku NO, Michie SA, Soetikno RM, et al. Susceptibility to hepatotoxicity in transgenic mice that express a dominant-negative human keratin 18 mutant. J Clin Invest 1996;98:1034–1046.
161. Liu J, Liu Y, Hartley D, Klaassen CD, Shehin-Johnson SE, Lucas A, Cohen SD. Metallothionein-I/II knockout mice are sensitive to acetaminophen-induced hepatotoxicity. J Pharmacol Exp Ther 1999;289:580–586.
162. Rofe AM, Barry EF, Shelton TL, Philcox JC, Coyle P. Paracetamol hepatotoxicity in metallothionein-null mice. Toxicology 1998;125:131–140.
163. Enomoto A, Itoh K, Nagayoshi E, et al. High sensitivity of Nrf2 knockout mice to acetaminophen hepatotoxicity associated with decreased expression of ARE-regulated drug metabolizing enzymes and antioxidant genes. Toxicol Sci 2001;59:169–177.
164. Lee JM, Calkins MJ, Chan K, Kan YW, Johnson JA. Identification of the NF-E2-related factor-2-dependent genes conferring protection against oxidative stress in primary cortical astrocytes using oligonucleotide microarray analysis. J Biol Chem 2003;278:12029–12038.
165. Bourdi M, Reilly TP, Elkahloun AG, George JW, Pohl LR. Macrophage migration inhibitory factor in drug-induced liver injury: a role in susceptibility and stress responsiveness. Biochem Biophys Res Commun 2002;294:225–230.
166. Boess F, Bopst M, Althaus R, et al. Acetaminophen hepatotoxicity in tumor necrosis factor/lymphotoxin-alpha gene knockout mice. Hepatology 1998;27:1021–1029.

9
Modulation of Drug Metabolism and Antiviral Therapies

Bernhard H. Lauterburg

Summary

Antiviral therapies are an important, emerging area of pharmaceutical research, particularly with the advent of the AIDS epidemic and the continued existence of other virally mediated diseases. This chapter focuses on pharmacological approaches to treat these diseases and summarizes the current classes of therapeutic agents. The concept of pharmacokinetic "boosting" in enhancing the efficacy of treatment is discussed, as is the interaction potential of clinically used antiviral agents and the role of intestinal metabolism and drug transporters, particularly the multidrug resistance proteins, in the handling of these drugs. Major classes of antiviral agents that are discussed include nucleoside and nucleotide analogs, other reverse-transcriptase inhibitors, protease inhibitors, fusion inhibitors, and interferons.

Key Words

Analogs: nucleoside; analogs: nucleotide; antiviral agents; cytochrome P450; CYP2D6; CYP3A4; HIV-protease inhibitors; interferons; intestinal metabolism; transport, multidrug resistance proteins; P-glycoprotein; reverse-transcriptase: nonnucleoside inhibitors,

1. THE CONCEPT OF PHARMACOKINETIC "BOOSTING"

Inadvertent pharmacokinetic drug interactions are a frequent cause of adverse drug reactions and, therefore, of concern to the treating physician. Yet, if intended, drug interactions may also be beneficial to the patient and can be exploited to improve the response to pharmacotherapy. This is not a new concept: probenecid, for example, which inhibits the renal excretion of penicillin, has been used for many years to achieve higher plasma concentrations and a longer duration of action of the antibiotic. Drug interactions at the level of biotransformation rather than the level of renal excretion can also be exploited to improve the bioavailability and delay the elimination of drugs, as demonstrated

From: *Methods in Pharmacology and Toxicology,*
Drug Metabolism and Transport: Molecular Methods and Mechanisms
Edited by: L. Lash © Humana Press Inc., Totowa, NJ

with potent inhibitors of the cytochrome P450 (P450) system, such as ketoconazole, itraconazole, or some macrolide antibiotics *(1–4)*. The boosting effect of the co-administration of an inhibitor of drug metabolism becomes most evident with drugs subjected to an extensive first-pass metabolism. In this situation, not only is the elimination delayed, but clinically often more importantly, there is a marked increase in bioavailability that is mainly due to inhibition of intestinal metabolism and interference with intestinal transport processes rather than hepatic metabolism.

Thus, coadministration of inhibitors of drug metabolism can increase the bioavailabilty and the exposure to other drugs. However, the use of a drug that inhibits drug metabolism but has a totally different therapeutic goal than the drug of interest (the therapeutic action of which it is supposed to boost) is not really rational pharmacotherapy. Why, for example, administer an antifungal agent such as itraconazole together with an immunosuppressant such as cyclosporine just in order to be able to lower the dose of cyclosporine? A potential economic benefit may be obtained at the cost of incurring an additional risk of adverse side effects, and the regimen for the patient is not simplified; at best it saves him or his insurance company some money.

There was renewed enthusiasm for the concept of deliberate inhibition of drug metabolism when it was observed that grapefruit juice can inhibit the intestinal biotransformation and transport of some compounds and markedly increase their bioavailability *(5)*. Grapefruit juice as a natural compound is acceptable to most patients; it is inexpensive and no significant adverse effects are to be expected. Unfortunately, the effect is quite variable from patient to patient and from batch to batch of juice, so that the boosting effect is not reproducible and this approach has not found any widespread clinical application.

This has changed with the advent of novel treatment regimens for human immunodeficiency virus (HIV) infection. Because patients with HIV infection often require several drugs for the treatment of associated problems, one soon became aware of the potent in vivo inhibitory and inducing effects on drug metabolism of some of the new antiviral compounds. It also became evident that combinations of drugs with different modes of action were required for successful treatment of the infection. In the case of HIV therapy, the concept of boosting is, therefore, much more attractive because the two or more interacting drugs all serve the same purpose, that is, inhibiting viral replication, and act synergistically toward the same therapeutic goal. Because two or more drugs are needed for therapeutic success in any event, there is no additional risk of boosting drug combinations for adverse effects. Thus, the co-administration of an HIV protease inhibitor with another protease inhibitor that is a potent inhibitor of P450 in often subtherapeutic doses has found widespread clinical application and results in marked increases in systemic exposure to active drugs. The drug combinations are not necessarily less expensive, but they are effective and may greatly simplify the otherwise quite complicated regimen for the patient and thereby improve compliance and finally therapeutic success.

2. INTERACTION POTENTIAL OF CLINICALLY USED ANTIVIRAL AGENTS

Until nonnucleoside antiretroviral agents and protease inhibitors became available, drugs for the treatment of viral infections were more or less limited to nucleoside analogs that interfered with viral replication. These compounds are generally not dependent on P450 for metabolism to a significant extent and therefore are not associated with clinically relevant drug interactions. This changed with the development of newer drugs used in the treatment of HIV infection (Table 1). All protease inhibitors and nonnucleoside reverse transcriptase inhibitors are substrates and in part potent inhibitors and/or inducers of the P450 system. Interactions among themselves and other drugs are therefore common and are actually exploited to improve current treatment schedules of HIV infection *(6)*.

3. NUCLEOSIDE ANALOGS

Nucleoside analogs are not substrates for P450 to a significant extent. They are, however, substrates of various transporters that will influence their renal excretion and their distribution in the organism, in particular their passage through the blood–brain barrier. They may inhibit the elimination of other drugs by interfering with these transport processes or indirectly by inhibiting mitochondrial function.

The nucleoside reverse transcriptase inhibitors zidovudine, didanosine, lamivudine, zalcitabine, and sanilvudine do not inhibit the transport of model compounds by P-glycoprotein *(7)*. They are, however, substrates for MRP4 *(8)* and organic anion transporters that will in part determine their rate of renal excretion and their distribution across the blood–brain barrier *(9,10)*. Overexpression and amplification of the MRP4 gene correlates with ATP-dependent efflux of azidothymidine monophosphate from cells and impairs the antiviral efficacy of azidothymidine and other nucleoside analogs *(8)*. Tubular secretion of some of the compounds may be impaired by the concomitant administration of probenecid or trimethoprim that are competitive inhibitors of renal tubular-secretion. Probenecid increases the plasma concentrations of acyclovir, and trimethoprim–sulfamethoxazole increases the plasma concentrations of lamivu-

Table 1
Cytochrome P450 and Antiviral Drugs

Substrates for cytochrome P450 isozymes

1A2	2B6	2C19	2C9	2D6	2E1	3A4,5,7
	Efavirenz	Nelfinavir				Indinavir
						Nelfinavir
						Ritonavir
						Saquinavir

Inhibitors of cytochrome P450 isozymes

1A2	2B6	2C19	2C9	2D6	2E1	3A4,5,7
Interferon				Ritonavir		Delaviridine
						Indinavir
						Nelfinavir
						Ritonavir
						Saquinavir

Inducers of cytochrome P450 isozymes

1A2	2B6	2C19	2C9	2D6	2E1	3A4,5,7
						Efavirenz
						Nevirapine

dine *(11–13)*. Both of these interactions are not clinically important and do not require dose adjustment. Probenecid also inhibits the glucuronidation of zidovudine and increases its plasma concentrations. The clinical importance of this increase is unknown.

Nucleoside analogs are phosphorylated to the active triphosphates, which inhibit reverse transcription in the case of HIV infection or replication of viral DNA. They may interact with drugs that compete for the same intracellular activation pathway. Ribavirin, for example, decreases the phosphorylation of zidovudine and stavudine in vitro, resulting in decreased concentrations of the active compound *(14)*. Zidovudine in turn may impair the intracellular phosphorylation of stavudine, and lamivudine inhibits the phosphorylation of zalcitabine *(15–17)*.

Other intracellular interactions may increase the activity of nucleoside reverse-transcriptase inhibitors. Hydroxyurea, an inhibitor of the enzyme ribonucleotide reductase, which is involved in the formation of deoxynucleotides, increases the antiviral action of didanosine *(18)*. One possible mechanism for this effect involves a decrease in the intracellular pool of 2′-deoxyadenosine-5′-triphosphate (dATP), which competes with 2′,3′-dideoxyadenosine-5′-triphosphate (ddATP), the active metabolite of didanosine, for incorporation into viral DNA. As a result, the intracellular ratio of ddATP to dATP is increased, improving the antiviral potency of didanosine. However, the long-term clinical benefits of hydroxyurea-containing combinations are unclear, because hydroxyurea blunts the increase in CD4 cells that occurs in response to antiretroviral therapy and has numerous adverse effects, including hepatitis, pancreatitis, and bone marrow toxicity.

Antiviral nucleoside analogs can impair mitochondrial function and will then indirectly impair the metabolism of other drugs. The first example of drug-induced mitochondrial dysfunction was fialuridine, which was studied in the treatment of hepatitis B. The compound has a preserved 3′-hydroxyl group and is incorporated into and persists in mitochondrial DNA. It has led to lactic acidosis, microvesicular steatosis, and hepatic failure *(19–21)*. The reverse transcriptase inhibitors used in the treatment of HIV infection, such as lamivudine, abacavir, and tenofovir, are chain terminators; deplete mtDNA to a lesser extent, and are less likely to disturb mitochondrial function. Nevertheless, nucleoside-analog reverse transcriptase inhibitors can result in mitochondrial dysfunction in HIV-infected patients. The most plausible explanation for this adverse effect is that nucleoside analogs inhibit mitochondrial DNA (mtDNA) polymerase and thereby impair mitochondrial function, resulting in lactic acidosis, hepatic steatosis, and occasionally hepatic failure *(22)*. These mechanisms include inhibition of specific enzymes in the tricarboxylic acid cycle and electron transport chain as well as inhibition of mitochondrial adenylate kinase and the ADP/ATP translocase. Alternate mechanisms for modification of mitochondrial DNA by nucleoside-analog reverse transcriptase inhibitors may involve the generation of reactive oxygen species. Exposure of cultured human lymphoid cell lines to clinically relevant concentrations of zidovudine depletes glutathione and increases mtDNA damage, effects that are prevented by *N*-acetylcysteine *(23)*.

4. NUCLEOTIDE ANALOGS

Adefovir and cidovofir are renally excreted and their excretion is inhibited by probenecid, which also reduces their nephrotoxicity *(24)*.

5. NONNUCLEOSIDE REVERSE TRANSCRIPTASE INHIBITORS

Nonnucleoside reverse-transcriptase inhibitors are structurally heterogenous. They are substrates of P450 and can inhibit or induce P450 activity *(25)*. Nevirapine and efavirenz are weak inducers of CYP3A4. They reduce the plasma concentrations of methadone by about 50% and can lead to opiate withdrawal symptoms in patients on methadone *(26–28)*. Nevirapine also decreases the plasma concentrations of indinavir and saquinavir. It does not, however, affect the pharmacokinetics of nelfinavir and ritonavir in a clinically relevant way. The latter drugs are not exclusively metabolized by CYP3A4. Moreover, they induce their own metabolism such that further induction may not become clinically evident. Nevirapine decreases the area under the plasma concentration time curve (AUC) of indinavir by approx 50% *(29)*. Efavirenz induces CYP3A4 activity but inhibits the activity of other P450 isoforms. It decreases the plasma concentrations of indinavir, lopinavir, saquinavir, and amprenavir, but increases the plasma concentrations of ritonavir and nelfinavir possibly through inhibition of CYP2C9 or CYP2C19 *(30)*. Effects of efavirenz on the plasma concentration of, for example, saquinavir can be counterbalanced by the administration of ritonavir *(31)*.

Delavirdine is a potent inhibitor of CYP3A4 and serious toxic effects may occur if it is administered with calcium-channel blockers, sedative or hypnotic drugs, antiarrhythmic drugs, or quinidine *(32)*. The administration of delavirdine with vasoconstrictor drugs such as ergotamine can lead to peripheral ischemia and can increase the toxicity of certain chemotherapeutic drugs, such as etoposide and paclitaxel. Delavirdine will also increase the plasma concentrations of protease inhibitors *(33,34)*.

6. HIV PROTEASE INHIBITORS

All of the available HIV protease inhibitors are characterized by low and variable bioavailability and by a relatively short plasma half-life, which requires frequent dosing to keep the plasma concentrations of the drug above effective inhibiting concentrations. They are extensively metabolized by P450 and are substrates for drug transporters. Many of this class of compounds such as ritonavir and nelfinavir are not only substrates for P450 but are at the same time inhibitors and/or inducers of P450 and each of these drugs may alter the metabolism of other antiretroviral and concomitantly administered drugs. The principal enzyme involved is CYP3A4, but other P450 enzymes, such as CYP2D6, may contribute as in the case of nelfinavir and ritonavir.

Ritonavir is principally metabolized by CYP3A4, with a minor contribution from CYP2D6 *(35)*. Ritonavir is a potent inhibitor of CYP3A4 *(36)* and inhibits the metabolism of indinavir and other HIV-protease inhibitors *(37,38)*. The potent inhibitory effect of ritonavir is associated with its metabolism and probably attributable to formation of reactive intermediates that inactivate CYP3A, possibly a fragment containing the 2-(1-methylethyl)thiazolyl group *(39)*. Other P450 enzymes and glucuronosyltransferases do not appear to be important in metabolism in humans. Ritonavir is a potent inhibitor of CYP3A4 and, to a lesser extent, CYP2D6. In addition to inhibiting P450 enzymes, ritonavir has enzyme-inducing properties, even inducing its own metabolism in a dose-dependent manner during the first 14 d of therapy *(40)*. Ritonavir partly offsets the enzyme-inducing effects of efavirenz and nevirapine. Nevertheless, addition of efavirenz or nevirapine to a combination of indinavir and ritonavir decreased the steady state concentration of indinavir by approx 50% *(41)*. Ritonavir decreases the plasma concentrations of theophylline, probably through the induction of CYP1A2. Contrary to the expectations based on in vitro data, the combination of ritonavir and saquinavir increases the clearance of methadone in humans, probably owing to displacement of methadone from plasma protein-binding sites and owing to induction of the metabolism of primarily the inactive *S*-methadone by inducing CYP2B6 *(42)*. Ritonavir and nelfinavir also increase glucuronosyltransferase activity, which may partly explain the substantial decreases in plasma ethinyl estradiol concentrations during concurrent therapy with these protease inhibitors *(43)*.

Saquinavir undergoes extensive first-pass gastrointestinal and hepatic metabolism, primarily by CYP3A4. Therefore, the oral bioavailability amounts to only about 4% and is highly susceptible to inhibition of CYP3A4 by other drugs, such as ritonavir *(37,44)* (Fig. 1).

Indinavir is extensively metabolized by CYP3A *(45)*. Seven metabolites have been identified, one glucuronide conjugate and six oxidative metabolites, after incubation with human liver microsomes. Experiments with recombinant P450 enzymes show that CYP3A4 produces most of the metabolites and that CYP2D6 can produce three of the metabolites, as well as a *cis*-diol—a metabolite that is not observed in vivo. *O*- and *N*-Glucuronidation are minor routes of elimination for indinavir and nelfinavir. Inhibition of CYP3A4 by ritonavir markedly increases the plasma concentration of indinavir *(38)*.

Nelfinavir is principally metabolized by CYP3A4 and CYP2C19 *(46)*. Therefore, its plasma concentration does not increase markedly when administered in combination with ritonavir *(47)*. In vitro experiments with various substrates indicate that nelfinavir can inhibit CYP3A, with little effects on the other P450 enzymes. However, although nelfinavir is an inhibitor of CYP3A4 and reportedly decreases the plasma concentrations of phenytoin, probably through the induction of its CYP2C9-mediated metabolism, nelfinavir is reported to have no effect on the disposition of nucleoside reverse transcriptase inhibitors, such as lamivudine and ddI.

Lopinavir inhibits CYP3A consistent with mechanism-based inhibition *(48)*.

Amprenavir inhibits CYP3A4 and 2C19 in human liver microsomes. A comparative study with other protease inhibitors in human liver microsomes shows the following rank order of P450 inhibition: ritonavir >> indinavir > nelfinavir > amprenavir > saquinavir.

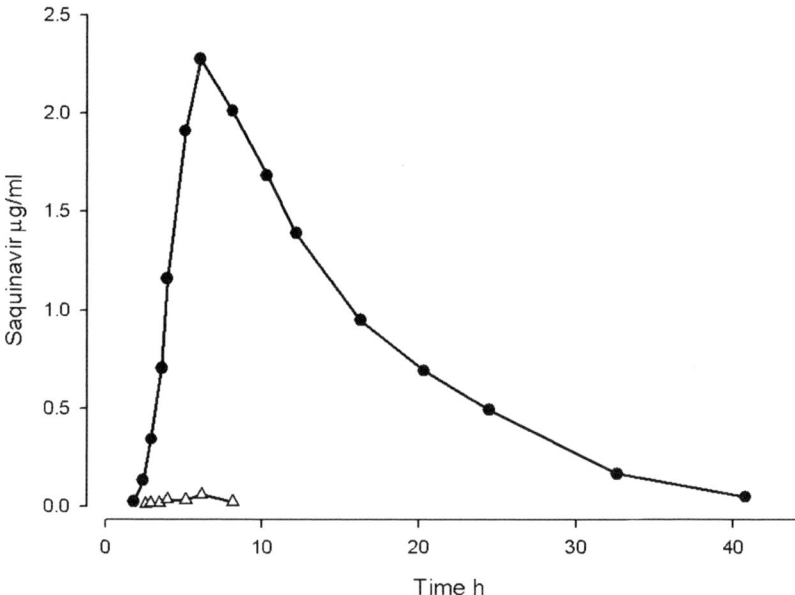

Fig. 1. Average plasma concentration of saquinavir in healthy subjects after administration of 400 mg saquinavir *(open triangles)* and 400 mg of saquinavir and 600 mg of ritonavir *(closed circles)*. (Redrawn from Hsu et al. *[44]*).

7. ROLE OF INTESTINAL METABOLISM AND DRUG TRANSPORTERS

In addition to being substrates for P450, most HIV-protease inhibitors are also substrates for and inhibitors of P-glycoprotein *(49)*. P-glycoprotein is present at numerous sites in the body. Its presence in renal tubular cells and hepatocytes results in increased drug excretion in urine and bile. P-glycoprotein in the endothelial cells of the blood–brain barrier prevents the entry of certain drugs into the central nervous system *(50,51)*. Most drugs that modulate CYP3A4 activity also modulate P-glycoprotein *(52)*. Interaction of the drug with the orphan nuclear receptor SXR upregulates drug elimination by modulating the efflux of intact drug from cells mediated by P-glycoprotein and its metabolism by P450 *(53)*. This signaling system protects the body from exposure to toxic compounds; however, it can also pose a severe barrier to drug therapy. The HIV-protease inhibitor ritonavir binds to SXR and activates its target genes. Other protease inhibitors are weaker (saquinavir) or unable to activate SXR (nelfinavir, indinavir). Interestingly, HIV-protease inhibitors are distinct from previously known SXR ligands in that they are peptide mimetic compounds. SXR ligands can also activate expression of multidrug resistance protein 2 (MRP2), a critical regulator of bile flow and biliary drug excretion *(54)*.

Ritonavir and saquinavir are both substrates for an efflux mechanism in the gut, most likely P-glycoprotein *(55)*. Ritonavir and to a lesser extent saquinavir inhibit the export of model substrates for P-glycoprotein and MRP2 *(56)*. Ritonavir is the most potent inhibitor *(57)*. Nevertheless, even in the presence of ritonavir, P-glycoprotein still limits the oral bioavailability of saquinavir and its penetration into brain and the fetus in vivo, as demonstrated in P-glycoprotein-deficient mice *(58)*. Metabolites of indinavir, even relatively polar ones, are also substrates for P-glycoprotein *(59)*. Other transporters, such as MRP2, but not MRP1, MRP3, MRP5, or the breast cancer resistance protein 1, also efficiently transport saquinavir, ritonavir, and indinavir *(60)*.

Inhibition of intestinal P450 enzymes and P-glycoprotein will primarily affect the rate and extent of drug absorption and can markedly increase the bioavailability of concomitantly administered drugs. However, the overlap of tissue distribution and substrate specificity of CYP3A4 and P-glycoprotein makes it difficult to define the specific mechanisms of some drug interactions and predict the plasma concentrations of certain drug combinations. Moreover, findings in vitro and in experimental animals cannot be readily extrapolated to man and the involvement of CYP3A4 and P-glycoprotein in drug interactions is not always complementary. For example, plasma indinavir concentrations either do not change or are decreased by the ingestion of grapefruit juice, suggesting that the activation of P-glycoprotein may compensate for the inhibition of CYP3A4 *(61)*. In any case, the inhibition of CYP3A4, P-glycoprotein, or both in the gut wall may have a substantial effect on plasma concentrations of many anti-HIV drugs. Inhibition of P-glycoprotein will also markedly influence the distribution of protease inhibitors. Thus, ketoconazole, an inhibitor of both CYP3A4 and P-glycoprotein, causes a large increase in cerebrospinal fluid concentrations of saquinavir and ritonavir, suggesting that the inhibition of efflux transporters can be used to target therapy to the central nervous system *(62)*.

In patients exhibiting the 3435C→T polymorphism in the ABCB1 gene encoding for the multidrug resistance transporter P-glycoprotein (MDR1), the plasma concentrations of nelfinavir and efavirenz tend to be lower *(63)*. Contrary to expectation, the recovery of the CD4 cell count, however, is faster and greater in the TT genotype. If this phenomenon is not a chance association, a possible explanation may be that the polymorphism causes decreased efflux of drugs from CD4 cells.

8. FUSION INHIBITORS

The first marketed viral fusion inhibitor is enfuvirtide (T-20), a 36-amino-acid peptide derived from the HR2 sequence of a laboratory strain of HIV-1 *(64)*. The drug does not appear to affect P450 enzymes. No drug interactions have been reported so far.

9. INTERFERONS

Interferons are used primarily as antiviral agents in the treatment of hepatitis C and B. In the course of an acute viral respiratory infection, the plasma levels of interferon-α (IFN-α) and IFN-γ increase during the symptomatic interval and there is a concomitant decrease in the clearance of antipyrine *(65)*. That this may be attributable to interferon is supported by the observation that the administration of exogenous IFN-α also decreases the clearance of model compounds such as theophylline, antipyrine, and aminopyrine, but not of hexobarbitone *(66,67)*. The metabolism of substrates of CYP1A2 is also inhibited, whereas substrates of CYP2E1 are not affected *(68)*. N-Acetyltransferase 2 (NAT2) is not affected by interferon *(69)*. In some studies, an association was found between the magnitude of P450 inhibition and the occurrence of side effects of interferon, such as fever and neurological toxicity *(68)*. Elevated concentrations of C-reactive protein in serum and elevated concentrations of IL-6 in patients with cancer were found to be associated with a decreased activity of P450, as evidenced by a decreased exhalation of labeled CO_2 after administration of labeled erythromycin *(70)*. The inhibition of drug metabolism following the administration of interferon, however, is not associated with increases in serum cytokines or acute phase proteins, suggesting that the mechanism by which IFN-α inhibits P450 activities in vivo does not involve inflammatory mediators such as tumor necrosis factor (TNF), interleukin (IL)-1, or IL-6 *(66)*. On the other hand, long-term administration of interferon to patients with hepatitis C does not change the activity of CYP1A2 and CYP3A, as indicated by the metabolism of caffeine and the urinary excretion of 6-β-hydrocortisol *(71)*. The mechanisms underlying the inhibition of drug metabolism by IFN may be the downregulation of the synthesis of various cytochromes by IFN-α and -β *(72–74)*. Overall, IFN-α tends to inhibit the hepatic clearance in humans of some but not all drugs to a highly variable and clinically usually not relevant extent.

10. THERAPEUTICALLY EXPLOITED DRUG INTERACTIONS

Interactions between various drugs can be exploited to improve therapeutic response. The concept of using drug interactions to the patient's benefit has been the focus of much research *(75)*. The administration of P450 inhibitors with other drugs can reduce the pill burden, increase plasma concentrations, simplify the dosing schedule, and circumvent drug interactions. Two strategies can be pursued: the combination of two antiviral drugs, that is, two protease inhibitors, at therapeutic doses, or the combination of a protease inhibitor with a low, therapeutically ineffective but still inhibiting dose of ritonavir, the most potent P450 inhibitor of the class. The first approach is known as *dual protease inhibition*, the latter as *low-dose boosting*. Thus, ritonavir is often co-administered with saquinavir, indinavir, or amprenavir to increase their

Table 2
Clinically Relevant Interactions Between Antiviral Drugs

Interacting drugs		Consequence
Amprenavir	Lopinavir-ritonavir	AUC amprenavir ⇑
Indinavir	Ritonavir	AUC indinavir ⇑ (~ threefold)
Indinavir	Delavirdine	AUC indinavir ⇑
Indinavir	Lopinavir-ritonavir	AUC indinavir ⇑
Saquinavir	Lopinavir-ritonavir	AUC saquinavir ⇑
Saquinavir	Nelfinavir	AUC saquinavir ⇑ (~ 5- to 12-fold)
Saquinavir	Ritonavir	Steady-state concentration of saquinavir ⇑ >20-fold)
Saquinavir	Delavirdine	AUC saquinavir ⇑ (~ 5-fold)

plasma concentration *(76)* (Table 2). The co-administration of ritonavir with saquinavir increases the AUC of saquinavir up to 60-fold without affecting the AUC of ritonavir. The extent of pharmacokinetic enhancement depends markedly on the timing of the administration of potentially interacting compounds *(77)*.

The bioavailability of saquinavir is low and up to 18 capsules per day must be given to achieve effective plasma concentrations. When ritonavir is co-administered with saquinavir the steady-state plasma concentrations of saquinavir increase by a factor of 20 and the dose of saquinavir can be reduced from 1200 mg every 8 h to 400 mg twice daily, decreasing the number of saquinavir capsules that must be taken from 18 to 4 per day. Similarly, co-administration of nelfinavir increases plasma saquinavir concentrations by a factor of about 12. Another example is indinavir which must be taken every 8 h on an empty stomach or with a meal that is low in fat to achieve therapeutically effective plasma concentrations. Such a drug schedule interferes substantially with the usual lifestyle. Concomitant administration of ritonavir increases the AUC and the trough plasma concentration of indinavir approx threefold. This allows for a decrease in dosing from three times daily without food to twice daily with food. With the addition of ritonavir to a treatment schedule, even once-daily regimens are feasible and have been shown to be clinically effective *(78)*.

The reduction in plasma amprenavir or saquinavir concentrations produced by efavirenz can be circumvented by the addition of ritonavir. Plasma saquinavir concentrations are not affected by efavirenz in patients who are also taking 400 mg of ritonavir twice daily. Ritonavir partly offsets the enzyme-inducing effects of efavirenz and nevirapine. Nevertheless, addition of efavirenz or nevirapine to a combination of indinavir and ritonavir decreased the steady-state concentration of indinavir by approx 50% *(41)*. Lopinavir relies on the inhibitory effects of ritonavir that increases the AUC for lopinavir by a factor of 20 to achieve plasma concentrations above the IC_{90} value for wild-type HIV. The inhibition of CYP3A4 by nelfinavir and indinavir, for example, can be balanced by the induction of the enzymes by other drugs such as efavirenz *(79)*.

Pharmacokinetic interactions between protease inhibitors other than ritonavir are generally more modest, corresponding to their less potent CYP3A inhibition. Indinavir increases the AUC of nelfinavir by less than twofold and that of saquinavir by 7.2-fold. In turn, nelfinavir increases the AUC of indinavir by about 50% and total and peak plasma exposures of saquinavir by a factor of approx 10. Co-administration of amprenavir with indinavir results in an increase in the AUC of amprenavir of 64% with no change in indinavir AUC.

11. POTENTIALLY DELETERIOUS DRUG INTERACTIONS

Not surprisingly, HIV-protease inhibitors are associated with numerous drug interactions that may lead to serious adverse events *(80)*. Known inducers of P450 activity will decrease the concentrations of protease inhibitors and may result in inadequate repression of viral replication. This risk exists when inducing antibiotics such as rifabutin must be administered for treatment of associated infections *(81,82)*. Inhibition of CYP3A4 by protease inhibitors may increase the plasma concentrations of other drugs and lead to adverse effects *(83)*. Critical drugs are certain anti-arrhythmics, sedatives and hypnotics, ergot derivatives, and 3-hydroxy-3-methylglutaryl coenzyme A reductase inhibitors such as lovastatin and simvastatin. The extent of inhibition follows the inhibitory potency observed in vitro, ritonavir being the most potent inhibitor followed by indinavir, amprenavir, nelfinavir, and saquinavir. However, interactions between protease inhibitors and other drugs are complex and often difficult to predict from in vitro or even in vivo studies. Depending on the duration of therapy, ritonavir may either inhibit or induce the metabolism of concomitantly administered drugs *(84)*. This phenomenon results from auto-induction of certain P450 enzymes *(40)*. Although studies in hepatocytes revealed no effect of rifampin on glucuronidation of zidovudine *(85)*, rifampin-induced glucuronidation of zidovudine is evident in vivo *(86)*.

Food supplements can affect the pharmacokinetics of antiviral drugs. Garlic supplements, for example, decrease the area under the plasma concentration time curve of saquinavir under controlled conditions in healthy volunteers by approx 50% *(87)*. Grapefruit juice in turn inhibits intestinal saquinavir metabolism and increases its bioavailability *(88,89)*. However, grapefruit juice cannot be relied on to consistently increase plasma concentrations of protease inhibitors, because the variations in the amounts of flavonoids and other potentially active substances varies among products.

Table 3
Internet Sites Focusing on Interactions Among Drugs Used in the Treatment of HIV Infection

http://www.medscape.com/px/hivscheduler
http://www.hiv-druginteractions.org/index.htm
http://www.tthhivclinic.com/interact_tables.html
http://www.aidsinfo.nih.gov/
http://hivinsite.ucsf.edu/InSite?page=ar-00-02
http://medicine.iupui.edu/flockhart/

Physicochemical interactions between drugs in the intestinal lumen may alter their absorption and can result in dramatic changes in plasma drug concentrations. For example, a formulation of didanosine that contains an aluminium–magnesium antacid buffer decreases the AUC for plasma ciprofloxacin by 80% *(90)*.

The administration of several antiviral drugs as used in the treatment of HIV infection results in a complex picture owing to inhibition and induction of P450 and drug transporters. Drug combinations can result in regimens with lower and less frequent dosing, enhancing patient adherence and thus reducing the likelihood of viral breakthrough. However, the interaction potential of drug combinations is considerable and may cause serious adverse advents. Unfortunately, most formal interaction studies in vivo and in vitro evaluate only two-drug regimens and may not be relevant for multidrug regimens that are frequently used. Therefore, reports on beneficial or adverse effects of drugs due to interactions with antiviral drugs keep appearing. A number of Internet sites focus on interactions with drugs used in the therapy of HIV infection and can be consulted for up-to-date information (Table 3).

REFERENCES

1. Tsunoda SM, Velez RL, von Moltke LL, Greenblatt DJ. Differentiation of intestinal and hepatic cytochrome P450 3A activity with use of midazolam as an in vivo probe: effect of ketoconazole. Clin Pharmacol Ther 1999;66:461–471.
2. Gorski JC, Jones DR, Haehner-Daniels BD, Hamman MA, O'Mara EM, Jr, Hall SD. The contribution of intestinal and hepatic CYP3A to the interaction between midazolam and clarithromycin. Clin Pharmacol Ther 1998;64:133–143.
3. Floren LC, Bekersky I, Benet LZ, et al. Tacrolimus oral bioavailability doubles with coadministration of ketoconazole. Clin Pharmacol Ther 1997;62:41–49.
4. Neuvonen PJ, Jalava KM. Itraconazole drastically increases plasma concentrations of lovastatin and lovastatin acid. Clin Pharmacol Ther 1996;60:54–61.
5. Kane GC, Lipsky JJ. Drug-grapefruit juice interactions. Mayo Clin Proc 2000;75: 933–942.

6. Plosker G, Scott L, Saquinavir. A review of its use in boosted regimens for treating HIV infection. Drugs 2003;63:1299–1324.
7. Shiraki N, Hamada A, Yasuda K, Fujii J, Arimori K, Nakano M. Inhibitory effect of human immunodeficiency virus protease inhibitors on multidrug resistance transporter P-glycoproteins. Biol Pharm Bull 2000;23:1528–1531.
8. Schuetz JD, Connelly MC, Sun D, et al. MRP4: a previously unidentified factor in resistance to nucleoside-based antiviral drugs. Nat Med 1999;5:1048–1051.
9. Takeda M, Khamdang S, Narikawa S, et al. Human organic anion transporters and human organic cation transporters mediate renal antiviral transport. J Pharmacol Exp Ther 2002;300:918–924.
10. Gibbs JE, Thomas SA. The distribution of the anti-HIV drug, 2'3'-dideoxycytidine (ddC), across the blood-brain and blood-cerebrospinal fluid barriers and the influence of organic anion transport inhibitors. J Neurochem 2002;80:392–404.
11. De Bony F, Tod M, Bidault R, On NT, Posner J, Rolan P. Multiple interactions of cimetidine and probenecid with valaciclovir and its metabolite acyclovir. Antimicrob Agents Chemother 2002;46:458–463.
12. Laskin OL, de Miranda P, King DH, et al. Effects of probenecid on the pharmacokinetics and elimination of acyclovir in humans. Antimicrob Agents Chemother 1982;21:804–807.
13. Sabo JP, Lamson MJ, Leitz G, Yong CL, MacGregor TR. Pharmacokinetics of nevirapine and lamivudine in patients with HIV-1 infection. AAPS Pharm Sci 2000;2:E1.
14. Sim SM, Hoggard PG, Sales SD, Phiboonbanakit D, Hart CA, Back DJ. Effect of ribavirin on zidovudine efficacy and toxicity in vitro: a concentration-dependent interaction. AIDS Res Hum Retrov 1998;14:1661–1667.
15. Hoggard PG, Kewn S, Barry MG, Khoo SH, Back DJ. Effects of drugs on 2',3'-dideoxy-2',3'-didehydrothymidine phosphorylation in vitro. Antimicrob Agents Chemother 1997;41:1231–1236.
16. Kewn S, Hoggard PG, Henry-Mowatt JS, et al. Intracellular activation of 2',3'-dideoxyinosine and drug interactions in vitro. AIDS Res Hum Retrov 1999;15:793–802.
17. Kewn S, Veal GJ, Hoggard PG, Barry MG, Back DJ. Lamivudine (3TC) phosphorylation and drug interactions in vitro. Biochem Pharmacol 1997;54:589–595.
18. Palmer S, Shafer RW, Merigan TC. Hydroxyurea enhances the activities of didanosine, 9-[2-(phosphonylmethoxy)ethyl]adenine, and 9-[2-(phosphonylmethoxy)propyl]adenine against drug-susceptible and drug-resistant human immunodeficiency virus isolates. Antimicrob Agents Chemother 1999;43:2046–2050.
19. McKenzie R, Fried MW, Sallie R, et al. Hepatic failure and lactic acidosis due to fialuridine (FIAU), an investigational nucleoside analog for chronic hepatitis B. N Engl J Med 1995;333:1099–1105.
20. Klecker RW, Katki AG, Collins JM. Toxicity, metabolism, DNA incorporation with lack of repair, and lactate production for 1-(2'-fluoro-2'-deoxy-beta-D-arabinofuranosyl)-5-iodouracil in U-937 and MOLT-4 cells. Mol Pharmacol 1994;46:1204–1209.

21. Lewis W, Levine ES, Griniuviene B, et al. Fialuridine and its metabolites inhibit DNA polymerase gamma at sites of multiple adjacent analog incorporation, decrease mtDNA abundance, and cause mitochondrial structural defects in cultured hepatoblasts. Proc Natl Acad Sci USA 1996;93:3592–3597.
22. Ogedegbe AE, Thomas DL, Diehl AM. Hyperlactataemia syndromes associated with HIV therapy. Lancet Infect Dis 2003;3:329–337.
23. Yamaguchi T, Katoh I, Kurata S. Azidothymidine causes functional and structural destruction of mitochondria, glutathione deficiency and HIV-1 promoter sensitization. Eur J Biochem 2002;269:2782–2788.
24. Cundy KC. Clinical pharmacokinetics of the antiviral nucleotide analogs cidofovir and adefovir. Clin Pharmacokinet 1999;36:127–143.
25. von Moltke LL, Greenblatt DJ, Granda BW, et al. Inhibition of human cytochrome P450 isoforms by nonnucleoside reverse transcriptase inhibitors. J Clin Pharmacol 2001;41:85–91.
26. Pinzani V, Faucherre V, Peyriere H, Blayac JP. Methadone withdrawal symptoms with nevirapine and efavirenz. Ann Pharmacother 2000;34:405–407.
27. Clarke SM, Mulcahy FM, Tjia J, et al. Pharmacokinetic interactions of nevirapine and methadone and guidelines for use of nevirapine to treat injection drug users. Clin Infect Dis 2001;33:1595–1597.
28. Altice FL, Friedland GH, Cooney EL. Nevirapine induced opiate withdrawal among injection drug users with HIV infection receiving methadone. AIDS 1999;13:957–962.
29. Murphy RL, Sommadossi JP, Lamson M, Hall DB, Myers M, Dusek A. Antiviral effect and pharmacokinetic interaction between nevirapine and indinavir in persons infected with human immunodeficiency virus type 1. J Infect Dis 1999;179:1116–1123.
30. Falloon J, Piscitelli S, Vogel S, et al. Combination therapy with amprenavir, abacavir, and efavirenz in human immunodeficiency virus (HIV)-infected patients failing a protease-inhibitor regimen: pharmacokinetic drug interactions and antiviral activity. Clin Infect Dis 2000;30:313–318.
31. Piketty C, Race E, Castiel P, et al. Efficacy of a five-drug combination including ritonavir, saquinavir and efavirenz in patients who failed on a conventional triple-drug regimen: phenotypic resistance to protease inhibitors predicts outcome of therapy. AIDS 1999;13:F71–F77.
32. Malaty LI, Kuper JJ. Drug interactions of HIV protease inhibitors. Drug Safety 1999;20:147–169.
33. Tran JQ, Petersen C, Garrett M, Hee B, Kerr BM. Pharmacokinetic interaction between amprenavir and delavirdine: evidence of induced clearance by amprenavir. Clin Pharmacol Ther 2002;72:615–626.
34. Ferry JJ, Herman BD, Carel BJ, Carlson GF, Batts DH. Pharmacokinetic drug–drug interaction study of delavirdine and indinavir in healthy volunteers. J Acquir Immune Defic Syndr Hum Retrovirol 1998;18:252–259.
35. Kumar GN, Rodrigues AD, Buko AM, Denissen JF. Cytochrome P450-mediated metabolism of the HIV-1 protease inhibitor ritonavir (ABT-538) in human liver microsomes. J Pharmacol Exp Ther 1996;277:423–431.

36. von Moltke LL, Greenblatt DJ, Grassi JM, et al. Protease inhibitors as inhibitors of human cytochromes P450: high risk associated with ritonavir. J Clin Pharmacol 1998;38:106–111.
37. Kempf DJ, Marsh KC, Kumar G, et al. Pharmacokinetic enhancement of inhibitors of the human immunodeficiency virus protease by coadministration with ritonavir. Antimicrob Agents Chemother 1997;41:654–660.
38. Saah AJ, Winchell GA, Nessly ML, Seniuk MA, Rhodes RR, Deutsch PJ. Pharmacokinetic profile and tolerability of indinavir-ritonavir combinations in healthy volunteers. Antimicrob Agents Chemother 2001;45:2710–2715.
39. Koudriakova T, Iatsimirskaia E, Utkin I, et al. Metabolism of the human immunodeficiency virus protease inhibitors indinavir and ritonavir by human intestinal microsomes and expressed cytochrome P4503A4/3A5: mechanism-based inactivation of cytochrome P4503A by ritonavir. Drug Metab Dispos 1998;26:552–561.
40. Hsu A, Granneman GR, Witt G, et al. Multiple-dose pharmacokinetics of ritonavir in human immunodeficiency virus-infected subjects. Antimicrob Agents Chemother 1997;41:898–905.
41. Aarnoutse RE, Grintjes KJ, Telgt DS, et al. The influence of efavirenz on the pharmacokinetics of a twice-daily combination of indinavir and low-dose ritonavir in healthy volunteers. Clin Pharmacol Ther 2002;71:57–67.
42. Gerber JG, Rosenkranz S, Segal Y, et al. ACTG 401 Study Team. Effect of ritonavir/saquinavir on stereoselective pharmacokinetics of methadone: results of AIDS Clinical Trials Group (ACTG) 401. J AIDS 2001;27:153–160.
43. Ouellet D, Hsu A, Qian J, et al. Effect of ritonavir on the pharmacokinetics of ethinyl oestradiol in healthy female volunteers. Br J Clin Pharmacol 1998;46:111–116.
44. Hsu A, Granneman GR, Cao G, et al. Pharmacokinetic interactions between two human immunodeficiency virus protease inhibitors, ritonavir and saquinavir. Clin Pharmacol Ther 1998;63:453–464.
45. Chiba M, Hensleigh M, Nishime JA, Balani SK, Lin JH. Role of cytochrome P450 3A4 in human metabolism of MK-639, a potent human immunodeficiency virus protease inhibitor. Drug Metab Dispos 1996;24:307–314.
46. Lillibridge JH, Liang BH, Kerr BM, et al. Characterization of the selectivity and mechanism of human cytochrome P450 inhibition by the human immunodeficiency virus-protease inhibitor nelfinavir mesylate. Drug Metab Dispos 1998;26:609–616.
47. Kurowski M, Kaeser B, Sawyer A, Popescu M, Mrozikiewicz A. Low-dose ritonavir moderately enhances nelfinavir exposure. Clin Pharmacol Ther 2002;72:123–132.
48. Weemhoff JL, von Moltke LL, Richert C, Hesse LM, Harmatz JS, Greenblatt DJ. Apparent mechanism-based inhibition of human CYP3A in-vitro by lopinavir. J Pharm Pharmacol 2003;55:381–386.
49. Lee CG, Gottesman MM, Cardarelli CO, et al. HIV-1 protease inhibitors are substrates for the MDR1 multidrug transporter. Biochemistry 1998;37:3594–3601.
50. Fromm MF. P-glycoprotein: a defense mechanism limiting oral bioavailability and CNS accumulation of drugs. Int J Clin Pharmacol Ther 2000;38:69–74.

51. Lin JH, Yamazaki M. Role of P-glycoprotein in pharmacokinetics: clinical implications. Clin Pharmacokinet 2003;42:59–98.
52. Kim RB, Wandel C, Leake B, et al. Interrelationship between substrates and inhibitors of human CYP3A and P-glycoprotein. Pharm Res 1999;16: 408–414.
53. Synold TW, Dussault I, Forman BM. The orphan nuclear receptor SXR coordinately regulates drug metabolism and efflux. Nat Med 2001;7:584–590.
54. Dussault I, Lin M, Hollister K, Wang EH, Synold TW, Forman BM. Peptide mimetic HIV protease inhibitors are ligands for the orphan receptor SXR. J Biol Chem 2001;276:33309–33312.
55. Alsenz J, Steffen H, Alex R. Active apical secretory efflux of the HIV protease inhibitors saquinavir and ritonavir in Caco-2 cell monolayers. Pharm Res 1998;15: 423–428.
56. Gutmann H, Fricker G, Drewe J, Toeroek M, Miller DS. Interactions of HIV protease inhibitors with ATP-dependent drug export proteins. Mol Pharmacol 1999;56: 383–389.
57. Drewe J, Gutmann H, Fricker G, Torok M, Beglinger C, Huwyler J. HIV protease inhibitor ritonavir: a more potent inhibitor of P-glycoprotein than the cyclosporine analog SDZ PSC 833. Biochem Pharmacol 1999;57:1147–1152.
58. Huisman MT, Smit JW, Wiltshire HR, Hoetelmans RM, Beijnen JH, Schinkel AH. P-glycoprotein limits oral availability, brain, and fetal penetration of saquinavir even with high doses of ritonavir. Mol Pharmacol 2001;59:806–813.
59. Hochman JH, Chiba M, Yamazaki M, Tang C, Lin JH. P-glycoprotein-mediated efflux of indinavir metabolites in Caco-2 cells expressing cytochrome P450 3A4. J Pharmacol Exp Ther 2001;298:323–330.
60. Huisman MT, Smit JW, Crommentuyn KM, et al. Multidrug resistance protein 2 (MRP2) transports HIV protease inhibitors, and transport can be enhanced by other drugs. AIDS 2002;16:2295–2301.
61. Soldner A, Christians U, Susanto M, Wacher VJ, Silverman JA, Benet LZ. Grapefruit juice activates P-glycoprotein-mediated drug transport. Pharm Res 1999;16: 478–485.
62. Khaliq Y, Gallicano K, Venance S, Kravcik S, Cameron DW. Effect of ketoconazole on ritonavir and saquinavir concentrations in plasma and cerebrospinal fluid from patients infected with human immunodeficiency virus. Clin Pharmacol Ther 2000;68:637–646.
63. Fellay J, Marzolini C, Meaden ER, et al. Swiss HIV Cohort Study. Response to antiretroviral treatment in HIV-1-infected individuals with allelic variants of the multidrug resistance transporter 1: a pharmacogenetics study. Lancet 2002; 359: 30–36.
64. Kilby JM, Eron JJ. Novel therapies based on mechanisms of HIV-1 cell entry. N Engl J Med 2003;348:2228–2238.
65. Brockmeyer NH, Mertins L, Spatz D, Tillmann I, Goos M. Endogenous interferon plasma levels and antipyrine pharmacokinetics in patients with viral infections. Int J Clin Pharmacol Ther Toxicol 1992;30:530–533.

66. Israel BC, Blouin RA, McIntyre W, Shedlofsky SI. Effects of interferon-alpha monotherapy on hepatic drug metabolism in cancer patients. Br J Clin Pharmacol 1993; 36:229–235.
67. Horsmans Y, Brenard R, Geubel AP. Short report: interferon-alpha decreases ^{14}C-aminopyrine breath test values in patients with chronic hepatitis C. Aliment Pharmacol Ther 1994;8:353–355.
68. Islam M, Frye RF, Richards TJ, et al. Differential effect of IFNalpha-2b on the cytochrome P450 enzyme system: a potential basis of IFN toxicity and its modulation by other drugs. Clin Cancer Res 2002;8:2480–2487.
69. Becquemont L, Chazouilleres O, Serfaty L, et al. Effect of interferon alpha-ribavirin bitherapy on cytochrome P450 1A2 and 2D6 and N-acetyltransferase-2 activities in patients with chronic active hepatitis C. Clin Pharmacol Ther 2002;71:488–495.
70. Rivory LP, Slaviero KA, Clarke SJ. Hepatic cytochrome P450 3A drug metabolism is reduced in cancer patients who have an acute-phase response. Br J Cancer 2002; 87:277–280.
71. Pageaux GP, le Bricquir Y, Berthou F, et al. Effects of interferon-alpha on cytochrome P-450 isoforms 1A2 and 3A activities in patients with chronic hepatitis C. Eur J Gastroenterol Hepatol 1998;10:491–495.
72. Cribb AE, Delaporte E, Kim SG, Novak RF, Renton KW. Regulation of cytochrome P-4501A and cytochrome P-4502E induction in the rat during the production of interferon alpha/beta. J Pharmacol Exp Ther 1994;268:487–494.
73. Stanley LA, Adams DJ, Balkwill FR, Griffin D, Wolf CR. Differential effects of recombinant interferon alpha on constitutive and inducible cytochrome P450 isozymes in mouse liver. Biochem Pharmacol 1991;42:311–320.
74. Carelli M, Porras MC, Rizzardini M, Cantoni L. Modulation of constitutive and inducible hepatic cytochrome(s) P-450 by interferon beta in mice. J Hepatol 1996; 24:230–237.
75. Piscitelli SC, Gallicano KD. Interactions among drugs for HIV and opportunistic infections. N Engl J Med 2001;344:984–996.
76. Furlan V, Taburet AM. Drug interactions with antiretroviral agents. Therapie 2001;56:267–271.
77. Washington CB, Flexner C, Sheiner LB, et al. AIDS Clinical Trials Group Protocol (ACTG 378) Study Team. Effect of simultaneous versus staggered dosing on pharmacokinetic interactions of protease inhibitors. Clin Pharmacol Ther 2003;73: 406–416.
78. Cooper CL, van Heeswijk RP, Gallicano K, Cameron DW. A review of low-dose ritonavir in protease inhibitor combination therapy. Clin Infect Dis 2003;36:1585–1592.
79. Pfister M, Labbe L, Lu JF, et al. AIDS Clinical Trial Group Protocol 398 Investigators. Effect of coadministration of nelfinavir, indinavir, and saquinavir on the pharmacokinetics of amprenavir. Clin Pharmacol Ther 2002;72:133–141.
80. de Maat MM, Ekhart GC, Huitema AD, Koks CH, Mulder JW, Beijnen JH. Drug interactions between antiretroviral drugs and comedicated agents. Clin Pharmacokinet 2003;42:223–282.

81. Hamzeh FM, Benson C, Gerber J, et al. AIDS Clinical Trials Group 365 Study Team. Steady-state pharmacokinetic interaction of modified-dose indinavir and rifabutin. Clin Pharmacol Ther 2003;73:159–169.
82. Polk RE, Crouch MA, Israel DS, et al. Pharmacokinetic interaction between ketoconazole and amprenavir after single doses in healthy men. Pharmacotherapy 1999;19:1378–1384.
83. Cato A, III, Cavanaugh J, Shi H, Hsu A, Leonard J, Granneman R. The effect of multiple doses of ritonavir on the pharmacokinetics of rifabutin. Clin Pharmacol Ther 1998;63:414–421.
84. Greenblatt DJ, von Moltke LL, Harmatz JS, et al. Alprazolam-ritonavir interaction: implications for product labelling. Clin Pharmacol Ther 2000;67:335–341.
85. Li AP, Reith MK, Rasmussen A, et al. Primary human hepatocytes as a tool for the evaluation of structure-activity relationship in cytochrome P450 induction potential of xenobiotics: evaluation of rifampin, rifapentine and rifabutin. Chem Biol Interact 1997;107:17–30.
86. Gallicano KD, Sahai J, Shukla VK, et al. Induction of zidovudine glucuronidation and amination pathways by rifampicin in HIV-infected patients. Br J Clin Pharmacol 1999;48:168–179.
87. Piscitelli SC, Burstein AH, Welden N, Gallicano KD, Falloon J. The effect of garlic supplements on the pharmacokinetics of saquinavir. Clin Infect Dis 2002;34: 234–238.
88. Eagling VA, Profit L, Back DJ. Inhibition of the CYP3A4-mediated metabolism and P-glycoprotein-mediated transport of the HIV-1 protease inhibitor saquinavir by grapefruit juice components. Br J Clin Pharmacol 1999;48:543–552.
89. Kupferschmidt HH, Fattinger KE, Ha HR, Follath F, Krahenbuhl S. Grapefruit juice enhances the bioavailability of the HIV protease inhibitor saquinavir in man. Br J Clin Pharmacol 1998;45:355–359.
90. Sahai J, Gallicano K, Oliveras L, Khaliq S, Hawley-Foss N, Garber G. Cations in the didanosine tablet reduce ciprofloxacin bioavailability. Clin Pharmacol Ther 1993;53:292–297.

10

Modulation of Thiols and Other Low-Molecular-Weight Cofactors

Effects on Drug Metabolism and Disease Susceptibility

Charles V. Smith

Summary

A brief summary of the pioneering work of Brodie, Gillette, and coworkers on the discovery and development of the concept of chemically reactive intermediates serves as the backdrop for this chapter on approaches to studying how chemicals modify thiols and other cellular nucleophiles. As examples, work is presented on classic hepatotoxicants such as acetaminophen, bromobenzene, carbon tetrachloride, and diquat. Discussion focuses on illustrations of key data and methods to assess lipid peroxidation, oxidant stress, chemically induced depletion of glutathione and protein thiols, and oxidative modification of proteins. Further adaptation of the methodologies and approaches that are discussed to relevant human and live animal models of toxicant action and physiological responses are needed. These strategies and the data that the applications can provide are important, not only for characterization of specific human exposures and toxicities, but also for the evolution of important fundamental principles, concepts, and experimental approaches.

Key Words

Acetaminophen: overdose; acetaminophen: hepatic necrosis induced by; acetaminophen: protein adducts; acetaminophen: thioether conjugates; *N*-acetyl-*p*-benzoquinone imine; antioxidant defense mechanisms; bromobenzene; carbon tetrachloride; free radicals; glutathione; glutathione disulfide; glutathione reductase; hyperoxic lung injury; lipid peroxidation; oxidant stress; polyunsaturated fatty acids; protein thiols; reactive intermediates; reactive nitrogen species; thiol oxidation.

1. INTRODUCTION

To even begin to mention the vast expanse of topics and subject areas relevant to the title assigned for this chapter, within anything resembling the limitations

From: *Methods in Pharmacology and Toxicology,*
Drug Metabolism and Transport: Molecular Methods and Mechanisms
Edited by: L. Lash © Humana Press Inc., Totowa, NJ

of space and time reasonable for the document, or for the lifetime of the author, would require the thinnest of discussions of any specific ideas, and even this coverage would be incomplete. The second alternative for this discussion is to pick a much more narrow range of topics, thus offending those valiant investigators whose noble works and brilliant thoughts are so egregiously ignored, maybe offending the authors of the works ignored as much as those authors whose works are discussed. The approach presented uses a set of seemingly narrow discussions of a few specific examples to illustrate fundamental concepts and principles that can be applied to other specific questions that lie within the range spanned by the broader area defined by the title of the chapter.

The germ theory of disease, so commonly accepted today, was a major advancement in human health, in large part because attempts to understand, treat, and prevent many diseases could be focused by rational, testable hypotheses upon ultimately identifiable discrete pathogens and mechanisms (1). By disproving the concept of spontaneous generation, which at the time was well known to be true and was widely accepted, Louis Pasteur's research led to the recognition that many human diseases, as well as diseases affecting plants and nonhuman animals, were caused by specific bacteria or other living pathogens that were even smaller than he could observe directly. The advances in understanding the means by which diseases were transported from one person to another, and from one city to another, that were made possible by Pasteur's investigations greatly altered management of what we now call communicable diseases. His work not only defined the conceptual bases for but also effected the immediate and practical adoption of antiseptic surgical practices, vaccination, and, of course, pasteurization. Less well-recognized at the time, but of inestimable significance to the continuing progress of human civilization, the fundamental scientific principles illustrated by Pasteur's studies demonstrated that lines of investigation that were unlikely to be productive could be recognized more readily, further enhancing the rate at which meaningful progress could be achieved through scientifically and mechanistically rational lines of research. The results and implications of Pasteur's studies were also essential in the large scale brewing of beer and wine making, thus earning him the gratitude of even the otherwise healthy portion of most populations.

Similarly, the pioneering work by Brodie, Gillette, and their contemporaries led to the appreciation that chemically reactive intermediates mediate the toxicities of a number of drugs and environmental chemicals and contribute to the pathogeneses of many human diseases. In something of an analogy with the vague and mystic laws of spontaneous generation, the surprisingly limited appreciation of the specificities with which radicals, free radicals, reactive oxygen and nitrogen species, oxidants, electrophilic alkylating species, and other chemically reactive intermediates can act has contributed to considerable confusion and misinformation, with consequent adverse effects on research progress. Although broad-spectrum antibiotics can help with some infections, understanding that individual species of bacteria exhibit different host-dependent pathogenicities and susceptibilities to individual antibiotics has made possible far superior treatment and prevention of specific diseases. Similarly, nutriceutical supplements or generally nonspecific "antioxidant" therapies can afford net benefits in some circumstances, but optimal management of oxidant and other mechanisms of tissue damage will require equally specific understanding of the chemical species and their respective mechanisms of action.

2. REACTIVE INTERMEDIATES

The hepatotoxicities of bromobenzene and CCl_4 *(2)* in rodents were vital to the early studies of chemically reactive intermediates in drug toxicities, but the subsequent discovery that the widely used analgesic acetaminophen caused metabolism-dependent hepatic necrosis in experimental animals *(3)* led to increasing emphasis on studies of this drug, in part due to the more obvious direct relevance to human health. Unfortunately, the toxicological relevance of acetaminophen hepatotoxicity continues to the present. At Columbus Children's Hospital, from August 2001 through May 2002, for example, 54 patients were seen with acetaminophen overdose as a primary or secondary diagnosis.

Acetaminophen-induced hepatic necrosis in rodents is preceded by depletion of glutathione (GSH) *(4)* and has been inextricably linked with covalent binding to hepatic proteins of chemically reactive metabolites of the parent drug *(5,6)*. Several lines of evidence pointed toward *N*-acetyl-*p*-benzoquinone imine (NAPQI) as a metabolite of acetaminophen that is responsible for the toxic effects of acetaminophen (Fig. 1). In fact, NAPQI is cited as the chemically reactive metabolite of acetaminophen in most papers published on the topic. However, this attribution overlooks the fact that authentic NAPQI, prepared by chemical synthesis, reacts with thiols to produce the corresponding disulfides (Fig. 2), along with acetaminophen, as well as to produce the 3'-thioether conjugates *(7,8)*. Acetaminophen metabolism in vivo does not increase tissue levels or biliary efflux of glutathione disulfide (GSSG) *(7,9,10)*. The biliary efflux of GSSG is a particularly sensitive indicator of exposure of parenchymal hepatocytes to oxidants. Nevertheless, the stable thioether products of acetaminophen metabolism are rationalized quite nicely by NAPQI. In light of the evidence on the nature of the thioether products formed, but the absence of increases in oxidation of thiols in response to acetaminophen dosing

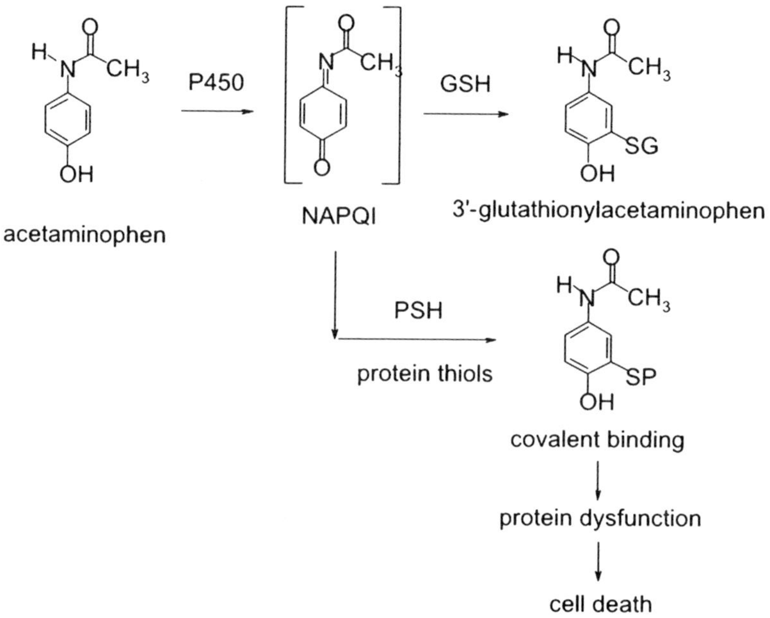

Fig. 1. Metabolic activation of acetaminophen. Metabolism of acetaminophen in vivo leads to an intermediate, thought by many to be NAPQI, that, in the presence of glutathione (GSH), forms the corresponding 3′-thioether adduct. The bracket in this and other figures indicates that in this scheme, NAPQI is postulated and has not been demonstrated conclusively. If demands on GSH exceed available cellular contents and synthetic capacities, alkylation of protein thiols, indicated here as PSH, is observed. The working hypothesis is that sufficient extents of alkylation of sufficiently critical protein thiols result in dysfunction of the respective proteins, which can lead to cell death. Although issues have been raised and persist over this working hypothesis, acetaminophen-induced hepatic necrosis in vivo has never been observed in the absence of covalent binding to protein, usually in the range of 1 nmol of drug bound per milligram of protein.

in vivo, we proposed the intermediacy of an adduct (Fig. 3), essentially a transport biosynthetic equivalent of NAPQI, that would not be subject to similar reduction by GSH or by ascorbate *(7)*.

Chen et al. *(8)* subsequently reported physical chemical evidence for formation of *ipso* and thiohemiketal adducts of NAPQI (Fig. 4), which are synthetically and functionally equivalent to the structure we proposed, for purposes of the effects on alkylation and oxidation of thiols that we were attempting to explain. Hepatotoxic doses of acetaminophen do increase hepatic contents of GSSG *(11–13)*, but late in the time course of initiation of hepatic damage. Chen proposed that NAPQI-protein thiol (PSH) *ipso* adducts could function as

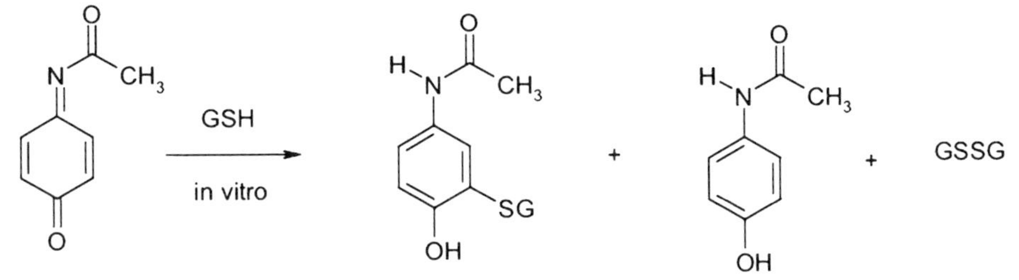

Modulation of Thiols and Other Cofactors

Fig. 2. Reactions of authentic NAPQI with GSH in vitro. Chemically synthesized NAPQI (hence no brackets in this figure, as opposed to the metabolic scheme in Fig. 1) reacts with GSH in vitro to produce the same 3′-thioether adduct as observed from metabolism in vivo; however, the reaction in vitro produces comparable amounts of acetaminophen and GSSG, which is not observed during peak acetaminophen metabolism in vivo.

storage or transport forms of NAPQI that would not be reduced by ascorbate, as is NAPQI, but would be reduced by GSH, once cellular GSH supplies recovered as a result of ongoing synthesis. These authors also postulated that such adducts could explain alkylations of nucleophilic sites outside of the endoplasmic reticular sites of generation and possibly provide a mechanism for transport of the alkylating species outside of the cells in which the reactive metabolite is generated. We interpreted the data as indicating that the oxidative processes reflected by the increased GSSG levels were results of organismal responses to cell damage. Both general processes may contribute to the observed late increases in hepatic GSSG contents, but whether any of the shifts in thiol/disulfide status indicated by these changes contribute meaningfully to acetaminophen-induced necrosis is a separate question.

This general principle of masked synthetic equivalent, namely a species that possesses some of the chemical properties associated with a specific species, but not the same molecule, has been proposed for other toxicants, such as methyl isocyanate *(14)* and 1,2-dibromoethane *(15)*. This general concept is important in reaching the levels of understanding on the actions of chemically reactive toxicants that will be needed to design rational approaches to the prevention of the respective toxicities, or for the optimal utilization of such toxicities in killing malignant cells or the cells of invading pathogens.

3. LIPID PEROXIDATION

Another example of the synthetic equivalent principle is the use of 1,1,3,3-tetramethoxypropane (TMP; or the analogous tetraethyoxy derivative, TEP) to generate standard curves for measurements of 1,3-malondialdehyde (MDA) as

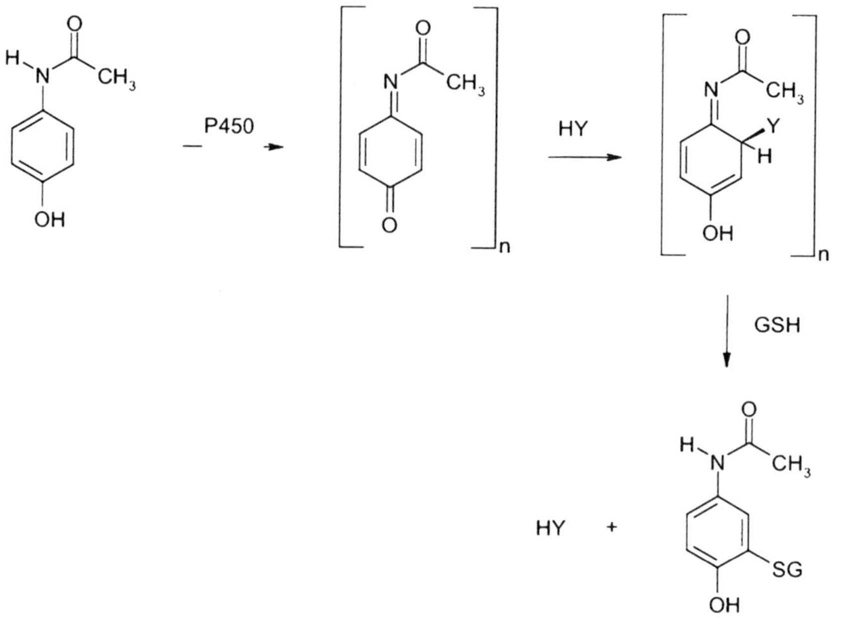

Fig. 3. A proposed mechanism for retention of alkylating properties of the chemically reactive metabolite of acetaminophen, in the absence of thiol oxidation. In the scheme depicted, an alternate nucleophile, HY, forms an sp^3 adduct with a NAPQI-like intermediate that is not active in the reduction reaction with GSH, but which reacts to give the 3'-thioether preferentially.

the thiobarbituric acid adduct (Fig. 5). Whether or not free, authentic MDA as such is a major intermediate in generation of the thiobarbituric acid adduct in vitro, the reactivities of MDA with molecules found in biological systems are such that little of what is measured as thiobarbituric acid-reactive substances (TBARS) is likely to represent MDA in the cells or tissues. As has been demonstrated by Kosugi and Kikugawa *(16)*, many other molecular species can give rise to the authentic adduct that is characteristic of MDA, or of TMP and TEP, under conditions of the TBARS test. However, authentication of the chemical identity of the adduct formed in the assay, as by high-performance liquid chromatography (HPLC) or even with mass spectrometry, does not establish that MDA was present in the biological matrix examined. The significance of this point is that the individual substances giving rise to the common adduct detected in the TBARS test will not necessarily exhibit identical chemistries or toxicities in the biological systems being probed.

In 1979, Wendel reported that fasted mice given hepatotoxic doses of acetaminophen exhaled markedly increased amounts of ethane *(17)*, which led to a

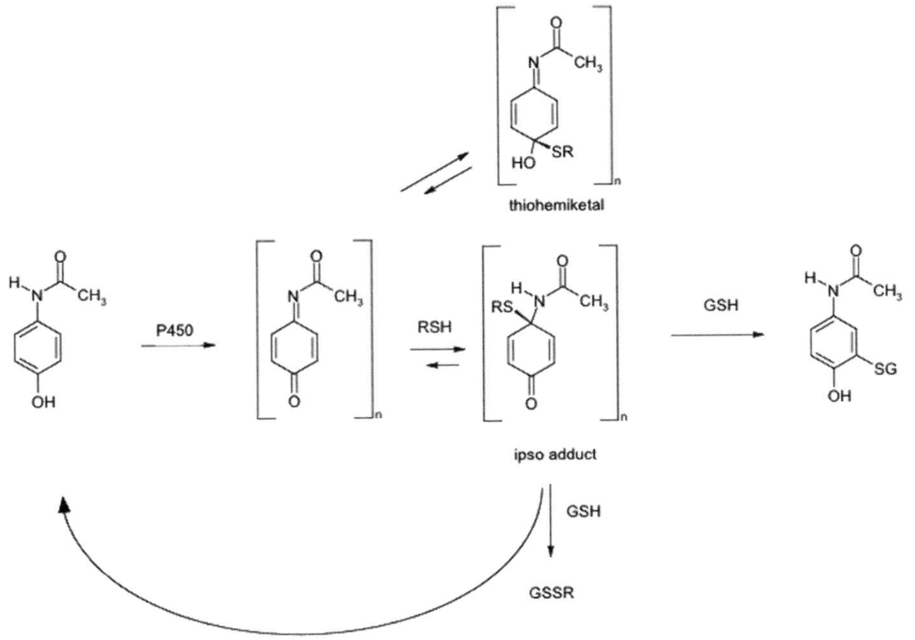

Fig. 4. Postulated formation of thiohemiketal and ipso adducts of NAPQI. In analogy with the scheme depicted in Fig. 3, the two adducts presented could explain some of the distinctions between the reactions observed in vitro and the effects observed in vivo.

flurry of interest in the role of lipid peroxidation in acetaminophen-induced injury, because of the presumed origination of ethane through β-scission of the corresponding hydroperoxides (LOOH) of the ω-3 series of polyunsaturated fatty acids (PUFA) *(18)*. We developed HPLC and gas chromatography–mass spectometry (GC–MS) methods for measurements of specific LOOHs and the corresponding lipid hydroxy acids (LOH) and found that hepatotoxic doses of acetaminophen did not increase hepatic LOOH or LOH contents measurably, in the same animals from which we observed dramatic increases in expiration of ethane and pentane *(19,20)*. The development and application of more chemically specific methods of analysis and use of selected experimental models (diethyl maleate [DEM], furosemide, CCl_4) as critical controls for mechanistic hypotheses indicated to us that the marked increases in ethane and pentane expiration in acetaminophen-treated mice did not signal substantive increases in peroxidation of hepatic lipids and did not suggest lipid peroxidation as a probable significant contributor to mechanisms of acetaminophen-induced liver injury. Subsequent studies of the effects of acetaminophen on formation of isoprostanes are consistent with our data and interpretations *(21)*.

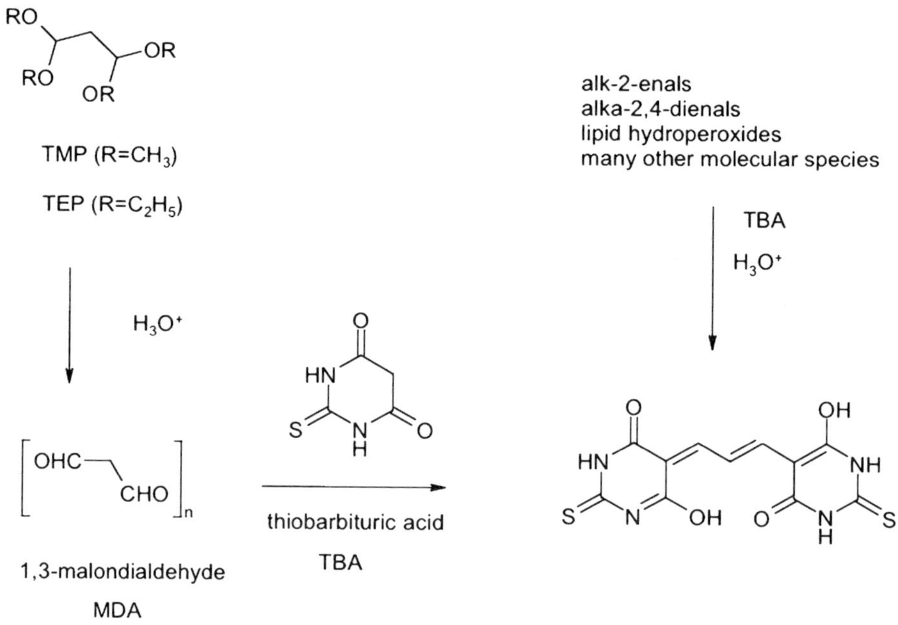

Fig. 5. Thiobarbituric acid reactive substances (TBARS). The TBA adduct commonly attributed to malondialdehyde (MDA) in efforts to quantitate lipid peroxidation in biological samples, can be derived from a wide range of specific substances, and even the authentic adduct cannot be interpreted with confidence as a measure of MDA content of the sample.

Although the research activities with lipid peroxidation and acetaminophen-induced hepatic necrosis died down considerably, the idea that "oxidant stress" contributed significantly to acetaminophen-induced necrosis arose. The ubiquity of O_2 in cells and tissues and of redox chemistry in normal cell metabolism dictate that reactive oxygen species and oxidant chemistries will "be involved" in some way in most toxicities. However, more specific questions regarding the toxicants and the molecular mechanisms through which they act are more likely to be useful. The term "oxidant stress" is not intrinsically well defined, and the oxidative transformations of biological molecules are not uniform across a range of toxicant challenges (18). The specific oxidative transformations associated with a toxicant challenge need to be identified, in part as a means of characterizing the reactive intermediates mediating the injury. Finding some evidence that is related in some way to some mode of oxidation does not define a mechanism of toxicant action at a level of specificity that is useful.

4. OXIDANT STRESS AND DEPLETION OF GSH AND PROTEIN THIOLS

Observations that the toxicities of many drugs were accompanied by decreases in tissue concentrations of GSH led some authors even to conclude that loss of GSH caused cell death. This hypothesis can be tested by producing similar extents and time courses of GSH depletion with agents, such as DEM, that do not cause hepatic necrosis *(10,22)*. Lethally injured cells may lose GSH, and diminished amounts of GSH available for cellular defense functions can exacerbate the effects of toxicant challenges, but hepatic GSH can be depleted substantially without initiation of acute lethal injury. With acetaminophen, the generation of a chemically reactive metabolite leads to utilization of GSH for synthesis of the thioether conjugate. If GSH supplies and synthetic capacities are exceeded, the normal route for disposition of the alkylating metabolites cannot function, resulting in alkylation of proteins (Fig. 1). Acute hepatic necrosis in acetaminophen-treated animals has never been observed in the absence of protein alkylation, and the levels of covalent binding with toxic doses, when measured, are usually in the range of 1 nmol of metabolite bound per mg of protein *(4,6)*. This level of protein alkylation would account for only about 1% of the total PSH content of rodent liver *(7,23–25)*, and this level of binding would not affect measurements of total tissue PSH status. However, hepatic PSH must be converted to other species, such as thioethers or disulfides. The characterization of the selective loss of a limited number of cysteine residues by alkylation, and any similarly restricted oxidation of potentially critical thiols will require the use of more selective methods of analysis than have been applied to the problem to date.

Investigation of this next level of specificity by treatment of hepatic subcellular fractions of saline- and acetaminophen-treated mice with monobromobimane (mBBr), which reacts readily with thiols to form highly fluorescent thioethers, revealed a single difference observable in the acetaminophen-treated animals, which was the loss of fluorescence intensity of a protein identified as carbamoyl phosphate synthetase-I (CPS-I) in the mitochondrial fractions of acetaminophen-treated mice *(26)*. CPS-I activities were diminished in parallel, and hyperammonemia was observed in the animals in which CPS-I activities were diminished. However, hepatic activities of glutamine synthetase, another major route for ammonia clearance, were decreased in these animals and probably contributed comparably to the hyperammonemia. Notably, glutamine synthetase was not identified as an affected protein with the mBBr–sodium dodecyl sulfate-polyacrylamide gel electrophoresis (SDS-PAGE) method, nor were the proteins identified by autoradiography of 2-D gels, with mass spectrometry

(27) or by western analyses with anti-acetaminophen–protein conjugate antibodies *(28–30)*. Even if a gel band or 2-D spot were a single protein, selective alkylation of a single cysteine on a protein that has multiple cysteine residues might not be detected by the mBBr–SDS-PAGE approach. If the affected cysteine residue is crucial for protein function, the pathological effects could be substantial. Alkylation and oxidation of low-abundance proteins, even at high fractional conversion, will be more difficult to detect and characterize by any method than will more modest percent conversion of an abundant protein; however modifications of low abundance proteins have great potential for effects on cell physiology and viability *(31)*. The experiments testing this hypothesis need to be conducted. At the very least, characterizations of the specific modifications caused by toxicants in vivo are needed to determine the kinds of transformations that are occurring and therefore may be affecting the lower abundance proteins similarly. The mechanistic clues provided by such studies, as well as the insights developed through continuing refinements in analytical methodologies, will be essential in achieving the analytical sophistication that will be needed for characterization of the more subtle molecular effects of toxicants.

GSH plays many critical roles in the highly integrated antioxidant defense mechanisms by which cells and tissues work to survive exposures to reactive oxygen species. Exposure of cells and tissues to reactive oxygen species often is characterized quantitatively through the measurement of GSSG, which is formed by the reduction of hydrogen peroxide or other peroxides at the expense of oxidation of GSH (Fig. 6) *(9,22)*. Subsequent thiol–disulfide exchange with protein thiols by the GSSG thus formed has been proposed as a mechanism for the initiation of cell dysfunction, through inactivation of enzymes by *S*-thiolation of critical sulfhydryl groups *(32–34)*. However, early studies of mechanisms of oxidant-induced cell injury were conducted largely in vitro. Initial efforts to study reactive oxygen-mediated hepatic necrosis in vivo were complicated by the fact that the agents that caused the greatest stimulation of production of reactive oxygen species, diquat, paraquat, and nitrofurantoin, simply did not cause cellular necrosis *(9)*. Conversely, agents that were acutely hepatotoxic, such as CCl_4, acetaminophen, and dimethylnitrosamine, caused no measurable increases in GSSG production or other oxidant stress responses. Hepatic necrosis could be produced by diquat in selenium-deficient animals, but excessive animal mortality and effects of dietary deficiency on other selenoproteins have limited studies of these models *(35,36)*.

5. GSSG REDUCTASE

Most GSSG produced in reduction of H_2O_2 or other oxidants is reduced back to GSH by glutathione reductase (GR) *(37)*. A significant role for GR in

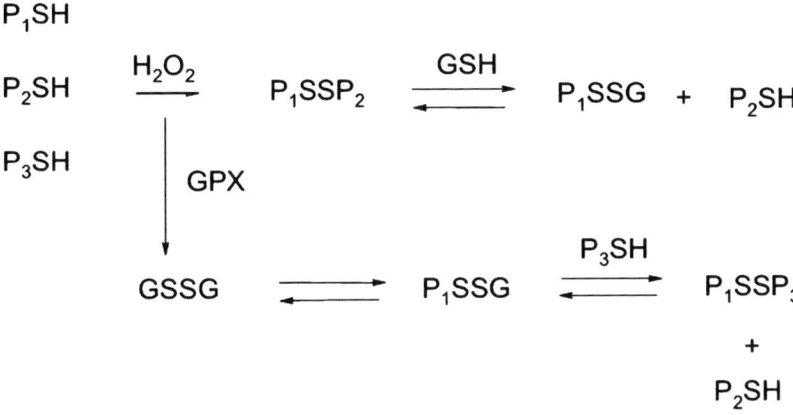

Fig. 6. Oxidation of protein thiols (PSH) to disulfides (PSSP). The protective effects of glutathione peroxidase (GPX) are not necessarily mediated by dissipation of the oxidative potential of oxidants, such as illustrated in this example by H_2O_2, because the GSSG formed retains the stoichiometric equivalency of the original oxidant. However, the potential to control and direct which specific thiol becomes S-thiolated, as through protein–protein interaction-derived specificities, has the potential to influence regulation of cell functions through thiol–disulfide redox interconversions.

antioxidant defense functions was deduced from studies in which animals and cells pretreated with 1,3-bis-(2-chloroethyl)-1-nitrosourea (BCNU), which inhibits GR, were found to be more susceptible to subsequent challenges by toxicants presumed to act through oxidant mechanisms. Potentiation of injury by BCNU is often cited as evidence that oxidant mechanisms are involved in the injury (38–41). Although BCNU does inhibit GR, the enhanced cytotoxicities of other toxicants in BCNU-pretreated cells are more closely correlated with the DNA crosslinks that BCNU forms than with inhibition of GR, unless the time between BCNU treatment and toxicant challenge is sufficient (12–24 h) to allow for repair of the DNA lesions, which is more rapid than is recovery of GR activities (42,43). Even so, the implication of enhancement of toxicity through inhibition of GR would be that failure to adequately reduce GSSG either permits GSH to be depleted, thus allowing the oxidation of other biomolecules by H_2O_2 not reduced by GSH, or that increased steady-state concentrations of GSSG lead to S-thiolation of critical proteins. Although thoroughly logical and supported by earlier studies of cell killing in vitro (33,34), we have found that acute hepatic necrosis initiated by reactive oxygen species in vivo was not accompanied by similar depletion of either GSH or of PSH contents (44).

6. OXIDATIVE MODIFICATION OF PROTEINS

In a number of experimental models, cellular damage by reactive oxygen species correlates more closely with oxidative transformations that are more characteristic of reactions catalyzed by redox-active metal chelates than with changes in thiol status *(45–53)*. Products of oxidation of lipids, nucleic acids, and proteins have been observed, in addition to products from oxidation of low-molecular-weight molecules such as GSH. We have studied each of these classes of potential target molecules *(19,20,54–56)*, and each offers advantages and challenges. The focus of the present proposal on protein oxidation is based on the potential for specific products of oxidation of specific proteins to provide better insight into the molecular mechanisms through which the oxidative alterations are mediated and to the subcellular compartments in which the transformations occur.

In most studies conducted to date, total contents of "protein carbonyls" are usually measured by radiolabel incorporation following reduction with $NaB[^3H]_4$ or by increased absorbance at 365 nm following derivatization with 2,4-dinitrophenylhydrazine (DNPH) *(47,48,57,58)*. Both reactions are designed to detect aldehydes and ketones not present in native proteins, but formed by oxidation *(59)*. Identification of specific proteins affected by oxidation offers considerably greater understanding of the mechanisms active in the disease or toxicity being studied. The DNP moiety is strongly immunogenic, and western analyses using antibodies against DNP-derivatized proteins has enabled investigators to identify proteins that are oxidized preferentially in human patients as well as in experimental models in vivo and in vitro. In rats exposed to hyperoxia, we identified anti-DNP-immunoreactive β-casein, which led us to the novel observation of accumulation of cytotoxic T-lymphocytes early in the course of hyperoxic lung injury *(60)*. Similarly, anti-DNP Western analyses of tracheal aspirate fluids from ventilated prematurely born infants revealed that oxidation and DNP-reactivity of a specific protein, which we identified as Clara cell secreted protein (CCSP), correlated with a much greater risk for development of bronchopulmonary dysplasia (BPD), which implies a potentially pivotal role for CCSP and/or Clara cell damage in the pathogenesis of BPD *(61)*. A most important point to be made regarding this latter study is that the CCSP-derived product is not quantitatively a major band in the anti-DNP Western analyses. Identification of this product by our experimental approach has provided insights that have significant implications for mechanisms contributing to BPD and has suggested approaches to the prevention and treatment of an important human disease.

More recently, the possible contributions of reactive nitrogen species (RNS), such as peroxynitrite ($ONOO^-$), have been implicated as contributors to acetaminophen-induced hepatic necrosis *(62–64)*. Although much of the data published to date are reminiscent of the alkane expiration studies discussed in the preceding, the observation by Knight et al. *(64)* of increases in protein nitration as early as 0.5 h post dose suggests potential contributions to causative mechanisms, rather than markers of phagocytic cleanup of damaged tissue pieces. The antinitrotyrosine staining early after acetaminophen is expressed principally in the vascular space, whereas the later immunoreactivity is observed in the parenchymal hepatocytes. Prevention of acetaminophen-induced hepatic necrosis by pretreatment with macrophage inactivators ($GdCl_2$) has been reported, but the plasma alanine aminotransferase (ALT) activities reported in this study (28 ± 1, $n = 5$) are quite inconsistent with the massive centrilobular hepatic necrosis evident in the histological section (Fig. 4B of the report cited) presented of an animal pretreated with $GdCl_2$ prior to acetaminophen *(63)*. Controversies also have arisen even as to the role of peroxynitrite in protein nitration *(65,66)*, but increased protein nitration in association with acetaminophen-induced hepatic necrosis appears to be well documented, and protein nitration clearly should have the capacity to contribute to cell damage. Protection against acetaminophen-induced necrosis by a superoxide dismutase (SOD) mimetic has been reported as well *(67)*, but the effects of this mimetic on acetaminophen metabolism was investigated at a much lower dose (50 mg/kg) than was used for the toxicity studies (1000 mg/kg), so possible effects on acetaminophen metabolism were not precluded.

Other investigators have assessed oxidatively modified amino acids in protein hydrolysates using GC–MS as biomarkers of protein oxidation *(68,69)*. However, experimental approaches that do not retain the identities of the proteins that were oxidatively modified, the specific amino acid residues (meaning position in primary sequence in the intact protein) affected, and the specific manner in which the residue has been modified do not take full advantage of the potential for specific, molecular information on the mechanisms operative in the oxidant stresses under study. Although such approaches are difficult, substantial progress has been made on the development and application of analytical methods for characterization of oxidized proteins at this level of specificity *(70–74)*.

7. CONCLUSIONS

Some of the strongest evidence suggesting that iron-mediated oxidative reactions are more significant determinants of oxidant cell damage than are thiol/disulfide shifts come from the resistance to diquat-induced hepatic necrosis of Sprague–Dawley (SD) rats, which show little hepatic damage even when pretreated with BCNU, despite massive increases in biliary efflux of GSSG in response to diquat (75). The failure of BCNU to make SD rats susceptible to hepatic damage by diquat and the lack of depletion of hepatic protein thiol contents in diquat-treated Fischer-344 (F344) rats that do sustain necrotic injury, even those F344 rats pretreated with BCNU, support the idea that thiol–disulfide shifts are not critical in this model of tissue injury. However, diquat-induced hepatic injury is enhanced in BCNU-pretreated F344 rats, which is not consistent with the hypothesis that thiols are unimportant. The absence of measurable PSH depletion in relevant models of oxidant injury simply does not support nonspecific thiol/disulfide shifts or oxidation mechanisms in injury, whereas the effects of modulation of GR activities by the molecular methods that have been studied to date suggest strong support for thiol/disulfide mechanisms in oxidant cell injury. Subcellular compartmentation and molecular specificity, at the level we discuss above for protein carbonyl analyses, are likely to be at the basis of these apparent contradictions in the toxicological relevance of toxicant-initiated alterations in cellular thiol/disulfide status (76,77). The seemingly conflicting interpretations of the data presently available provide a very strong rationale for the difficult studies that will be essential to characterize mechanisms of toxicant actions at the necessary levels of molecular specificity. Oxidations of both the thiol-disulfide nature and of the non-thiol-disulfide types are likely to contribute to mechanisms of oxidant injury, but the elucidation of the relevant mechanisms will require chemically specific methods of the sort we describe.

Direct measurements of the oxidation to disulfides, sulfenic, sulfinic or sulfonic acids, or alkylation to thioethers, of specific cysteine residues on specific proteins are needed to elucidate the molecular mechanisms of oxidant injuries and to test such hypotheses. The recent studies by Cotgreave and his colleagues are particularly noteworthy as systematic approaches to methods capable of providing the data at the necessary level of specificity (78,79). Further adaptation of these methodologies and approaches to relevant human and live animal models of toxicant action and physiological responses are needed. These strategies and the data that the applications can provide are important, not only for characterization of specific human exposures and toxicities, but also for the evolution of important fundamental principles, concepts, and experimental approaches.

ACKNOWLEDGMENT

The support of National Institutes of Health Grants GM44262, HL068948, and HL63364 is gratefully recognized.

REFERENCES

1. Pasteur L. The germ theory and its applications to medicine and surgery. Compt Acad Sci 1878;1037–1043.

2. Plaa GL. Chlorinated methanes and liver injury: highlights of the past 50 years. Annu Rev Pharmacol Toxicol 2000;40:42–65.
3. Mitchell JR, Jollow DJ, Potter WZ, Davis DC, Gillette JR, Brodie BB. Acetaminophen-induced hepatic necrosis. I. Role of drug metabolism. J Pharmacol Exp Ther 1973;187:185–194.
4. Jollow DJ, Mitchell JR, Potter WZ, Davis DC, Gillette JR, Brodie BB. Acetaminophen-induced hepatic necrosis. II. Role of covalent binding in vivo. J Pharmacol Exp Ther 1973;187:195–202.
5. Mitchell JR, Jollow DJ, Potter WZ, Gillette JR, Brodie BB. Acetaminophen-induced hepatic necrosis. IV. Protective role of glutathione. J Pharmacol Exp Ther 1973;187:211–217.
6. Smith CV, Lauterburg BH, Mitchell JR. Covalent binding and acute lethal injury in vivo: How has the hypothesis survived a decade of critical examination? In: Wilkinson G, Rawlins MD, eds. Drug Metabolism and Disposition: Considerations in Clinical Pharmacology. London: MTP Press, 1985:161–181.
7. Smith CV, Mitchell JR. Acetaminophen hepatotoxicity in vivo is not accompanied by oxidant stress. Biochem Biophys Res Commun 1985;133:329–336.
8. Chen W, Shockcor JP, Tonge R, Hunter A, Gartner C, Nelson SD. Protein and nonprotein cysteinyl thiol modification by N-acetyl-p-benzoquinone imine via a novel ipso adduct. Biochem 1999;38:8159–8166.
9. Lauterburg BH, Smith CV, Hughes H, Mitchell JR. Biliary excretion of glutathione and glutathione disulfide in the rat: regulation and response to oxidative stress. J Clin Invest 1984;73:124–133.
10. Smith CV, Jaeschke H. Effect of acetaminophen on hepatic content and biliary efflux of glutathione disulfide in mice. Chem Biol Interact 1989;70:241–248.
11. Jaeschke H. Glutathione disulfide formation and oxidant stress during acetaminophen-induced hepatotoxicity in mice in vivo: the protective effect of allopurinol. J Pharmacol Exp Ther 1990;255:935–941.
12. Tirmenstein MA, Nelson SD. Acetaminophen-induced oxidation of protein thiols. Contribution of impaired thiol-metabolizing enzymes and the breakdown of adenine nucleotides. J Biol Chem 1990;265:3059–3065.
13. Rogers LK, Valentine CJ, Szczypka M, Smith CV. Effects of hepatotoxic doses of acetaminophen and furosemide on tissue concentrations of CoASH and CoASSG in vivo. Chem Res Toxicol 2000;13:873–882.
14. Slatter JG, Rashed MS, Pearson PG, Han DH, Baillie TA. Biotransformation of methyl isocyanate in the rat. Evidence for glutathione conjugation as a major pathway of metabolism and implications for isocyanate-mediated toxicities. Chem Res Toxicol 1991;4:157–161.
15. Jean PA, Reed DJ. Utilization of glutathione during 1,2-dihaloethane metabolism in rat hepatocytes. Chem Res Toxicol 1992;5:386–391.
16. Kosugi H, Kikugawa K. Potential thiobarbituric acid-reactive substances in peroxidized lipids. Free Rad Biol Med 1989;7:205–207.
17. Wendel A, Feuerstein S, Konz K-H. Acute paracetamol intoxication of starved mice leads to lipid peroxidation in vivo. Biochem Pharmacol 1979;28:2051–2055.

18. Smith CV. Correlations and apparent contradictions in assessment of oxidant stress status in vivo. Free Rad Biol Med 1991;10:217–224.
19. Hughes H, Smith CV, Horning EC, Mitchell JR. High performance liquid chromatography and gas chromatography-mass spectrometry determination of specific lipid peroxidation products in vivo. Anal Biochem 1983;130:431–436.
20. Hughes H, Smith CV, Mitchell JR. Quantitation of lipid peroxidation products by gas chromatography-mass spectrometry. Anal Biochem 1986;152:107–112.
21. Morrow JD, Awad JA, Kato T, et al. Formation of novel non-cyclooxygenase-derived prostanoids (F2-isoprostanes) in carbon tetrachloride hepatotoxicity. An animal model of lipid peroxidation. J Clin Invest 1992;90:2502–2507.
22. Smith CV, Mitchell JR. Pharmacological aspects of glutathione in drug metabolism. In: Dolphin D, Poulson R, Avramovic O, eds. Coenzymes and Cofactors. New York: John Wiley;1989:1–44.
23. Smith CV, Todd EL, Hughes H, Mitchell JR. Isolation and identification of specific products of alkylation of hepatic protein in vivo by reactive metabolites of acetaminophen and bromobenzene. Fed Proc 1984;41:361.
24. Smith CV, Hughes H, Lauterburg BH, Mitchell JR. Oxidant stress and hepatic necrosis in rats treated with diquat. J Pharmacol Exp Ther 1985;235:172–177.
25. Hoffmann K-J, Streeter AJ, Axworthy DB, Baillie TA. Identification of the major covalent adduct formed in vitro and in vivo between acetaminophen and mouse liver proteins. Mol Pharmacol 1985;27:566–573.
26. Gupta S, Rogers LK, Taylor SK, Smith CV. Inhibition of carbamyl phosphate synthetase-I and glutamine synthetase by hepatotoxic doses of acetaminophen in mice. Toxicol Appl Pharmacol 1997;146:317–327.
27. Qiu Y, Benet LZ, Burlingame AL. Identification of the hepatic protein targets of reactive metabolites of acetaminophen in vivo in mice using two-dimensional gel electrophoresis and mass spectrometry. J Biol Chem 1998;273:17940–17953.
28. Bulera SJ, Birge RB, Cohen SD, Khairallah EA. Identification of the mouse liver 44-kDa acetaminophen-binding protein as a subunit of glutamine synthetase. Toxicol Appl Pharmacol 1995;134:313–320.
29. Pumford NR, Halmes NC, Martin BM, Cook RJ, Wagner C, Hinson JA. Covalent binding of acetaminophen to N-10-formyltetrahydrofolate dehydrogenase in mice. J Pharmacol Exp Ther 1997;280:501–505.
30. Halmes NC, Hinson JA, Martin BM, Pumford NR. Glutamate dehydrogenase covalently binds to a reactive metabolite of acetaminophen. Chem Res Toxicol 1996;9:541–546.
31. Gygi SP, Corthals GL, Zhang Y, Rochon Y, Aebersold R. Evaluation of two-dimensional gel electrophoresis-based proteome analysis technology. Proc Natl Acad Sci USA 2000;97:9390–9395.
32. Jones DP, Thor H, Smith MT, Jewell SA, Orrenius S. Inhibition of ATP-dependent microsomal Ca^{2+} sequestration during oxidative stress and its prevention by glutathione. J Biol Chem 1983;258:6390–6393.

33. Di Monte D, Bellomo G, Thor H, Nicotera P, Orrenius S. Menadione-induced cytotoxicity is associated with protein thiol oxidation and alteration in intracellular Ca^{2+} homostasis. Arch Biochem Biophys 1984;235:343–350.
34. Di Monte D, Ross G, Bellomo G, Elkow L, Orrenius S. Alterations in intracellular thiol homeostasis during the metabolism of menadione by isolated rat hepatocytes. Arch Biochem Biophys 1984;235:334–342.
35. Burk RF, Lawrence RA, Lane JM. Liver necrosis and lipid peroxidation in the rat as a result of paraquat and diquat administration. Effect of selenium deficiency. J Clin Invest 1980;65:1024–1031.
36. Burk RF, Lane JM. Ethane production and liver necrosis in rats after administration of drugs and other chemicals. Toxicol Appl Pharmacol 1979;50:467–478.
37. Spalding DJM, Mitchell JR, Jaeschke H, Smith CV. Diquat hepatotoxicity in the Fischer-344 rat: the role of covalent binding to tissue proteins and lipids. Toxicol Appl Pharmacol 1989;101:319–327.
38. Kehrer JP. The effect of BCNU (carmustine) on tissue glutathione reductase activity. Toxicol Lett 1983;17:63–68.
39. Kehrer JP, Haschek W, Witschi H. The influence of hyperoxia on the acute toxicity of paraquat and diquat. Drug Chem Toxicol 1979;2:397–408.
40. Kehrer JP, Paraidathathu T. Enhanced oxygen toxicity following treatment with 1,3-bis(2-chloroethyl)-1-nitrosourea. Fund Appl Toxicol 1984;4:760–767.
41. Smith CV, Hughes H, Lauterburg BH, Mitchell JR. Chemical nature of reactive metabolites determines their biological interactions with glutathione. In: Larsson A, Orrenius S, Holmgren A, Mannervik B, eds. Functions of Glutathione: Biochemical, Physiological, Toxicological, and Clinical Aspects. New York: Raven Press, 1983:125–138.
42. Bodell WJ, Aida T, Berger MS, Rosenblum ML. Increased repair of O^6-alkylguanine DNA adducts in glioma-derived human cells resistant to the cytotoxic and cytogenetic effects of 1,3-bis(2-chloroethyl)-1-nitrosourea. Carcinogenesis 1986;7:879–883.
43. Mulligan M, Althaus B, Linder MC. Non-ferritin, non-heme iron pools in rat tissues. Int J Biochem 1986;18:791–798.
44. Smith CV, Hughes H, Lauterburg BH, Mitchell JR. Oxidant stress and hepatic necrosis in rats treated with diquat. J Pharmacol Exp Ther 1985;235:172–177.
45. Smith CV. Evidence for the participation of lipid peroxidation and iron in diquat-induced hepatic necrosis *in vivo*. Mol Pharmacol 1987;32:417–422.
46. Gupta S, Rogers LK, Smith CV. Biliary excretion of lysosomal enzymes, iron, and oxidized protein in Fischer-344 and Sprague–Dawley rats and the effects of diquat and acetaminophen. Toxicol Appl Pharmacol 1994;125:42–50.
47. Khan MF, Wu X, Alcock NW, Boor PJ, Ansari GA. Iron exacerbates aniline-associated splenic toxicity. J Toxicol Environ Health A 1999;57:173–184.
48. Khan MF, Wu X, Boor PJ, Ansari GA. Oxidative modification of lipids and proteins in aniline-induced splenic toxicity. Toxicol Sci 1999;48:134–140.
49. Khan MF, Boor PJ, Gu Y, Alcock NW, Ansari GA. Oxidative stress in the splenotoxicity of aniline. Fund Appl Toxicol 1997;35:22–30.

50. Rikans LE, Ardinska V, Hornbrook KR. Age-associated increase in ferritin content of male rat liver: implication for diquat-mediated oxidative injury. Arch Biochem Biophys 1997;344:85–93.
51. Rikans LE, Cai Y, Kosanke SD, Venkataraman PS. Redox cycling and hepatotoxicity of diquat in aging male Fischer 344 rats. Drug Metab Dispos 1993;21:605–610.
52. Mertens JJ, Gibson NW, Lau SS, Monks TJ. Reactive oxygen species and DNA damage in 2-bromo-(glutathion-S-yl) hydroquinone-mediated cytotoxicity. Arch Biochem Biophys 1995;320:51–58.
53. Bolton JL, Trush MA, Penning TM, Dryhurst G, Monks TJ. Role of quinones in toxicology. Chem Res Toxicol 2000;13:135–160.
54. Vulimiri SV, Gupta S, Smith CV, Moorthy B, Randerath K. Rapid decreases in indigenous covalent modifications (I-compounds) of male F-344 rat liver DNA by diquat treatment. Chem Biol Interact 1995;95:1–16.
55. Randerath K, Randerath E, Smith CV, Chang J. Structural origins of bulky oxidative DNA adducts (type III-compounds) as deduced by oxidation of oligonucleotides of known sequence. Chem Res Toxicol 1996;9:247–254.
56. Gupta S, Kleiner HE, Rogers LK, Lau SS, Smith CV. Redox stress and hepatic DNA fragmentation induced by diquat *in vivo* are not accompanied by increased 8-hydroxydeoxyguanosine contents. Redox Rep 1997;3:31–39.
57. Winterbourn CC, Chan T, Buss IH, Inder TE, Mogridge N, Darlow BA. Protein carbonyls and lipid peroxidation products as oxidation markers in preterm infant plasma: associations with chronic lung disease and retinopathy and effects of selenium supplementation. Pediatr Res 2000;48:84–90.
58. Buss IH, Darlow BA, Winterbourn CC. Elevated protein carbonyls and lipid peroxidation products correlating with myeloperoxidase in tracheal aspirates from premature infants. Pediatr Res 2000;47:640–645.
59. Stadtman ER, Berlett BS. Reactive oxygen-mediated protein oxidation in aging and disease. Chem Res Toxicol 1997;10:485–494.
60. Knight SA, Smith CV, Welty SE. Iron and oxidized β-casein in the lavages of hyperoxic Fischer-344 rats. Life Sci 1998;62:165–176.
61. Ramsay PL, DeMayo FJ, Hegemier SE, Wearden ME, Smith CV, Welty SE. Clara cell secretory protein oxidation and expression in premature infants who develop bronchopulmonary dysplasia. Am J Respir Crit Care Med 2001;164:155–161.
62. Hinson JA, Pike SL, Pumford NR, Mayeux PR. Nitrotyrosine-protein adducts in hepatic centrilobular areas following toxic doses of acetaminophen in mice. Chem Res Toxicol 1998;11:604–607.
63. Michael SL, Pumford NR, Mayeux PR, Niesman MR, Hinson JA. Pretreatment of mice with macrophage inactivators decreases acetaminophen hepatotoxicity and the formation of reactive oxygen and nitrogen species. Hepatology 1999;30:186–195.
64. Knight TR, Kurtz A, Bajt ML, Hinson JA, Jaeschke H. Vascular and hepatocellular peroxynitrite formation during acetaminophen toxicity: role of mitochondrial oxidant stress. Toxicol Sci 2001;62:212–220.

65. Schramm L, La M, Heidbreder E, et al. L-Arginine deficiency and supplementation in experimental acute renal failure and in human kidney transplantation. Kidney Int 2002;61:1423–1432.
66. Beckman JS. –OONO: rebounding from nitric oxide. Circ Res 2001;89:295–297.
67. Ferret PJ, Hammoud R, Tulliez M, et al. Detoxification of reactive oxygen species by a nonpeptidyl mimic of superoxide dismutase cures acetaminophen-induced acute liver failure in the mouse. Hepatology 2001;33:1173–1180.
68. Davies MJ, Fu S, Wang H, Dean RT. Stable markers of oxidant damage to proteins and their application in the study of human disease. Free Rad Biol Med 1999;27:1151–1163.
69. Leeuwenburgh C, Rasmussen JE, Hsu FF, Mueller DM, Pennathur S, Heinecke JW. Mass spectrometric quantification of markers for protein oxidation by tyrosyl radical, copper, and hydroxyl radical in low density lipoptotein isolated from human atherosclerotic plaques. J Biol Chem 1997;272:3520–3526.
70. Yang C-Y, Gu Z-W, Yang H-X, et al. Oxidation of bovine β-casein by hypochlorite. Free Rad Biol Med 1997;22:1235–1240.
71. Yang C-Y, Gu Z-W, Yang H-X, Gotto AM Jr, Smith CV. Oxidative modifications of apoB-100 by exposure of low density lipoproteins to HOCl in vitro. Free Rad Biol Med 1997;23:82–89.
72. Yang C-Y, Gu Z-W, Yang M, et al. Selective modification of apoB-100 in the oxidation of low density lipoproteins by myeloperoxidase *in vitro*. J Lipid Res 1999;40:686–698.
73. Yang C-Y, Gu Z-W, Yang M, Lin S-N, Siuzdak G, Smith CV. Identification of modified tryptophan residues in apolipoprotein B-100 derived from copper ion-oxidized low-density lipoprotein. Biochemistry 1999;38:15903–15908.
74. Yang C-Y, Wang J, Krutchinsky AN, Chait BT, Morrisett JD, Smith CV. Selective oxidation in vitro by myeloperoxidase of the N-terminal amine in apolipoprotein B-100. J Lipid Res 2001;42:1891–1896.
75. Smith CV. Effect of BCNU pretreatment on diquat-induced oxidant stress and hepatotoxicity. Biochem Biophys Res Commun 1987;144:415–421.
76. Hwang C, Sinskey AJ, Lodish HF. Oxidized redox state of glutathione in the endoplasmic reticulum. Science 1992;257:1496–1502.
77. Smith CV, Jones DP, Guenthner TM, Lash LH, Lauterburg BH. Compartmentation of glutathione. Implications for the study of toxicity and disease. Toxicol Appl Pharmacol 1996;140:1–12.
78. Lind C, Gerdes R, Hamnell Y, et al. Identification of *S*-glutathionylated cellular proteins during oxidative stress and constitutive metabolism by affinity purification and proteomic analysis. Arch Biochem Biophys 2002;406:229–240.
79. Dandrea T, Bajak E, Warngard L, Cotgreave IA. Protein *S*-glutathionylation correlates to selective stress gene expression and cytoprotection. Arch Biochem Biophys 2002;406:241–252.

11

Multidrug Resistance Proteins and Hepatic Transport of Endo- and Xenobiotics

Phillip M. Gerk and Mary Vore

Summary

Transporters that use ATP are called ATP-binding cassette (ABC) transporters. One family of ABC transporters that plays a major role in the ability of the liver to eliminate various drugs is the multidrug resistance proteins (MRPs). There are nine cloned genes in the MRP (ABCC) subfamily. Generally, these carriers transport diverse sulfate, glutathione, or glucuronide conjugates of endogenous compounds like estrogen and bilirubin, as well as drugs and toxins. Although all of the MRPs mediate ATP-dependent efflux, their tissue expression and cellular localization vary. MRP2 is most highly expressed in the liver at the canalicular domain and is the primary focus of this chapter. Several in vitro approaches to study drug transport in the liver are discussed. Although these approaches have been described in detail elsewhere, the authors present their own perspectives, with particular emphasis on the baculovirus expression vector system. Additional methods and approaches that are discussed include the choice of animal tissue preparation, expression system to be used, and experimental paradigms, including uptake in membrane vesicles, cell monolayers, and procedures to measure ATPase activity and its relationship to transport.

Key Words

ATPase activity; ATP-binding cassette transporters; baculovirus expression; expression systems; hepatocytes; liver; membrane vesicles; multidrug resistance associated proteins; Sf9 cell culture, Sf9 membrane vesicle preparation.

1. INTRODUCTION

Most biologically active compounds can be described in terms of their degree of lipophilicity or hydrophilicity. Lipophilic compounds can pass through lipid membranes rapidly, so movement is limited by aqueous diffusion. Hydrophilic compounds do not pass through membranes easily, and thus

From: *Methods in Pharmacology and Toxicology,*
Drug Metabolism and Transport: Molecular Methods and Mechanisms
Edited by: L. Lash © Humana Press Inc., Totowa, NJ

require a transporter to facilitate their movement into and out of cells *(1)*. Of course, many compounds fall in between these extremes, and the need for protein-mediated transport is determined by the mass movement required to obtain or avoid their physiologic, pharmacologic, or toxicologic activities, as the case may be. This review focuses on protein-mediated transport processes rather than simple diffusion.

Protein-mediated transport is accomplished by channels and transporters. Channels serve as gated pores that regulate the rapid movement of ions across membranes, and are not further discussed in this chapter. Transporters fall into several categories, which are all saturable. Facilitated diffusion carriers do not require energy and simply accelerate the diffusion of their substrates down their electrochemical potential gradient (downhill transport). In contrast, active transporters can build and maintain concentration gradients (uphill transport). Primary active transporters use nucleotides like ATP (or rarely, light) as an energy source, using the release of energy to drive the conformational change that translocates the transport substrate. Allocrite is another formal term used to describe the transported compound (informally referred to as "substrate"), to distinguish it from ATP, which is a true substrate hydrolyzed by ATP-dependent transporters *(2)*. Secondary (and tertiary) active transporters use the change in free energy from the downhill transport of one compound to drive the uphill transport of another. The general properties of transporters have been described in greater detail by Stein *(1,3)*.

Recently, transporters have been classified into two superfamilies. Transporters that use ATP are called ATP-binding cassette (ABC) transporters and have been recently reviewed *(4,5)*. All other transporters are classified in the solute carrier (SLC) superfamily. More information on nomenclature, classification, and functions of transporters can be found at the websites in Table 1.

Clearly, the liver plays a major role in drug elimination, both through metabolism and transport. Several important hepatic transporters are shown in Fig. 1 *(5,6)*. The main movement of solutes is from the basolateral side (where uptake transporters predominate) to the canalicular (apical) side (where efflux transporters predominate). The solutes will then flow with bile through the bile ducts and eventually to the intestine. Thus, the liver has two related transport functions: bile formation and excretion. Bile formation results from the transport of osmotically active solutes into the confined space of the canaliculus, followed by the passive movement of water until equilibrium is reached *(7)*. Osmolytes present in bile include bile acids, which are transported into the canaliculus by the bile salt export pump (Bsep, Abcb11); the accompanying counterion, Na^+, along with the bile acids contribute a major component of bile flow, termed *bile*

Table 1
Useful Websites for Studying Hepatic Transport

Website address	Description
http://bigfoot.med.unc.edu/watkinsLab/	Substrates, inhibitors, and inducers of human hepatocyte and enterocyte transporters
http://www.gene.ucl.ac.uk/nomenclature/genefamily.shtml	Nomenclature of human genes including transporters
http://nutrigene.4t.com/humanabc.htm	Information and classification on ABC transporters
http://www.biology.ucsd.edu/~msaier/transport	Milton Saier's transport protein database
http://www.gentest.com/	Source of expressed MDR1, "transportocytes," and hepatocytes; ATPase protocol
http://www.invitrogen.com	Source of Bac-to-Bac and BaculoDirect Expression systems
http://www.med.rug.nl/mdl/english/tab3.htm	Information and classification on SLC 10, 21, 22, ABCB, and ABCC transporters
http://www.pharmingen.com	Source of BaculoGold Expression System
http://www.solvobiotech.com/	Source of expressed ABC transporters, transport and ATPase protocols

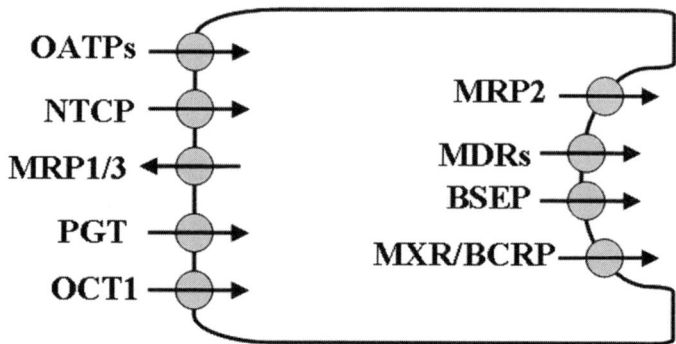

Fig. 1. Basolateral and canalicular hepatic transporters. Basolateral transporters are shown on the left, canalicular transporters are shown on the right. BSEP, Bile salt export pump; MDRs, multidrug resistance transporter (including human MDR1 and MDR3 and their rat homologues Mdr1a/1b and Mdr2); MRP, multidrug resistance-associated protein; MXR/BCRP, mitoxantrone resistance transporter/breast cancer resistance protein; NTCP, sodium-taurocholate cotransporting protein; OATP, organic anion transporting polypeptides; OCT1, organic cation transporter 1; PGT, prostaglandin transporter.

acid dependent bile flow (7). The significantly decreased bile flow in TR⁻ rats, deficient in multidrug resistance associated protein 2 (Mrp2, Abcc2; discussed in greater detail below) provides significant support to the theory that Mrp2 substrates, including glutathione and glucuronide conjugates, are also important osmolytes in bile that are responsible for *bile acid independent bile flow (8)*. Glutathione, an Mrp2 substrate, is considered to be the single most important osmolyte contributing to bile acid independent bile flow *(8)*. Thus, the transport functions of the liver are not independent of, but rather interactive with, metabolism, as demonstrated with Mrp2 in the following subheading.

2. MRPS: FUNCTIONS AND MECHANISMS

There are nine cloned genes in the MRP (ABCC) subfamily. Generally, these transporters transport diverse sulfate, glutathione, or glucuronide conjugates of endogenous compounds like estrogen and bilirubin, as well as drugs and toxins *(6,9)*. For example, MRP1-4 all transport β-estradiol-17-(β-D-glucuronide) ($E_2$17G), but with differing efficiencies *(6)*. Although all of the MRPs mediate ATP-dependent efflux, their tissue expression and cellular localization vary. MRP2 is most highly expressed in the liver at the canalicular domain, so this chapter focuses on MRP2. Genetic deficiency of MRP2 causes Dubin–Johnson syndrome, resulting in hyperbilirubinemia, decreased bile flow, decreased excretion of many endo- and xenobiotics, and deposition of a dark pigment in the

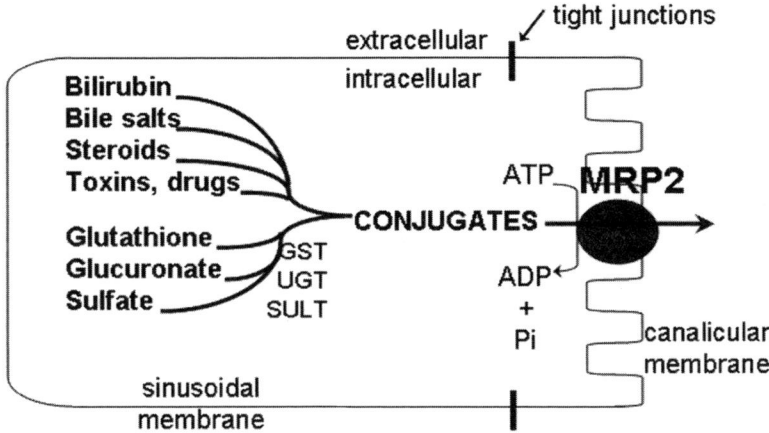

Fig. 2. Function of MRP2 in the hepatocyte. Various compounds can be conjugated by intracellular enzymes including glutathione-*S*-transferases (GST), UDP-glucuronosyltransferases (UGT), and sulfotransferases (SULT). Many of these conjugates are then effluxed across the canalicular membrane in an ATP-dependent manner by MRP2. (Adapted from ref. *10*.)

liver. Like other MRPs, MRP2 mediates the excretion of conjugates (Fig. 2), but MRP2 shows less dependence on glutathione cotransport, compared to MRP1.

Mrp2 expression can be altered by pathologic states such as renal failure, pregnancy, cholestasis, and acute phase response *(9)*. However, MRP3 is expressed on the basolateral membrane, and its expression can be induced by cholestasis, serving as a potential protective mechanism against the intracellular accumulation of toxic compounds and metabolites in the hepatocyte *(11,12)*. In addition, farnesoid X receptor, pregnane X receptor, and constitutive androstane receptor ligands, and several drugs can alter Mrp2 expression. Expression may be altered at the level of transcription, translation, and posttranslation through endocytic retrieval *(9)*.

3. METHODS (IN VITRO)

This chapter outlines several in vitro approaches to study drug transport in the liver. Although these approaches have been described in detail elsewhere, here we present our perspectives, with particular emphasis on the baculovirus expression vector system.

3.1. Animal Tissue Preparations

In addition to in vivo studies in animals, several preparations can be used for in vitro experiments. The perfused liver is useful to examine hepatic extraction, metabolism, and biliary excretion, and most closely simulates physiologic conditions *(13)*. Uptake and/or efflux can be examined in isolated rat or human hepatocytes. Hepatocyte preparations have been described elsewhere; in addition, they are available from Gentest. Next, it is possible to isolate canalicular and basolateral membrane vesicles, which can then be used for vesicular uptake studies. The preparation and use of these vesicles has also been described *(14,15)*. Furthermore, the comparison of biliary excretion or canalicular membrane transport activities between normal rats and Mrp2-deficient rats (Groningen yellow/TR⁻ or Eisai hyperbilirubinemic rats) has facilitated the identification of Mrp2 substrates and its impact on their transport *(16)*.

3.2. Expression Systems

As shown in Fig. 1, there are several ABC transporters expressed at the canalicular membrane, and these have overlapping substrating specificities. One of the serious limitations of animal tissue preparations is the difficulty in determining the contribution from individual transporters. To overcome this problem, these transporters can be overexpressed to study their functions independently. They can be expressed transiently, by injecting oocytes with cRNA or transfecting yeast with an expression plasmid. However, injection of oocytes is tedious, and subject to seasonal variations in the harvest of oocytes. Yeast expression also faces limiting factors, including difficulty harvesting protein and the low level of posttranslational modifications. Alternatively, transporters have been stably transfected and expressed in several different mammalian cell lines, including MDCK cells *(17)*, HeLa cells *(18)*, COS-7 cells *(19)*, CHO cells *(20)*, HEK293 cells *(21)*, and others. Through stable transfections, proteins can be expressed in a mammalian environment, with appropriate posttranslational modifications. However, a long selection process is often required; furthermore, MRP2 is not efficiently routed to the plasma membrane *(22)*.

In addition to these methods, virus-mediated expression has been shown to be an effective approach. Commonly, the genes are inserted into the baculovirus, which is then used to infect insect cells. Alternatively, genes can be inserted into adenoviruses, and then used to infect certain cell lines. In either case, the cell machinery is then conscripted to overexpress the protein of interest. Cell membranes can then be harvested, and vesicular uptake experiments can be performed, as described in Subheading 3.3.1. Several commercially available products are marketed for baculovirus-mediated expression, which accelerate and simplify insertion of the gene of interest into the baculovirus vector. One product with which we have extensive experience is from Gibco (now Invitrogen), called the Bac-to-Bac Baculovirus Expression Vector System, and is described below. In brief, this system involves inserting the cDNA of interest into a shuttle vector (pFastBac1), which is then transformed into DH10Bac cells containing the circular baculovirus genome (bacmid) and a transposition helper plasmid. Transposition takes place, resulting in the insertion of the cDNA into the bacmid, and loss of β-galactosidase activity, allowing white colonies to be selected on plates containing Blue-gal. Bacmid DNA is then isolated and used to transfect Sf9 cells, which then produce the recombinant baculovirus. The baculovirus is then amplified, titered, and used to infect Sf9 cells for protein production. Another product, from Pharmingen, called BaculoGold, uses recombination in insect cells under the selective pressure of antibiotics. More conventional methods have been described in an extensive and informative manual *(23)*. Most recently, Invitrogen has produced another product, BaculoDirect, which allows the above mentioned transposition event to occur enzymatically. This product offers the advantage of speed and convenience, but it is quite expensive. More information on these products can be found on the websites for these companies in Table 1.

3.3. Experimental Paradigms

The hypothesis to be tested determines which functional approach is most appropriate. In this brief overview, we discuss uptake into membrane vesicles, transport across a cell monolayer, and ATPase activity.

3.3.1. Membrane Vesicle Uptake

The preparation and use of membrane vesicles has facilitated numerous investigations not possible with living cells, tissues, or organisms. In this in vitro preparation, the experimental conditions can, therefore, be modified without concerns regarding cell viability. Although preparation of isolated basolateral or canalicular membrane vesicles from rat liver is tedious and gives a low yield, the technique is ideally suited for use with expression systems.

Membrane vesicles are a mixture of inside-out and right-side out orientations, but only the inside-out vesicles have access to ATP and thus can transport the substrate, as the ATP-binding cassettes are intracellular-facing. We assume that ATP diffusion across the membranes is negligible, so the observed ATP-dependent transport represents activity of only the inside-out membrane vesicles. For comparison, membrane vesicles from Sf9 cells are reported to be approx 65% inside-out *(24)*; canalicular membrane vesicles are 32 ± 5% inside-out *(25)*; membranes prepared from LLC-PK$_1$ cells are 49% inside-out *(26)*.

Transport experiments are performed in a Tris-sucrose buffer *(27)*, containing ATP or AMP, MgCl$_2$, an ATP-regenerating system, with unlabeled agents in either dimethyl sulfoxide (0.5%) or vehicle (2% of 10:4:1 Tris-sucrose buffer–propylene glycol–ethanol). Preliminary studies showed that the choice of vehicle had no effect on transport. ATP-dependent transport of [^{3}H]E$_2$17G into membrane vesicles (10 µg/20 µL) is measured by incubating at 37°C for 2–5 min in 12 × 75 mm polystyrene tubes (Sarstedt), then stopped with

3.5 mL (a P5000 pipetter is useful for speed) of ice-cold stop buffer *(27)*; the mixture is then quickly filtered by transferring to a Millipore 15-mL filter funnel and collected on 25 mm Durapore 0.4-µm filters (Millipore). These filters were selected due to their minimal binding of $E_2 17G$ at low (90 nM) or high (100 µM) concentrations; binding was less than that to HAWP or nitrocellulose filters, and similar to that to Whatman glass fiber type A/E filters (unpublished data). The tubes are rinsed once with 3.5 mL of stop buffer, then the funnel is rinsed again with 3.5 mL of stop buffer, as described *(14)*. Filters are collected in 7-mL scintillation vials, and radioactivity is dissolved (several hours or overnight) in scintillation counting cocktail (Bio-Safe II, RPI, Mt. Prospect, IL). Liquid scintillation counting is performed to detect ^{3}H. Data obtained in the presence of AMP should be subtracted from that in the presence of ATP; furthermore, data should be corrected for background transport by endogenous transporters. We prefer nonlinear regression for analysis of Michaelis–Menten saturation curves, and we typically use a weighting scheme of $1/y^2$, because the variability tends to increase with transport rates.

Similar protocols for MRP1/2 mediated transport into membrane vesicles are available at www.solvo.com. In addition, this method has recently been adapted for use in the 96-well format, and is likely to be useful for high-throughput screening for the pharmaceutical industry *(28)*. However, it requires expensive equipment and this level of throughput is generally not necessary for academic research laboratories.

3.3.2. Transmonolayer Flux

Using cell monolayers derived from tissues of interest (as in the Caco-2, MDCKII or other cell models), one can obtain transcellular transport parameters, which may be helpful in understanding the vectorial transport of substrates across an epithelium *(29,30)*. Typically, cells are grown to confluence on transwell filters, and passage of substrate from one side to the other is analyzed, either by liquid scintillation counting, or photometrically. In addition, the use of a side by side diffusion chamber system (Fig. 3) has been described previously in detail *(31)*. The advantage of the latter over the commonly used transwell system is the ability to obtain a more accurate estimate of transport parameters (especially for lipophilic compounds) by minimizing the influence of the unstirred layers in both fluid chambers *(32,33)*. The disadvantages include having a more complex system of transporters and enzymes to study, and the difficulty and time required to produce cells grown to confluence on these filters.

3.3.3. ATPase Activity

In addition to transport function, it may also be desirable to examine another biochemical function of ABC transporters, namely ATPase activity.

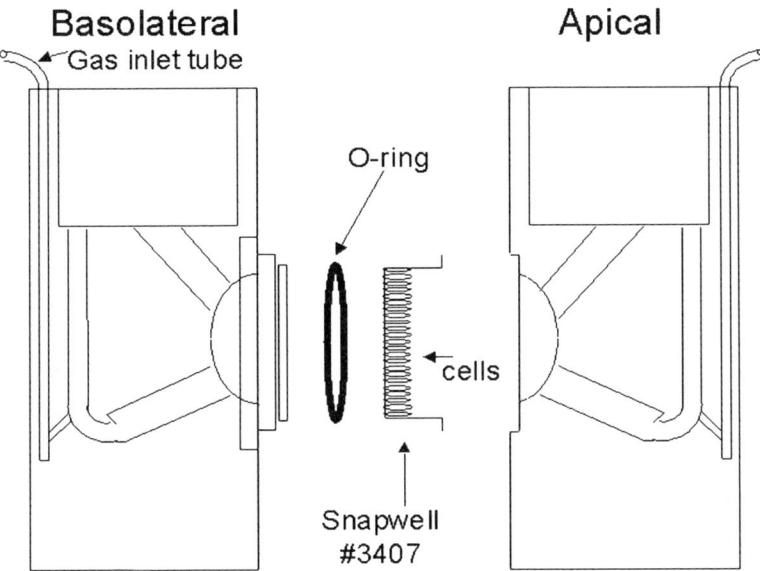

Fig. 3. Snapwell diffusion chambers. The chambers consist of the basolateral (**left**) compartment, the apical (**right**) compartment, the cells grown on a snapwell filter, and an O-ring to form a seal. Gas is bubbled at 25–30 mL/min through both gas inlet tubes, resulting in a lifting action that creates linear fluid movement through each chamber, thus minimizing the unstirred layers on both sides. Samples can be drawn at any time without disruption.

Typically, this is done using membranes prepared from cells expressing the ABC transporter of interest. ATPase activity can be used to screen interactions between compounds of interest and ABC transporters of concern. However, negative results may not necessarily indicate a lack of interaction, nor does a positive result indicate that a compound is a transport substrate *(34)*. ATPase activity data can be used to discern the biochemical functions of ABC transporters *(2)*.

ATPase activity stimulation by a compound is not strictly correlated with its transport activity *(34)*. For example, a stimulatory (or inhibitory) effect on ATPase activity indicates an interaction between the compound and the ABC transporter; however, a lack of an effect does not indicate a lack of interaction. Part of the discrepancy between ATPase stimulation and transport activity may be related to the baseline ATPase activity of these transporters. In the absence of added substrates, MDR1 exhibits idle ATPase cycling *(35)*, which may occur with other ABC transporters as well. Idle cycling may make it difficult to observe a net change in ATPase activity, as follows. If a known transport substrate is added to an ABC transporter, it binds to an ABC transporter; ATP is hydrolyzed, and a conformational change occurs resulting in transport; the transporter may then return to its original state, completing the cycle *(2)*. ATPase activity due to the interaction between a substrate and the ABC transporter must be greater than the baseline ATPase activity, to observe a measurable change in net ATPase activity. However, the presence of added substrate(s) may also alter the rate of ATPase idle cycling, which could result in a decreased sensitivity of the ATPase assay to detect ATPase stimulation due to transport substrates.

ATPase activity is measured by determining the liberation of inorganic phosphate from ATP with a colorimetric reaction *(36)*. This reaction uses zinc acetate and ammonium molybdate to form a complex with inorganic phosphate; the complex is then reduced using ascorbate. We have found this method robust to changes in the incubation buffer, sensitive to low amounts of inorganic phosphate, and very reproducible. Other detection methods can also be used but are not discussed here.

The incubation media contains 10 mM $MgCl_2$, 40 mM 2-(*N*-morpholino)-ethanesulfonic acid, 40 mM tris-(hydroxymethyl)-aminomethane, 5 mM dithiothreitol, 50 mM KCl, 0.1 mM ethylene glycol tetraacetate, 4 mM sodium azide, 1 mM ouabain, and 5 mM MgATP, as described *(37)*. The crude protein concentration is 50 µg/100 µL, and the incubation time is 30 min at 37°C. The assay is optimized with regards to time and protein by comparing probenecid-stimulated ATPase activity to control (in the case of Mrp2). Reactions are stopped by adding 100 µL of 5% sodium lauryl sulfate, and liberated inorganic phosphate is measured colorimetrically as mentioned above (λ = 850 nm) *(36)*. Data obtained in the presence of vanadate (0.3 mM) are subtracted from each determination to establish the vanadate-sensitive ATPase activity. Appropriate statistical comparisons can then be performed.

ATPase activity assays have also been adapted for 96-well systems *(38)*. The limiting factor with this adaptation is the availability of an accurate and reliable plate reader. This is in part due to the limitations of most plate readers, which read absorbance at a maximum wavelength of 600 nm, which is below the peak sensitivity of 850 nm *(38)*. Nonetheless, this technique can be used successfully. Detailed protocols for this method are available at www.gentest.com. or www.solvo.com.

In conclusion, there are many techniques currently available to study the function of hepatic transporters. The key is to choose an appropriate system for the experimental questions and hypotheses at hand. Many investigators are using the baculovirus expression vector system due to its relative ease and low cost. In the following subheadings are detailed the protocols we have found to be effective in characterizing Mrp2 function.

4. PROTOCOL 1: SF9 CELL CULTURE

4.1. Background

Sf9 cells grow well in suspension or attached to plastic. In suspension culture, cells double about every 20–24 h, and viability (by trypan blue exclusion) is >97%. Cells can be seen mostly as singlets and doublets, but a few triplets and quadruplets (and a few small groups) can be observed. Uncommonly larger clusters can be seen. Cultures having these characteristics (doubling time, viability, minimal clumping) are considered "healthy cultures." Some investigators use "impeller" flasks, in which a magnetic impeller directly contacts the liquid culture. However, these flasks are expensive, difficult to clean, and relatively easily contaminated. A more practical and convenient method uses shaking cultures, in which cells are grown in polymethylpentene (PMP, available from Nalgene) Erlenmeyer flasks shaken continuously.

4.2. Recovery of Cells From Liquid Nitrogen (or –80°C)

1. Warm 16 mL of the medium to 27°C in a 125-mL PMP flask (Nalgene). We use SF900 II SFM (serum-free medium) from Invitrogen. This medium allows us to more easily perform transfections and viral plaque assays, both of which must be performed in the absence of serum. The cost is high, but other common media (such as Grace's medium with 10% fetal bovine serum) are slightly more expensive due to the current high cost of fetal bovine serum. Furthermore, the manufacturer states that the saturation density in SF900 II SFM is higher than other media, potentially allowing a longer log growth phase.
2. Warm the cells to 37°C quickly in a water bath, continually checking to determine when the aliquot is nearly melted.
3. Wipe the tube with alcohol, transfer contents to flask.
4. Shake at 130–150 rpm on a platform shaker (Lab-Line, available through Fisher) at 27°C, 1–4 d until cell counts are approx 1.5–2×10^6 cells/mL.
5. Split again to 0.6×10^6 cells/mL and allow to grow as described in step 1.
6. Split cells again as in step 5, but let them grow to 3–4×10^6 cells/mL.
7. Culture as described in Subheading 4.3.

4.3. Routine Subculture

1. The medium is warmed to 27°C.
2. Wipe gloved hands and flask with alcohol. Gently swirl flask, and use yellow 1-mL disposable pipets to draw 0.2 mL of cells. Take two samples for each flask, and place in 1.5-mL Eppendorf tubes.
3. Promptly return flask to incubator shaker (27°C, 130–150 rpm).
4. Add 0.2 mL of trypan blue to the tube, invert several times to mix.
5. Place approx 10 µL of the mix onto the hemacytometer. Under ×10 magnification, count the total number of cells and the number of dark (dead) cells in the middle set of squares.

6. Count two aliquots per tube, two tubes per flask.
7. Determine the total number of cells and the number of dead cells and calculate the percentage of viable cells. Multiply this percentage by the total number of cells, and then multiply by 5000 to obtain the cell density. Example: 510 total cells counted, 10 dead cells: 98% viable, 2.5×10^6 viable cells/mL.
8. Seed the cells at $0.6–0.75 \times 10^6$ viable cells/mL, 25–50 mL per 125-mL flask, or 50–100 mL per 250-mL flask, or 100–200 mL per 500-mL flask.
9. Let the cells grow 2 d, or until they reach a cell density of $3–4.5 \times 10^6$ viable cells/mL.

4.4. Cryogenic Storage of Sf9 Cells

1. Centrifuge approx 30 mL of cells ($3–4.5 \times 10^6$ viable cells/mL) at 100 RCF for 5 min.
2. Aspirate supernatant, resuspend to $1–1.5 \times 10^7$ viable cells/mL in 7.5% DMSO–92.5% SFM II 900 medium chilled on ice.
3. Aliquot into 1-mL cryovials labeled with the date, passage number, and type of cells. Place at –80°C overnight in cryogenic freezing container (Nalgene), then transfer to liquid nitrogen if desired, or retain at –80°C. Our experience shows that cells retain viability even after several months at –80°C.

5. PROTOCOL 2: SUCROSE-FRACTIONATED SF9 MEMBRANE VESICLE PREPARATION FROM CELLS INFECTED WITH MRP2-BACULOVIRUS

Steps 1–3 are based on ref. *39* and steps 4–20 are adapted from ref. *27*.

1. Grow Sf9 cells in suspension culture with Gibco SFM II-900 serum-free insect cell medium to a concentration of $3–4 \times 10^6$ viable cells/mL.
2. Infect cells with titered viral stock ($10^7–10^8$ pfu/mL) at multiplicity of infection = 3, as 80- to 100-mL cultures containing 1×10^6 viable cells/mL, in 250-mL polymethylpentene (PMP) screw-capped flasks.
3. At 64–68 h postinfection, harvest $1.5–2 \times 10^8$ Sf9 cells by centrifugation (500*g*, 4°C, 5 min) using 200-mL Nalgene conical centrifuge tubes.
4. Withdraw or aspirate supernatant, and resuspend pellet in 10 mL of hypotonic lysis buffer (1 m*M* TrisCl, 0.1 m*M* EDTA, pH 7.4, at 4°C, with 1 m*M* phenylmethylsulfonyl fluoride (stock = 100 m*M* in isopropyl alcohol), 5 µg/mL of leupeptin, 1 µg/mL of pepstatin (stock = 5 mg/mL in dimethyl sulfoxide), 5 µg/mL of aprotinin.
5. Determine the total volume of cell suspension minus 10 mL to estimate the volume of the cell pellet. Add more lysis buffer to reach a total volume of 40 times the cell pellet volume.
6. Incubate cells on ice for 60 min with gentle occasional swirling. Subsequent steps are carried out in the cold room at 4°C.
7. Centrifuge cell lysate at 27,500 rpm in a Beckman SW28 rotor ($100,000g_{av}$) at 4°C for 40 min.

8. Withdraw or aspirate supernatant, resuspend the pellet in 10 mL of isotonic TS buffer containing 10 mM Tris-Cl, 250 mM sucrose, pH 7.4, at 4°C.
9. Homogenize 10–15 mL in a 15-mL Dounce B tight homogenizer (glass/glass, tight pestle, 30 strokes = cycles) on ice in the cold room. Be careful not to introduce air bubbles.
10. Slowly, gently, and carefully overlay homogenate on 2 mL of 38% (w/v) sucrose solution in 5 mM Tris-HEPES, pH 7.4, at 4°C in 12 mL of Beckman Ultra-Clear centrifuge tubes. Bring the volume to the bottom of the word "Beckman" on the tubes with homogenate or TS buffer.
11. Carefully place tubes in SW41 or TH641 rotor and centrifuge for 60 min at 39,000 rpm (255,000g) at 4°C.
12. Collect the turbid layer at the interface and dilute to 35 mL with TS buffer and centrifuge 27,500 rpm (100,000g) for 40 min at 4°C in an SW28 rotor. Alternatively, dilute to 23–24 mL and load into tubes for the SW41 rotor and centrifuge for 40 min at 4°C at 100,000g.
13. Aspirate supernatant, resuspend with 300–400 µL of TS buffer first using P1000 pipet, then connect P200 pipet tip to the end of P1000 tip until all the mass is uniformly resuspended.
14. Vesiculate by passing the suspension 30 times (= 15 cycles) through a 25-gauge needle on the end of a 1-mL syringe. Avoid making bubbles or foam.
15. Aliquot into labeled tubes and drop tubes into liquid nitrogen for about 5–10 min, then transfer to –80°C.
16. Measure protein concentration by the Lowry method, bovine albumin as the standard. Usually protein concentration is about 3–5 µg/µL or higher.
17. Total processing time from infected cells in suspension culture to vesicles in liquid nitrogen should be about 6 h or less.
18. To use membranes, remove from –80°C and place in 37°C water bath for 1–2 min, then put on ice for at least 2 min.
19. If desired, revesiculate by passing vesicles diluted to 2.5 µg/µL again 30 times through a 25-gauge needle as described in step 14. This part is not mentioned in the literature for Sf9 vesicles but it is commonly performed for liver membrane vesicles. We include this every time and obtain reproducible results (CV ± 10%).
20. Keep the tube on ice and complete the experiments within 2–3 h after thawing. Use 4 µL to deliver 10 µg per replicate. Before withdrawing each sample, gently flick the tube two or three times to stir the membranes, to improve uniformity.
21. We typically use the membranes within 3 wk of production. However, Solvo Biotechnology (Budapest, Hungary) adds protease inhibitors and extends storage at –80°C to 2 yr.

6. PROTOCOL 3: SF9 CRUDE MEMBRANE VESICLE PREPARATION FROM BACULOVIRUS-INFECTED CELLS

1. Grow Sf9 cells in suspension culture with Gibco SFM II-900 serum-free insect cell medium to a concentration of 3–4 × 10^6 viable cells/mL.

2. Infect cells with titered viral stock ($\geq 10^8$ pfu/mL) at an appropriate multiplicity of infection (MOI), as 80- to 100-mL cultures containing 1×10^6 viable cells/mL, in 250-mL polymethylpentene (PMP) screw-capped flasks (Nalgene).
3. At the desired time post-infection, harvest 1.5–2×10^8 Sf9 cells by centrifugation ($500g$, 4°C, 5–6 min) using 200-mL Nalgene conical centrifuge tubes.
4. Withdraw or aspirate supernatant, and resuspend pellet in 10 mL of hypotonic lysis buffer (1 mM Tris-Cl, 0.1 mM ethylenediamine tetraacetate, pH 7.4, at 4°C, with 1 mM phenylmethylsulfonyl fluoride (stock = 100 mM in isopropyl alcohol), 5 µg/mL of leupeptin, 1 µg/mL of pepstatin (stock = 5 mg/mL in dimethyl sulfoxide), and 5 µg/mL of aprotinin.
5. Determine the difference in the total volume of cell suspension minus 10 mL to estimate the volume of the cell pellet. Multiply the total volume of cell pellets by 40 and add more lysis buffer to reach this value in milliliters.
6. Incubate cells on ice for 60 min with gentle occasional swirling.
7. Homogenize 10–15 mL in a 15-mL Dounce B tight homogenizer (glass/glass, tight pestle, 30 strokes = cycles) on ice. Be careful not to introduce air bubbles.
8. Centrifuge cell lysate at $500g$ in a 15- or 50-mL conical bottom tube at 4°C for 5–6 min.
9. Transfer supernatant to ultracentrifuge tubes and centrifuge at $100,000g_{av}$ (25,000 rpm in an SW41 rotor, or 27,500 rpm in an SW28 rotor) 30 min at 4°C.
10. Aspirate supernatant, resuspend the pellet with 300–400 µL of TS buffer first using a P1000 pipet, then connect P200 pipet tip to the end of P1000 tip until all the mass is uniformly resuspended.
11. Vesiculate by passing the suspension 30 times (= 15 cycles) through a 25-gauge needle on the end of a 1-mL syringe.
12. Aliquot into labeled tubes and drop tubes into liquid nitrogen for about 5–10 min, then transfer to –80°C.
13. Measure protein concentration by the Lowry method *(40)*, using bovine albumin as the standard. Usually protein concentration is about 6–10 µg/µL or higher.
14. Total processing time from infected cells in suspension culture to vesicles in liquid nitrogen should be about 5 h or less.
15. To use membranes, remove from –80°C and place in 37°C water bath for 1–2 min, then put on ice for at least 2 min.
16. If desired, revesiculate by passing diluted vesicles again 30 times through a 25-gauge needle as above.
17. Keep the tube on ice and use within 2–3 h after thawing. Before withdrawing each sample, gently flick the tube two or three times to stir the membranes, to help with uniformity.

7. SUMMARY AND CONCLUSIONS

Transport of endo- and xenobiotics is an important hepatocellular function, which serves two roles: bile formation and excretion. The MRPs in particular mediate the efflux of diverse sulfate, glutathione, or glucuronide conjugates of endogenous compounds like estrogen and bilirubin, as well as drugs and toxins from the hepatocyte. MRP2 in particular contributes importantly to both excretion and bile formation. Several in vitro approaches may be used to characterize hepatic transport processes. Because the main hepatic transporters have been cloned, it is possible to examine the function and mechanism of isolated transporters in expression systems. This chapter particularly emphasizes use of the baculovirus expression vector system to express MRP2 in Sf9 insect cells.

REFERENCES

1. Stein WD. Channels, Carriers, and Pumps: An Introduction to Membrane Transport. San Diego: Academic Press; 1990.
2. Holland IB, Blight MA. ABC-ATPases, adaptable energy generators fuelling transmembrane movement of a variety of molecules in organisms from bacteria to humans. J Mol Biol 1999;293:381–399.
3. Stein WD. Transport and Diffusion Across Cell Membranes. San Diego: Academic Press; 1986.
4. Dean M, Rzhetsky A, Allikmets R. The human ATP-binding cassette (ABC) transporter superfamily. Genome Res 2001;11:1156–1166.
5. Borst P, Elferink RO. Mammalian ABC transporters in health and disease. Annu Rev Biochem 2002;71:537–592.
6. Faber KN, Muller M, Jansen PL. Drug transport proteins in the liver. Adv Drug Deliv Rev 2003;55:107–124.
7. Trauner M, Boyer JL. Bile salt transporters: molecular characterization, function, and regulation. Physiol Rev 2003;83:633–671.
8. Ballatori N, Rebbeor JF. Roles of MRP2 and oatp1 in hepatocellular export of reduced glutathione. Semin Liver Dis 1998;18:377–387.
9. Gerk PM, Vore M. Regulation of expression of the multidrug resistance-associated protein 2 (MRP2) and its role in drug disposition. J Pharmacol Exp Ther 2002;302:407–415.
10. Keppler D, Leier I, Jedlitschky G. Transport of glutathione conjugates and glucuronides by the multidrug resistance proteins MRP1 and MRP2. Biol Chem 1997; 378:787–791.
11. Shoda J, Kano M, Oda K, et al. The expression levels of plasma membrane transporters in the cholestatic liver of patients undergoing biliary drainage and their association with the impairment of biliary secretory function. Am J Gastroenterol 2001;96:3368–3378.
12. Kullak-Ublick GA, Stieger B, Hagenbuch B, Meier PJ. Hepatic transport of bile salts. Semin Liver Dis 2000;20:273–292.
13. Huang L, Smit JW, Meijer DK, Vore M. Mrp2 is essential for estradiol-17β(β-D-glucuronide)-induced cholestasis in rats. Hepatology 2000;32:66–72.
14. Boyer JL, Meier PJ. Characterizing mechanisms of hepatic bile acid transport utilizing isolated membrane vesicles. Methods Enzymol 1990;192:517–533.
15. Meier PJ, Boyer JL. Preparation of basolateral (sinusoidal) and canalicular plasma membrane vesicles for the study of hepatic transport processes. Methods Enzymol 1990;192:534–545.

16. Suzuki H, Sugiyama Y. Transporters for bile acids and organic anions. Pharm Biotechnol 1999;12:387–439.
17. Evers R, de Haas M, Sparidans R, et al. Vinblastine and sulfinpyrazone export by the multidrug resistance protein MRP2 is associated with glutathione export. Br J Cancer 2000;83:375–383.
18. Loe DW, Almquist KC, Cole SP, Deeley RG. ATP-dependent 17 β-estradiol 17-(β-D-glucuronide) transport by multidrug resistance protein (MRP). Inhibition by cholestatic steroids. J Biol Chem 1996;271:9683–9689.
19. Ryu S, Kawabe T, Nada S, Yamaguchi A. Identification of basic residues involved in drug export function of human multidrug resistance-associated protein 2. J Biol Chem 2000;275:39617–39624.
20. Shapiro AB, Ling V. ATPase activity of purified and reconstituted P-glycoprotein from Chinese hamster ovary cells. J Biol Chem 1994;269:3745–3754.
21. Hagmann W, Nies AT, Konig J, Frey M, Zentgraf H, Keppler D. Purification of the human apical conjugate export pump MRP2 reconstitution and functional characterization as substrate-stimulated ATPase. Eur J Biochem 1999;265:281–289.
22. Borst P, Evers R, Kool M, Wijnholds J. The multidrug resistance protein family. Biochim Biophys Acta 1999;1461:347–357.
23. O'Reilly DR, Miller LK, Luckow VA. Baculovirus expression vectors: a laboratory manual. New York: Oxford University Press; 1994.
24. van Aubel RA, van Kuijck MA, Koenderink JB, Deen PM, van Os CH, Russel FG. Adenosine triphosphate-dependent transport of anionic conjugates by the rabbit multidrug resistance-associated protein Mrp2 expressed in insect cells. Mol Pharmacol 1998;53:1062–1067.
25. Bohme M, Muller M, Leier I, Jedlitschky G, Keppler D. Cholestasis caused by inhibition of the adenosine triphosphate-dependent bile salt transport in rat liver. Gastroenterology 1994;107:255–265.
26. Konno T, Ebihara T, Hisaeda K, et al. Identification of domains participating in the substrate specificity and subcellular localization of the multidrug resistance proteins MRP1 and MRP2. J Biol Chem 2003;278:22908–22917.
27. Ito K, Suzuki H, Sugiyama Y. Single amino acid substitution of rat MRP2 results in acquired transport activity for taurocholate. Am J Physiol 2001;281:G1034–G1043.
28. Tabas LB, Dantzig AH. A high-throughput assay for measurement of multidrug resistance protein-mediated transport of leukotriene C_4 into membrane vesicles. Anal Biochem 2002;310:61–66.
29. Akita H, Suzuki H, Ito K, et al. Characterization of bile acid transport mediated by multidrug resistance associated protein 2 and bile salt export pump. Biochim Biophys Acta 2001;1511:7–16.
30. Cui Y, Konig J, Keppler D. Vectorial transport by double-transfected cells expressing the human uptake transporter SLC21A8 and the apical export pump ABCC2. Mol Pharmacol 2001;60:934–943.
31. Hidalgo IJ, Hillgren KM, Grass GM, Borchardt RT. A new side-by-side diffusion cell for studying transport across epithelial cell monolayers. In Vitro Cell Dev Biol 1992;28A:578–580.

32. Hidalgo IJ, Hillgren KM, Grass GM, Borchardt RT. Characterization of the unstirred water layer in Caco-2 cell monolayers using a novel diffusion apparatus. Pharm Res 1991;8:222–227.
33. Yu H, Sinko PJ. Influence of the microporous substratum and hydrodynamics on resistances to drug transport in cell culture systems: calculation of intrinsic transport parameters. J Pharm Sci 1997;86:1448–1457.
34. Polli JW, Wring SA, Humphreys JE, et al. Rational use of in vitro P-glycoprotein assays in drug discovery. J Pharmacol Exp Ther 2001;299:620–628.
35. Litman T, Druley TE, Stein WD, Bates SE. From MDR to MXR: new understanding of multidrug resistance systems, their properties and clinical significance. Cell Mol Life Sci 2001;58:931–959.
36. Saheki S, Takeda A, Shimazu T. Assay of inorganic phosphate in the mild pH range, suitable for measurement of glycogen phosphorylase activity. Anal Biochem 1985;148:277–281.
37. Bakos E, Evers R, Sinko E, Varadi A, Borst P, Sarkadi B. Interactions of the human multidrug resistance proteins MRP1 and MRP2 with organic anions. Mol Pharmacol 2000;57:760–768.
38. Drueckes P, Schinzel R, Palm D. Photometric microtiter assay of inorganic phosphate in the presence of acid-labile organic phosphates. Anal Biochem 1995;230: 173–177.
39. Van Aubel RA, Peters JG, Masereeuw R, Van Os CH, Russel FG. Multidrug resistance protein mrp2 mediates ATP-dependent transport of classic renal organic anion p-aminohippurate. Am J Physiol 2000;279:F713–F717.
40. Lowry OH, Rosebrough NJ, Farr AL, Randall RJ. Protein measurement with the folin phenol reagent. J Biol Chem 1951;193:265–275.

12

Structural Determinants of Folate and Antifolate Membrane Transport by the Reduced Folate Carrier

Wei Cao and Larry H. Matherly

Summary

Besides its important role in folate homeostasis, membrane transport is a critical determinant of the antitumor activities of *anti*folate therapeutics used in cancer chemotherapy, such as methotrexate (MTX) and an exciting new generation of antifolates typified by Tomudex and Pemetrexed. Further, impaired cellular uptake of antifolates is a frequent mode of drug resistance. The ubiquitously expressed transporter termed the reduced folate carrier (RFC) is the best characterized of the folate transport systems in mammalian cells. This chapter summarizes recent significant advances involving the molecular structure of the RFC protein, including its topology and glycosylation, as well as identification of its functionally and structurally important domains and amino acids. Insights into these features have been gleaned by epitope insertion and accessibility methods, and by mutating specific amino acids, through selection of antifolate resistant cells with impaired RFC function, and by site-directed mutagenesis. The recent expression of a functional "cysteine-less" human RFC has permitted the use of scanning cysteine mutagenesis and thiol modification techniques for mapping membrane topology and surface accessibilities, and for identifying functionally important domains in the RFC protein.

Key Words

Antifolate; epitope insertion; hydropathy analysis; K562 human erythroleukemia cells; L1210 murine leukemia cells; 3-(*N*-Maleimidylpropionyl)biocytin; methanethiosulfonate; methotrexate; mutagenesis: deletional; mutagenesis: insertional; mutagenesis: scanning cysteine; mutagenesis: scanning glycosylation; mutagenesis: site-directed; photoaffinity labeling; reduced folate carrier; transmembrane domains.

1. INTRODUCTION

Folate is a generic term for the water-soluble members of the B class of vitamins that are essential for normal growth and development of all tissues *(1)*.

From: *Methods in Pharmacology and Toxicology,*
Drug Metabolism and Transport: Molecular Methods and Mechanisms
Edited by: L. Lash © Humana Press Inc., Totowa, NJ

Folic acid is the stable, synthetic parent structure of the biologically important folates that differ in the oxidation state of the pteridine ring, the nature of the one-carbon substituent at positions N5 and N10, and the presence of additional (generally two to eight) γ-linked glutamyl residues. Folate deficiency contributes to chromosomal instability and malignant transformation, and plays an important role in the development of cardiovascular disease and fetal abnormalities *(1)*. These effects may result from impaired nucleotide biosynthesis and repair of DNA damage, and/or DNA hypomethylation caused by decreased *S*-adenosylmethionine.

Chemically, folate monoglutamates are hydrophilic structures (Fig. 1) that because of their anionic character exhibit limited capacities to cross biological membranes by diffusion alone. Mammalian cells have evolved sophisticated uptake processes for facilitating membrane transport of folate cofactors *(2,3)*. One or more of these transport systems must be present in mammalian cells to provide sufficient folate cofactors to support synthesis of purine nucleotides, thymidylate, serine, and methionine for cell proliferation. Moreover, these systems also participate in specialized tissue functions, including absorption across the intestinal luminal epithelium, reabsorption in the proximal tubules of the kidney, and transplacental folate uptake *(2,3)*.

In addition to its important role in folate homeostasis, membrane transport is a critical determinant of the antitumor activities of *anti*folate therapeutics used in cancer chemotherapy, such as methotrexate (MTX) and an exciting new generation of antifolates typified by Tomudex and Pemetrexed *(4–7)* (Fig. 1). Further, impaired cellular uptake of antifolates is a frequent mode of drug resistance *(8–13)*.

The ubiquitously expressed transporter termed the reduced folate carrier (RFC) is the best characterized of the folate transport systems in mammalian cells *(2,3)*. The transport properties of RFC were first described more than 35 yr ago in murine leukemia cells *(14,15)*. Since the cloning of rodent RFCs in 1994 *(16,17)*, there have been a number of significant advances involving the molecular structure of the RFC protein, including its topology, glycosylation, and the identification of functionally and structurally important domains and amino acids. Insights into these features have been gleaned by epitope insertion and accessibility methods, and by mutating specific amino acids, through selection of drug-resistant cells with antifolate drugs and targeting specific amino acids for site-directed mutagenesis based on homology and topology considerations. The recent expression of a functional cysteine-less human RFC has permitted the introduction of scanning cysteine mutagenesis and thiol-modification techniques for mapping the membrane

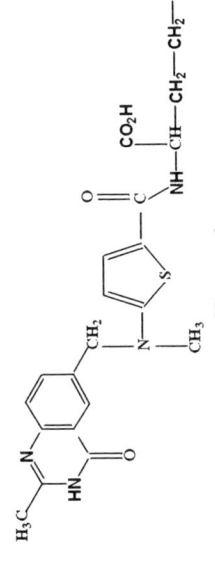

Fig. 1. Folate and antifolate substrates for RFC.

topology and surface accessibility, and for identifying functionally important domains. In this review, we summarize the major recent developments in characterizing RFC structure and function.

2. FUNCTIONAL PROPERTIES OF RFC

Reduced folates such as 5-methyltetrahydrofolate and classical antifolates such as MTX (Fig. 1) are actively transported into mammalian cells by the same facilitated transport process termed the reduced folate carrier or RFC *(2–6)*. For tetrahydrofolate cofactors, adequate rates of intracellular delivery are essential for DNA synthesis and cell proliferation. For MTX, membrane transport is critical to antitumor effects because of its role in generating sufficient unbound intracellular antifolate to sustain maximal dihydrofolate reductase (DHFR) inhibition and synthesis of MTX polyglutamates *(7)*. A number of other antifolate chemotherapy drugs (e.g., Pemetrexed, Tomudex, GW1843U89, and 5,10-dideazatetrahydrofolate) are also excellent substrates for RFC *(5–7)*. Some of these structures are shown in Fig. 1.

Studies of the functional characteristics of RFC date back to the late 1960s *(14,15)*. Most of these studies used murine (L1210) leukemia cells and radioactive MTX as a surrogate for reduced folates, because MTX transport was unidirectional over short intervals, reflecting its rapid and tight binding to cellular DHFR *(14,18)*. Moreover, unlike reduced folates, metabolism of MTX was nominal over the short intervals used for transport assays. At steady state, bound MTX can be distinguished from free MTX by efflux into drug-free media, thus permitting calculation of transmembrane gradients and uphill transport from the membrane potential *(14,18)*.

The functional properties of RFC-mediated transport have been exhaustively characterized for both rodent and human tumor models in culture and, with only a few exceptions (*see* later), these have been remarkably uniform *(3)*. Thus, MTX transport by RFC is temperature-dependent, sodium-independent, and is sensitive to competitive inhibition by other transport substrates *(2–5)*. Although a neutral pH is optimal for RFC in leukemia cells *(19)*, in other models (intestinal epithelial and prostate carcinoma cells) *(20–22)*, an acidic pH optimum is observed. The basis for this is unclear.

RFC-mediated uptake is saturable at low micromolar concentrations (K_t ~1–5 μM) for most tetrahydrofolate and many antifolate substrates *(2–6)*. By contrast, folic acid is typically a poor substrate for RFC (K_t > 100 μM). Transport of reduced folates by RFC is not stereospecific for 5-methyltetrahydrofolate, as the K_t values for the natural (6S) and unnatural (6R) stereoisomers are similar *(23)*. Conversely, the (6R) isomer of 5-formyltetrahydrofolate has a far lower affinity than the natural (6S) stereoisomer *(24)*. Interestingly, the benzoquinazoline antifolate, GW1843U89, is a surprisingly poor substrate for the murine RFC ($V_{max}/K_t = 0.25$) and one of the best known substrates for the human carrier ($V_{max}/K_t = 20.3$) *(25)*.

RFC is highly sensitive to its anionic environment. Thus, replacing extracellular anions with nonanionic N-(2-hydroxyethyl)piperazine-N'-2-ethanesulfonic acid (HEPES)–sucrose buffers results in a highly concentrative uptake of MTX *(26)*. This partly reflects the decreased competition for substrate binding to RFC in anion-free buffers, because MTX influx is competitively inhibited by assorted inorganic anions (e.g., chloride, bicarbonate, phosphate) in physiological buffers, and the K_t values for MTX influx are reduced nearly 10-fold in the absence of anions *(26)*. Moreover, in studies with membrane vesicles *trans*-loaded with sulfate or phosphate anions, the influx V_{max} for MTX was increased twofold *(27)*. Transport of antifolates via RFC can occur bidirectionally *(2–6)*; however, under physiologic conditions, the actual outward flux through RFC is small compared to other modes of efflux, such as that mediated by the multidrug-resistance-associated proteins (MRPs) *(28)*. In physiologic buffers, influx of radiolabeled MTX by RFC is significantly enhanced ("*trans*-stimulated") in cells preloaded with high concentrations of 5-formyl or 5-methyltetrahydrofolate *(29,30)* and is inhibited by a variety of structurally diverse organic anions (e.g., organic phosphates, including adenine nucleotides and thiamine phosphates) *(30)*. Interestingly, in anion-free buffers without glucose, the rate of MTX efflux is inhibited. Efflux can be stimulated with physiologic anion-containing buffers including both inorganic and organic anions (folic acid, 5-formyltetrahydrofolate, AMP, ADP, thiamine pyrophosphate, phosphate, sulfate, and chloride) *(31–33)*. The anion concentrations required for half-maximal stimulation of efflux are similar to their K_i values for inhibition of influx by RFC.

Thus, large electrochemical anion gradients appear to accelerate the movement of RFC within the plasma membrane and thus are likely to provide the driving force for the concentrative uptake of folate by the carrier *(30–33)*. Most probably, this involves an extrusion of intracellular organic anions into the extracellular medium and down a concentration gradient that drives uptake of folate substrates into cells. Consistent with this model are recent studies with phosphorylated derivatives of thiamine that show that these anionic species are good substrates for RFC in L1210 cells, and that efflux of these forms is dramatically enhanced in cells with increased expression of RFC *(34)*. However, neither the nature of the actual physiologic counter-anion nor the properties of the binding site(s) for dianionic folate substrates or the putative transport counteranion on the RFC molecule are established.

3. PROPERTIES OF THE HRFC PROTEIN AND ISOLATION AND CHARACTERIZATION OF HRFC CDNAS

3.1. Biochemical Properties of Endogenously Expressed RFC Protein

Biochemical studies of the RFC protein were not possible for many years due to its low endogenous level of expression in cultured mammalian cells. However, beginning in the early 1980s, a number of innovative approaches were developed to circumvent this limitation.

In 1984, Sirotnak and coworkers developed a strategy to select L1210 murine leukemia cells with upregulated RFC *(35)*. Selection was based on the notion that carrier-mediated uptake of tetrahydrofolate cofactors is rate limiting to their biosynthetic utilization and involved growing cultures in folate-free medium containing growth-limiting concentrations of (6*R*,*S*) 5-formyltetrahydrofolate. Under these conditions only cell variants that possessed elevated transport capacities for reduced folates were capable of sustained growth. By this approach, L1210 variants with 3- to 40-fold increased RFC were selected. Similarly, transport-upregulated CCRF-CEM *(36)*, K562 *(37)*, and HL60 *(38)* human leukemia sublines were generated by selection under folate-restrictive conditions.

Another important advance was the development of strategies for identifying and quantitating low levels of RFC protein. Specific binding of radiolabeled RFC substrates (5-methyltetrahydrofolate, methotrexate, or aminopterin) to surface RFCs at 0°C (performed in the presence and absence of high concentrations of a competing unlabeled ligand) in intact cells provides an overall estimate of carrier levels *(39)*. However, it was not until the development of affinity ligands that the molecular properties of the protein could be studied. A number of agents have been used to covalently label the RFC protein, including 8-azidoadenosine-5'-monophosphate *(40)*, 4,4'-diisothiocyanostilbene-2,2'-disulfonate *(41)*, carbodiimide-activated antifolates *(42)*, 3,3'-dithiobissulfosuccinimidyl propionate *(43)*, *N*-hydroxysuccinimide (NHS) MTX ester *(44)*, and N^{α}-(4-amino-4-deoxy-10-methylpteroyl)-N^{ε}-4-azido-5-salicylyl)-L-lysine (APA-ASA-Lys) *(45)*. While these reagents all irreversibly inhibited [^{3}H]MTX uptake into cell cultures, only NHS-MTX and APA-ASA-Lys showed the sensitivity and specificity needed for radioaffinity labeling of the carrier.

NHS-[^{3}H]MTX and NHS-[^{3}H]aminopterin have been extensively used for covalently radiolabeling the carrier *(8,37,38,44)* because they are easily synthesized from NHS and commercially available tritiated antifolates and exhibit a relatively high specificity for the transporter in both cultured murine and human cells. The reactive forms of these NHS-activated antifolate esters have not been identified, but they presumably represent either NHS α- or γ-antifolate esters. The stable covalent adduct(s) generated between the RFC protein and these tritiated affinity inhibitors have not been characterized.

Structure–Function of Reduced Folate Carrier

In our studies of transport-upregulated K562 human erythroleukemia cells (designated K562.4CF) treated with NHS-[^{3}H]HMTX, tritium was incorporated into a broadly migrating approx 76- to 85-kDa band that was increased (~7-fold) over parental K562 cells and could be completely blocked by unlabeled MTX or (6S) 5-formyltetrahydrofolate, establishing specificity *(37)*. In additional experiments, we confirmed that the affinity labeled protein was glycosylated as treatment of K562.4CF plasma membranes with endo-β-galactosidase resulted in a shift of the labeled band to a substantially lower molecular weight species (~57,800 ± 7730; $n = 5$). Conversely, the mouse RFC from L1210 leukemia cells treated with NHS-[^{3}H]MTX or NHS-[^{3}H]aminopterin typically migrated on sodium dodecyl sulfate (SDS) gels or gel filtration (with 0.1% SDS) as a 42- to 48-kDa species *(8)*. However, more recent studies with antibodies to the mouse RFC identified a 58-kDa RFC protein *(46)*, suggesting that the smaller molecular mass species may have arisen from proteolytic degradation of the larger RFC form.

APA-[^{125}I]-ASA-Lys is a radioiodinated photoaffinity ligand originally used for labeling DHFR *(47)* that was subsequently adapted for labeling RFC *(45)*. Ultraviolet activation of a reactive nitrene in APA-[^{125}I]-ASA-Lys results in the covalent modification of proteins to which it is bound. The advantages of APA-^{125}I-ASA-Lys over NHS-[^{3}H]MTX include its increased specificity for MTX-binding proteins, resulting from its decreased reactivity in the absence of ultraviolet irradiation, and its far greater sensitivity, associated with incorporation of the ^{125}I radionuclide. Freisheim and coworkers used APA-[^{125}I]-ASA-Lys to label the approx 80- to 85-kDa glycosylated hRFC protein from transport-upregulated CCRF-CEM cells *(45)*.

3.2. Cloning of the RFC cDNAs That Restore Transport to Transport-Impaired Cultured Cells

A major step toward cloning the RFC was taken in 1992 when Flintoff and colleagues showed that tetrahydrofolate cofactor and MTX transport could be restored in transport-impaired Chinese hamster ovary (CHO) cells by transfections with CHO genomic DNA cosmid clones *(48)*. By 1994, a mouse RFC cDNA was isolated by expression cloning and found to restore MTX transport function and MTX sensitivity to transport-impaired ZR75-1 human breast carcinoma cells *(16)*. Subsequently, Flintoff and coworkers described a homologous hamster cDNA that could restore MTX transport to transport-impaired CHO cells *(17)*. By 1995, there were four published reports on the properties of the homologous human RFC cDNAs *(49–52)*. This was followed in 1997 by a report of a nearly identical cDNA clone from human intestine *(53)*. These cDNAs consistently restored MTX sensitivities and major properties typical of endogenously expressed RFCs to transport-impaired mouse, human, and hamster cells, including characteristic patterns of uptake with radiolabeled folate and antifolate substrates *(49–54)*. Other properties included inhibition by known RFC transport substrate competitors (GW1843U89, folic acid, 5-formyltetrahydrofolate, Tomudex) and irreversible inhibition by NHS-MTX, and a capacity for *trans*-stimulation by preloading cells with reduced folates *(9)*.

Other transport characteristics, however, differed from those expected. For example, in transfected K562 cells, transport was only 3–30% of the levels expected based on the level of membrane hRFC by radioaffinity labeling or Western blotting assays *(9,55)*. In other studies, differences in substrate specificities or pH optima for transport were found for endogenous and ectopically expressed RFCs *(52,56,57)*. At least part of this difference was cell specific (and, presumably, involved tissue-specific modulators) as the same mouse cDNA restored transport with different properties in L1210 leukemia cells and immortalized IEC-6 intestinal epithelial cells *(57)*. The nature of these putative modulators is uncertain, but may involve posttranslational modifications of the RFC protein or, possibly, its association with other non-RFC transport proteins. Interestingly, when plasma membrane proteins from parental K562 cells were fractionated by Sephacryl S300 gel filtration under native conditions in the presence of *N*-dodecyl-β-maltoside, an hRFC fraction migrated as a high molecular mass species (250 kDa) kDa) (T.Witt, B.C. Ding, and L.H. Matherly, *unpublished observation*), suggesting either self association or complexation with other (possibly regulatory) proteins.

In our laboratory, a series of human cDNAs were isolated by screening a K562.4CF cDNA library with a fragment of murine RFC cDNA *(52)*. Three clones (i.e., KS6, KS32, and KS43) were isolated (1.4 kb, 2.5 kb, and 2.8 kb, respectively), the longest of which contained a 98-bp 5′-untranslated region (UTR), a 1776-bp open reading frame, and a 3′-UTR of 864 bp, followed by a poly(A) sequence (GenBank Accession No. U19720). From the predicted sequence for the 591-amino-acid protein, the molecular mass for hRFC is 64,873 Da. For transport-impaired CHO or K562 cells transfected with the KS43 cDNA, we detected a cDNA-encoded approx 85–92 kDa protein by photoaffinity labeling with APA-[^{125}I]-ASA-Lys *(9,52)* (Fig. 2). This form was deglycosylated by treatment with *N*-glycosidase F to approx 65 kDa, in close agreement with the predicted size of the full-length hRFC clone and deglycosylated NHS-[^{3}H]MTX-labeled protein in K562.4CF cells *(9)*.

By hydropathy analysis of amino acid character *(58)*, the KS43-encoded protein conformed to a computer model expected for an integral membrane protein, with up to 12 stretches of mostly hydrophobic, α-helix-promoting amino acids, internally oriented N- and C-terminal domains, an external *N*-glycosylation site at Asn58, and a large central linker connecting putative

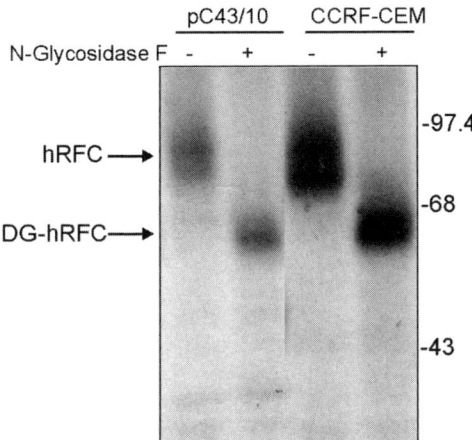

Fig. 2. Photoaffinity labeling with APA-[^{125}I]ASA-Lys. CHO (pC43/10) transfectants expressing hRFC and wild type CCRF-CEM T-ALL cells were treated with APA-[^{125}I]ASA-Lys, irradiated with long wavelength ultraviolet light, and radiolabeled proteins were extracted with 10 mM Tris-HCl (pH 7.0) and 1% Triton X-100. Aliquots were separated on SDS gels with and without pretreatment with N-glycosidase F. Untreated hRFC and deglycosylated hRFC (DG-hRFC) are indicated.

transmembrane domains (TMDs) 1–6 and 7–12 (Fig. 3). Portions of this topology model have been experimentally confirmed (*see* Subheading 4.1.). The predicted amino acid sequence for hRFC is 64–66% identical to the homologous rodent RFCs with homologies localized mostly in the TMDs (particularly for TMDs 1–5, 7, and 8; Figs. 3 and 4). There is little similarity in the N- or C-terminal regions or in the TMD6/7 linker domain. The human cDNA-encoded product contains 72–79 more amino acids than the rodent carriers. The predicted *N*-glycosylation site for hRFC (Asn58) is conserved for the rat and hamster proteins, but not in the mouse RFC. There is at least one additional consensus *N*-glycosylation site in the rodent RFCs not present in hRFC. A functional approx 65-kDa hRFC protein was detected on Western blots prepared from hRFC-null K562 cells transfected with Gln58 hRFC cDNA in which Asn58 is replaced by Gln *(55)*. Both wild-type and Gln58 hRFC with C-terminal hemagglutinin (HA) epitopes (YPYDVPDYASL) were also functional and were efficiently targeted to the plasma membrane by immunofluorescence staining with rhodamine-conjugated anti-HA antibody *(55)*. Thus, it appears that *N*-glycosylation of hRFC does not play a significant role in membrane targeting or transport function.

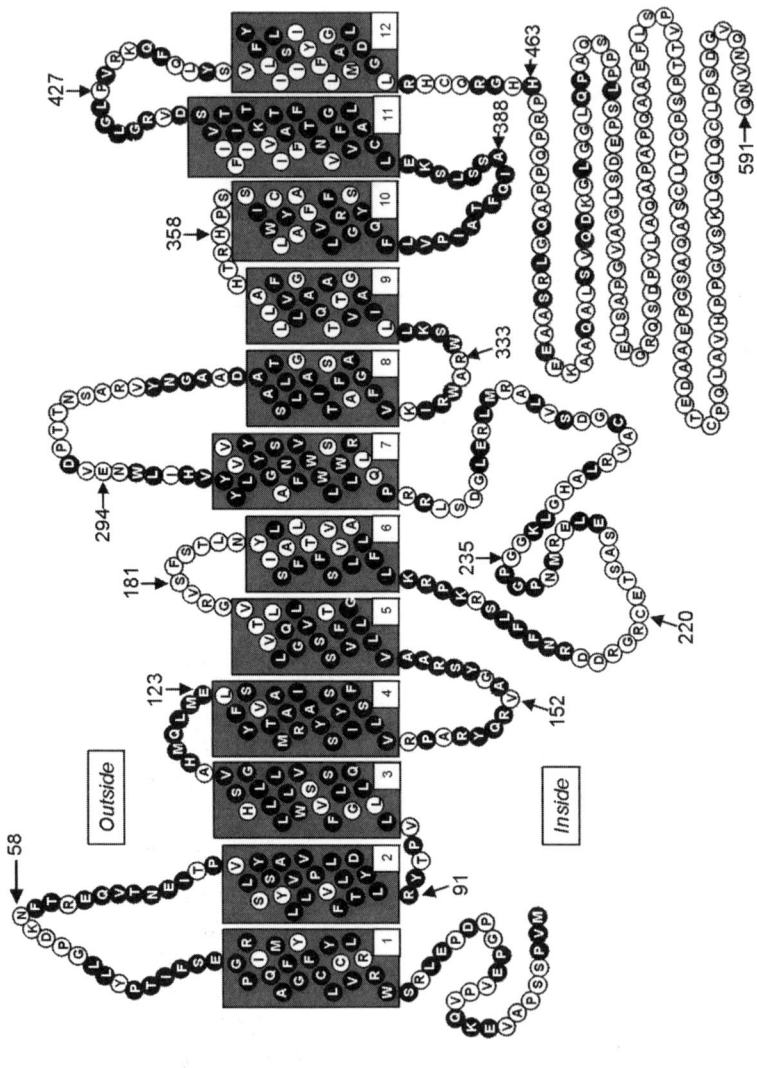

Fig. 3. Topology structure for hRFC based on hydropathy analysis. A computer-generated topology model (ref. 58), based on the predicted hRFC amino acid sequence is shown depicting 12 TMDs, internally oriented N- and C-terminal domains, and a cytosolic loop domain connecting TMDs 6 and 7. Amino acids are designated by the single-letter abbreviations. Conserved amino acids are designated by the *dark circles*.

4. STRUCTURE AND FUNCTION OF RFC

4.1. Analysis of hRFC Membrane Topology by HA Epitope Insertion and Scanning Glycosylation Mutagenesis

Although computer-generated analyses of membrane topology and secondary structure are important tools for interpreting structure and function information for membrane proteins, it is essential that these models be experimentally confirmed. In the original report by Cowan and coworkers *(16)*, murine RFC was suggested to conform to a 12 TMD topology model, resembling that for the glucose carrier (GLUT1). For hRFC, the demonstration of *N*-glycosylation at Asn58 for the endogenous *(37)* and ectopically expressed carrier *(9,55)* confirmed an extracellular orientation for the loop domain connecting TMDs 1 and 2. Moreover, immunofluorescence detection of the HA-epitope at the C-terminus (at Gln587) of hRFC expressed in transport-impaired K562 cells required membrane permeabilization with Triton X-100 (0.1%), thus confirming an intracellular orientation for this region *(55)*.

More recently, additional studies used analogous HA epitope accessibility methods to map the orientations of particular hRFC domains *(59,60)*. Thus, intracellular orientations were established by inserting HA epitopes into the hRFC N-terminus (Pro20, Gly17), the connecting loop between TMDs 6 and 7 (Ser225, Glu226) and TMDs 8 and 9 (Ala332), and treating with HA-specific antibody with and without permeabilization *(59,60)*. Because HA epitopes in connecting loops between TMDs 3 and 4 (Gln120) and between TMDs 7 and 8 (Glu294, Pro297) were accessible to antibody without permeabilization, these were identified as extracellular *(59,60)*. By *N*-glycosylation scanning mutagenesis, in which an *N*-glycosylation consensus sequence [NX(S/T)] is inserted into putative loop domains, followed by Western blotting of functional constructs to confirm glycosylation status, the TMD5/6 loop of hRFC was, likewise, confirmed as extracellular *(60)*.

Collectively, these studies verify portions of the computer-predicted topology model for hRFC including TMDs 1–8 and the N- and C-termini. However, the topology structure for TMDs 9–12 remained ambiguous owing to inherent limitations of these experimental approaches. For HA epitope accessibility methods, insertion of the 9-amino-acid HA epitope may not appreciably affect plasma membrane targeting of the ectopically expressed mutant carriers; however, transport function was frequently disrupted *(59,60)* due to protein misfolding and/or the generation of conformational states different from the wild-type RFC. In addition, for glycosylation scanning mutagenesis, it was not possible to distinguish a lack of glycosylation at inserted *N*-glycosylation sites due to their cytosolic orientations from spacial effects in which a consensus

```
Human    MVPSSPAVEKQVPVEPGPDPELRSWRRLVCYLCFYGFMAQIRPGESFITPYLLGPDKNFT    60
Mouse    ...TGQVA...AYE..RQ.H..K...C..F....F.....L.........F..--ERK..    58
Hamster  ...TGQVA...ACE..RQ.R..K...C..F....F.....L...........--QQ...    58
Rat      ...TGQVG...ACE..RQ.R..K...W..F....F.....L...........--ER...    58

Human    REQVTNEITPVLSYSYLAVLVPVFLLTDYLRYTPVLLLQGLSFVSVWLLLLLGHSVAHMQ    120
Mouse    K.......I.M.P..H................K...V..C....C........T..V...    118
Hamster  I.......I..P..H.....I.........K.I.I..C...MC........T..V...    118
Rat      K.......I.-MP..H.....I.........K.I.V..C...VC........T..V...    117

Human    LMELFYSVTMAARIAYSSYIFSLVRPARYQRVAGYSRAAVLLGVFTSSVLGQLLVTVGRV    180
Mouse    ...V......................H.S....M.S.............I......A.....HI    178
Hamster  ...V......................S....M.S..................V.WPLEQK    178
Rat      ...V...I..................Q.S....M.S.............I......V.VTLGGI    177

Human    SFST--LNYISLAFLTFSVVLALFLKRPKRSLFFNRDDRGRCETSASELERMNPGPG---    235
Mouse    .--.YT..CV..G.IL..L..S.............STLA.-GALPC..DQ.H...DRPE    235
Hamster  .QNSNM......G.II..LG.S.......H......SALVH-KALPC..DQ.H....RPE    237
Rat      .--TYM..C...G.IL..LG.S.......R......SALVQ-GALPC..DQ.H....RPE    234

Human    -GKLGHALRVACGDSVLARMLRELGDSLRRPQLRLWSLWWVFNSAGYYLVVYYVHILWNE    294
Mouse    TR..DRM.-GT.R..F.V...S...VENA.Q......C........S....IT....V..RS    294
Hamster  P...ERV.-GS.RN.F.VC..S...VGN..Q.HV...C.............I.....V..-S    295
Rat      PR..ERM.-GT.RD.F.V...S...VKNV.Q......C.............IT....V..KI    293

Human    VDPTTNSARVYNGAADAASTLLGAITSFAAGFVKIRWARWSKLLIAGVTATQAGLVF---    351
Mouse    T.SSLS----....V.......S.....S...LS...TL....V....I.I..S...CMF    350
Hamster  I.KNL.----....V.......S.....S.........L....V..S.I.I......CMY    351
Rat      TDSRL.----....V.......S...A.T....N....L....V..S.I.I......CMF    349

Human    LLAHTRHPSSIWLCYAAFVLFRGSYQFLVPIATFQIASSLSKELCALVFGVNTFFATIVK    411
Mouse    Q------IRD..V..VT......A..................I...L...AL.    404
Hamster  MVHYVTWVHK...VL.MTY......A..................I...L...AL.    411
Rat      QI------PD..VC.VTF.....A..................I...L...AL.    403

Human    TIITFIVSDVRGLGLPVRKQFQLYSVYFLILSIIYFLGAMLDGLRHCQRGHHPRQPPAQG    471
Mouse    .C..LV...K.....Q..D...RI.FI...M....TC.AW.G.....Y....R.QPLAQ..E    464
Hamster  .A..LV...K.....K.E....CI.....MV..V.C.V...V...V.Y.R..R.QPL.LP.E    471
Rat      .S..LV...K.....Q.HQ...RI.FM...T....CLAW.G.....YYR...R.QPLAQA.A    463

Human    LRSAAEEKAAQALSVQDKGLGGLQPAQSPPLSPEDSLGAVGPASLEQRQSDPYLAQAPAP    531
Mouse    ...PL.T-SV..I.L..GD.R.P...SAPQL..EDG-MEDDR.DLRVEAKA    512
Hamster  .-.PL.N-SV.VP.M..R.......SAPQL.PEDG-VEDSEASLRAEAKA    518
Rat      .-.PL.D-SV.AI.L..GD.RRP...SAPQL.PEDG.VEDGRADLRVEAKA    519

Human    QAAEFLSPVTTPSPCTLCSAQASGPEAADETCPQLAVHPPGVSKLGLQCLPSDGVQNVNQ    591
```

Fig. 4. Amino acid homologies for the human and rodent RFCs. Conserved amino acids in the rodent RFCs are indicated by a period. Gaps (noted with a dash) are introduced as needed for alignment.

sequence may be simply too close to the end of a transmembrane segment for proper *N*-glycosylation by oligosaccharyl transferase *(61)*. As described in Subheading 4.3.1., the use of scanning cysteine accessibility methods (SCAM) for mapping membrane topology has circumvented many of these limitations.

4.2. Insights Into Structural and Functional Determinants of Transport From Studies of Mutant RFCs

An important goal of RFC structural studies is to identify what amino acid residues or domains actually contribute to binding and translocation of anionic folate and antifolate substrates. Insights into these features have been gleaned from characterizing the functional consequences of mutating specific amino acids, by selection of drug-resistant cells with antifolate drugs (with or without pretreatment with a chemical mutagen), and by targeting specific amino acids for site-directed mutagenesis based on homology and toplogy considerations.

4.2.1. Role of TMD1

Particular attention has focused on residues in or flanking TMD1, based on findings that mutations of highly conserved residues result in profound effects on transport substrate binding and/or rates of carrier translocation. For instance, Gly44Arg was first identified in transport-impaired CCRF-CEM T-cell acute lymphoblastic leukemia cells (CEM/MTX-1) in our laboratory and was associated with an 11-fold increase in K_t for MTX *(62)*. The same mutation was reported in a separate CCRF-CEM subline selected for resistance to the hemiphthaloyl ornithine antifolate, PT523 *(63)*. Glu45Lys was first identified in MTX-resistant L1210 cells treated with *N*-methyl-*N*-nitrosourea and selected in the presence of MTX *(64)*. Glu45Lys-RFC exhibited a global decline in carrier mobility, decreased K_t values for folic acid and 5-formyltetrahydrofolate, an unchanged K_t for 5-methyltetrahydrofolate, and a markedly increased K_t for MTX. A nearly identical transport phenotype was attributed to Glu45Lys hRFC in separate CCRF-CEM sublines selected for MTX resistance *(10,65)* and in a number of CCRF-CEM cell lines selected for resistance to the benzoquinazoline antifolate, GW1843U89 *(63,66)*.

Interestingly, site-directed mutagenesis at position 45 increased affinities for 5-formyltetrahydrofolate and folic acid with some amino acid substitutions (Gln, Arg) but not others (Asp, Leu, Trp) *(67)*. This suggests that size rather than charge at position 45 is the major structural consideration for substrate specificity. Although all position 45 mutants were functional, there were substantial differences in maximal transport rates (V_{max}) for different substitutions *(67)*. These results are interesting in that they imply that Glu45 may not directly participate in substrate binding but, nonetheless, may exert an indirect effect and play an important role in generating an optimum conformation for substrate binding. This notion is further considered in Subheading 4.3.3.

Ser46 was also suggested to be important to RFC function, as Ser46Asn in MTX-resistant L1210 cells resulted in a decreased rate of carrier mobility (V_{max}) but no change in K_t *(68)*. The V_{max} effect was substantially greater for

MTX than for reduced folates. A Ser46Ile mutation in hRFC was detected in CCRF-CEM cells selected for resistance to GW1843U89 *(66)* and Ser46Asn was detected in a primary osteosarcoma specimen *(69)*. An Ile48Phe mutation was detected in the mouse RFC from L1210 cells selected for resistance to the glycinamideribonucleotide (GAR) formyltransferase inhibitor, 5,10-dideazatetrahydrofolate *(70)*. This mutation resulted in a marked increase in the accumulation of folic acid and expansion of cellular folate pools, owing to a selective decrease in the K_t for folic acid compared with antifolate transport substrates.

Collectively, these results seem to suggest a unique transport role for amino acids in or flanking TMD1 in RFC. In Subheading 4.3.2., we describe very recent results with scanning cysteine accessibility methods that further clarify the functional contributions of amino acids localized to this region.

4.2.2. Structural and Functional Roles of Other TMDs

Other functionally or structurally important regions from mutant studies include TMD8 (Ser309 [Ser313 in hRFC] *[71]* and Ser297 in murine RFC [not conserved in hRFC] *[72]*), TMD3 (Val104 in murine RFC [Val105 in hRFC] *[73]* and Trp105 in mRFC *[70]* [Trp108 in hRFC]), and TMD4 (Ser127 in hRFC *[62]*, Ala130 in murine RFC [Ala132 in hRFC] *[54]*). Effects of mutating these residues on transport parameters were variable and ranged from primary effects on carrier mobility without a change in MTX K_t (e.g., Ala130Pro in mouse RFC) *(54)* to decreases in both affinity (increased K_t) and V_{max} for MTX (Ser127Asn in hRFC) *(62)*, or selective effects on the observed transport phenotype for antifolate substrates (Trp105Gly and Ser309Phe in mouse RFC) compared to folates *(70,71)*. Trp105Gly increased the transport by mouse RFC of folic acid compared to 5,10-dideazatetrahydrofolate. Ser309Phe in mouse RFC resulted in increased (~5-fold) K_t values for MTX and 5-formyltetrahydrofolate without significant changes in affinities for folic acid and 5-methyltetrahydrofolate.

4.2.3. Roles of Conserved Charged Residues in RFC TMDs by Site-Directed Mutagenesis

From the predicted membrane topology and homology comparisons between hRFC and the rodent carriers (Figs. 3 and 4), potentially important charged residues in the hRFC TMDs were identified, including Asp88 (TMD2), Asp453 (TMD12), Arg133 (TMD4), Arg373 (TMD10), and Lys411 (TMD11). Substitution of the highly conserved Asp88 in hRFC with valine abolished transport of both MTX and 5-formyltetrahydrofolate *(74)*, suggesting an important structural or functional role for this residue. However, valine replacement of Asp453 had only a small effect on carrier activity. Transport activity for murine RFC was abolished by replacement of the conserved Arg131 (Arg133 in hRFC) and

Arg363 (Arg373 in hRFC) residues with leucines *(75)*. For hamster RFC, an important role for Arg373 was, likewise, suggested by the progressively decreased capacities of position 373 mutant RFCs (Arg373 ~ Lys > His > Gln > Ala) to complement a transport defective hamster phenotype in supporting colony formation on low levels of 5-formyltetrahydrofolate *(76)*. The effects of these substitutions at position 373 involved carrier translocation (decreased 16- to 50-fold) rather than substrate binding, mutant RFC stabilities, or intracellular trafficking *(76)*. For Lys404 in murine RFC (corresponding to Lys411 in hRFC), leucine substitution resulted in a selective loss of binding and transport of reduced folates over MTX *(75)*. Interestingly, in hRFC, replacement of Lys411 by leucine resulted in a significant loss of transport activity for both MTX and 5-formyltetrahydrofolate *(77)*, implying that the role of this residue in carrier function is somewhat different between the murine and human transporters.

4.2.4. Deletional and Insertional Mutagenesis of RFC

Deletional mutagenesis has been used to explore the structural determinants for plasma membrane targeting and transport of RFCs. Several of these studies have used enhanced green fluorescent protein (EGFP) C-tagged RFC constructs *(78,79)*. Thus, removal of 16 amino acids (residues 7–22) from the hamster RFC *(79)*, or 27 N-terminal (residues 1–27) or 139 C-terminal (453–591) amino acids from hRFC *(78)* did not appreciably affect membrane targeting or transport function. However, in other studies, C-terminal deletions of hamster RFC (residues 461–518) had a modest effect on surface targeting and transport *(79)*, whereas for murine RFC, loss of the C-terminus (residues 445–512) resulted in a complete loss of surface targeting *(80)*. Not surprisingly, large deletions (e.g., 302–591, 1–301) including TMDs completely abolished surface targeting of hRFC *(78)*.

The role of the central connecting loop between TMD6 and TMD7 of RFC has been the subject of considerable interest. Thus, deletion of up to 31 of 66 amino acids from the TMD6/TMD7 linker in murine RFC *(80)*, or up to 45 of 67 residues from this region in hamster RFC *(79)*, preserved membrane targeting and transport activity. Larger deletions (57 and 53–55 amino acids, respectively) abolished activity *(79,80)*. A critical requirement for carrier function suggested by these experiments involves a highly conserved stretch of 11 amino acids flanking TMD6 (positions 202–212 in mouse RFC and 204–214 in the hamster RFC and hRFC) (Figs. 3 and 4).

We recently studied the functional roles of the TMD6/TMD7 linker domain and the conserved Lys204–Arg214 peptide in hRFC by deletional and insertional mutagenesis and ectopic expression in transport-impaired K562 cells *(81)*. Deletions of 49 or 60 amino acids from the TMD6/7 linker (positions 215–263 and 204–263, respectively) completely abolished transport activity for both MTX and 5-formyltetrahydrofolate. However, replacement of the deleted segments with nonhomologous 73 or 84 amino acid segments of the structurally analogous thiamine transporter SLC19A2 (ThTr1; 18% homologous to hRFC for the TMD6/7 linker) restored transport, although maximal activity had an absolute requirement for the conserved 204–214 peptide *(81)*. Deletion of only the 204–214 peptide completely abolished transport. These studies suggest that the primary role of the connecting loop between TMDs 6 and 7 is to ensure the proper spacing between the two halves of the RFC protein for optimal function and that this is virtually independent of amino acid sequence. The stretch of 11 highly conserved amino acids from positions 204–214 in hRFC appears to be essential for high level RFC transport activity.

4.2.5. RFC Tertiary Structure

Characterization of conserved charged residues in or flanking TMDs by mutant analysis can shed light on the tertiary structural elements in membrane proteins including interactions between distal domains. Interpretation is, in part, based on the notion of an energetic unfavorability associated with uncompensated charged amino acids localized within the lipid bilayer that are inaccessible to the aqueous environment within the putative transmembrane-spanning channel. However, should there be a salt bridge between residues of opposite charge, charged amino acids localized to hydrophobic environments can be substantially stabilized *(82)*. Salt bridges between oppositely charged residues in separate domains can serve to orient TMDs for membrane insertion and/or for optimal transport function *(83,84)*.

For hRFC, neutralization of the charge on Arg133 (TMD4) by substitution with leucine or on Asp88 (TMD2) by replacement with valine abolished transport activity *(74)*. However, when both mutations were present in the same construct (i.e., Asp88Leu/Arg133Val), transport activity was restored. This suggests that disruption of the charge-pair by replacing either Arg133 or Asp88, individually, with a neutral amino acid results in an unstable, unpaired charge. However, simultaneous neutralization of both charged amino acids results in a nearly complete restoration of transport activity. These results strongly suggest that Arg133 and Asp88 form a salt bridge complex that stabilizes the association between TMDs 2 and 4 in the hRFC tertiary structure.

Other reports have also explored RFC tertiary structure. In murine RFC, a structural or functional interaction between Glu45 (flanks TMD1) and Lys404 (TMD11) was implied because the properties of the double Glu45Lys/Lys404Glu murine RFC mutant more closely resembled the properties of the Glu45Lys mutant than those for the Lys404Glu mutant *(85)*. Finally, a crosslinking analysis of the hamster RFC suggested that Arg373 (in TMD10) is in close proximity to Glu394 (flanks TMD11), implying juxtaposition of these domains *(76)*.

4.3. Scanning Cysteine Accessibility Methods for Determining Membrane Topology and Mapping Substrate Binding Sites

Because polytopic membrane proteins are notoriously difficult to crystallize, a number of innovative experimental strategies have been developed to obtain critical structural information not otherwise attainable. Of particular interest are "scanning cysteine accessibility methods" or SCAM, based on the availability of a series of unique thiol-targeted reagents (e.g., alkylthiosulfonates, maleimides) with reactivities amenable to use with intact cells *(86–88)*. Thus, by inserting cysteines into functional "cysteine-less" proteins generated by site-directed mutagenesis, and treating transfected cells expressing cysteine insertion mutants with thiol-reactive reagents, it is possible to establish membrane topologies *(89–91)*, identify amino acids that are aqueous accessible and/or contribute to substrate binding *(92–95)*, and also demonstrate spacial relationships between distal TMDs *(96,97)*. Recent studies from our laboratory have begun to use SCAM in combination with thiol-reactive reagents to probe hRFC structure and function *(98)*.

4.3.1. Characterization of a Cysteine-Less hRFC and Membrane Topology Mapping by SCAM

There are 11 cysteine residues in the hRFC protein. We found that 4 of 11 cysteines can be removed by deleting 56 C-terminal amino acids with only a modest effect on transport. We replaced the remaining 7 cysteines (Cys30, 33, 220, 246, 365, 396, 458) with serines. Myc-his$_6$ epitopes were added to the truncated C-terminus of the wild-type (hRFC-*wt*) and cysteine-less hRFC constructs (hRFC-*Cys-less*) to facilitate immunolocalization and immunoprecipitation of the ectopically expressed proteins with anti-his6 and anti-myc antibodies. Both hRFC-*wt* and hRFC-*Cys-less* constructs were transfected into transport-defective CHO cells, and found to exhibit normal membrane targeting and high levels of MTX uptake *(98)*.

The availability of a functional cysteine-less hRFC suggested an alternative approach for mapping the topology of TMDs 7–12, thus circumventing the limitations of prior HA-epitope insertion and glycosylation scanning mutagenesis methods (Subheading 4.1.). Accordingly, CHO cells expressing functional hRFC constructs including Ser301Cys (TMD7/8 loop), Ala332Cys (TMD8/9), Ser360Cys (TMD9/10), Ala388Cys (TMD10/11), Ser390Cys (TMD10/11), and Arg429Cys (TMD11/12) mutants (Fig. 3) were treated with thiol-reactive biotin maleimide [3-(*N*-maleimidylpropionyl)biocytin] with or without the membrane impermeant stilbenedisulfonate maleimide (4-acetamido-4′-maleimidylstilbene-2,2′-disulfonic acid). Plasma membrane proteins were solubilized and hRFC immunoprecipitated. The immunoprecipitates were fractionated on SDS gels, and biotinylated thiols detected with peroxidase-linked streptavidin, whereas total hRFC proteins were detected with hRFC-specific antibody. Consistent with their predicted extracellular orientations, the Ser301Cys, Ser360Cys, and Arg429Cys hRFC mutants were all highly reactive with biotin maleimide and labeling was significantly blocked with membrane impermeant stilbenedisulfonate maleimide (Figure 5 shows results for Ser301Cys). By HA-epitope accessibility methods (Subheading 4.1), the TMD8/9 loop domain including position 332 has a cytosolic orientation. While Ala332Cys was unreactive under conditions (200 μM, 30 min) that labeled extracellular cysteines (Fig. 5), a low level of labeling at this position was detected following sustained treatments (2 h) with a higher concentration of biotin maleimide (1 mM) in spite of its intracellular localization (not shown). While Ala388Cys and Ser390Cys mutants, located in the middle of the putative conserved TMD10-11 loop domain (Figs. 3 and 4), were completely unreactive under these conditions, these positions (as well as Ala332Cys) were labeled followed permeabilization with Streptolysin O (W. Cao and L.H. Matherly, *unpublished observation*).

These patterns of biotin maleimide reactivity and protection by stilbenedisulfonate maleimide for residues localized in the loop domains for TMDs 7–8, 9–10, and 11–12 are entirely consistent with their extracellular orientations, and the labeling characteristics of Ala332Cys in the TMD8–9 loop region and Ala388Cys and Ser390Cys in the TMD10–11 loop suggest that they are oriented in the cytoplasm. Thus, the SCAM results, combined with previous findings of *N*-glycosylation at Asn58 and the results of HA-insertion and scanning glycosylation mutagenesis experiments, strongly support a 12-TMD structure for hRFC with cytosolic orientations for the N- and C-termini and TMD6/7 loop domain.

4.3.2. Structure and Function of TMD1 and Flanking Domain by SCAM

As noted in Subheading 4.2.1., amino acids in or flanking TMD1 in RFC (e.g., Gly44, Glu45, Ser46, Ile48) have been of particular interest, as a disproportionate frequency of mutations that result in impaired carrier function and antifolate resistance have been localized to this region. The availability of a functional cysteine-less hRFC construct afforded us an opportunity to probe the functional and structural features of this region by SCAM.

Accordingly, we mutated each of the 24 residues from Trp25 to Ile48, including the entire predicted TMD1, to cysteine using the hRFC-*Cys-less* as template. All of the 24 cysteine mutants were expressed in transport-impaired CHO cells and, with the exception of Arg42Cys, were functional *(98)*. We found that by treating the transfected cells with the small, water-soluble membrane impermeant thiol regent, sodium (2-sulfonatoethyl)methanethiosulfonate (MTSES), transport of MTX by the Gln40Cys, Gly44Cys, Glu45Cys, and Ile48Cys mutants was significantly inhibited (>30%), and for Gln40Cys, Gly44Cys, and

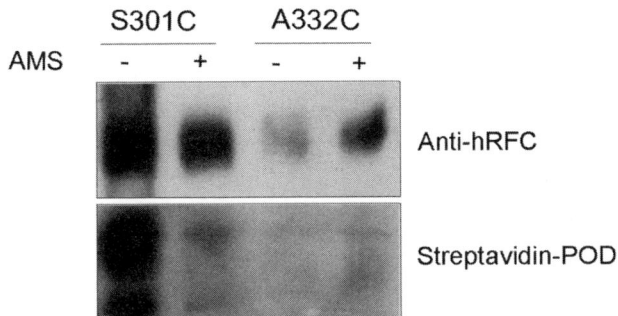

Fig. 5. Biotin maleimide reactivity with Ala332Cys (A332C) and Ser301Cys (S301C) mutants in hRFC. Cysteine mutants were treated with 200 µM biotin maleimide with and without 200 µM stilbenedisulfonate maleimide (AMS) for 15 min. Membrane proteins were immunoprecipitated with anti-myc antibody/protein G agarose, and analyzed on westerns with hRFC antibody (**upper panel**) and streptavidin-peroxidase (POD) (**lower**).

Ile48Cys, the MTSES inhibitions were protected by leucovorin ([6R,S]5-formyl tetrahydrofolate) *(98)*. These results imply that positions 40, 44, and 48 (but not positions 45 or 46) all lie in or near a substrate binding domain.

Additional studies were performed to characterize the TMD1-loop junction and establish the membrane localization of amino acids 40–48 *(98)*. CHO cells expressing single cysteine mutants from positions 37 to 43 spanning the predicted TMD1-exofacial loop boundary (Figs. 3 and 4) were treated with membrane-impermeant MTSEA-biotin ([N-biotinylaminoethyl] methanethiosulfonate), followed by immunoprecipitation and detection of surface biotinylated cysteines by western blotting with peroxidase-linked streptavidin. Pro43Cys, Arg42Cys, Ile41Cys, and Gln40Cys mutants were labeled, thus demonstrating their aqueous exposures and accessibility to MTSEA-biotin and probable extracellular localizations. However, no labeling of Ala39Cys, Met38Cys, and Phe37Cys mutants was detected, establishing their inaccessibility and probable membrane localizations. These results strongly suggest that the membrane boundary for TMD1 lies between positions 39 and 40.

To further confirm the localization of positions 44, 45, 46, and 48 in hRFC, we treated CHO transfectants expressing the Gly44Cys, Glu45Cys, Ser46Cys, and Ile48Cys mutant hRFCs with biotin maleimide under conditions that label extracellular cysteines, in the presence and absence of membrane impermeant stilbenedisulfonate maleimide, followed by immunoprecipitation and Western blotting with peroxidase–streptavidin *(98)*. All these positions were labeled with biotin maleimide, and biotinylation was significantly blocked by pretreatment with stilbenedisufonate maleimide, confirming that positions 44, 45, 46, and 48 are exposed to aqueous solvent and that they lie in the exofacial loop domain connecting TMDs 1 and 2 rather within TMD1.

4.3.3. Role of TMD1 in hRFC Function

The role of TMD1, in general, and amino acids 40, 44, 45, 46, and 48, in particular, in RFC transport remains a paradox. Whereas previous mutant studies seemed to suggest a possible functional importance for positions 44, 45, 46, and 48 by SCAM, only positions 40, 44, and 48 were unequivocally identified as contributing to substrate binding. The lack of a significant inhibition by MTSES at position 45 that was protected by leucovorin was particularly notable, because Glu45Lys is a frequent RFC mutation in transport-impaired cells and this phenotype involves dramatic (and opposite) effects on binding affinities for MTX vs folic acid and reduced folates *(10,64,65)* (Subheading 4.2.1.).

What is apparent, however, is that none of the residues from positions 40–48 are structural components of the putative aqueous transmembrane channel for anionic folate and antifolate substrates. Thus, any role for this segment would seem to be indirect and involve effects on carrier conformation and/or maintenance of charge states for amino acids directly involved in the uptake process. Alternatively, a more direct "scaffolding" role can be envisaged, in which substrate binding to this segment occurs at the exofacial membrane surface, followed by its transfer to the putative aqueous transmembrane channel. While the TMDs lining the putative transmembrane channel have not been identified, from the lack of MTSES reactivity at positions 25–39 in TMD1, it seems probable that TMD1 is not involved.

5. SUMMARY AND FUTURE DIRECTIONS

The chapter attempts to summarize recent significant advances in the understanding of the molecular determinants of RFC structure and function. Based on cumulative results of a host of experimental approaches with RFCs from different species, a picture of RFC structure has emerged that suggests its similarity to other members of the Major Facilitator superfamily of transporters *(99)* to which it belongs. The data convincingly argue for a symmetrical topologic structure in which two groups of six TMDs are connected by a large cytosolic loop domain whose primary role is to provide sufficient spacing for optimal carrier function. Neither the cytosolic facing N- nor C-termini are directly involved in transport function, and they appear to only slightly influence RFC membrane targeting. By analogy with other transporters, it is assumed that the 12 individual TMDs associate with one another to form a entity resembling an aqueous channel for transmembrane passage of charged folate and antifolate substrates, and that these associations may be fostered by the formation of critical salt bridges between charged residues localized within TMD domains such as that between Asp88 in TMD2 and Arg133 in TMD4 of hRFC.

An important goal of future structural studies of RFC involves further characterizing these TMD associations, and determining the critical structural domains and individual residues that contribute to substrate binding and membrane traverse of anionic folate and antifolate substrates. As uphill transport of folates and antifolates by RFC is believed to involve a physical transposition of the carrier within the membrane and an extrusion of organic anions down a large (intra- to extracellular) concentration gradient, mechanistic studies are also needed that identify the nature of the physiologic counteranion and the relationship between its binding site and that for folate substrates. Although reports have identified a number of conserved charged amino acids that may contribute to folate and antifolate substrate binding, a formidable task remains, namely discerning putative direct participation of these targeted residues in substrate (and/or anion) binding and translocation from possible indirect (e.g., conformational) effects. Answering many of these questions should be facilitated by the availability of an active cysteine-less hRFC *(98)* that permits the use of SCAM with thiol-reactive agents for probing key structural and functional features of the hRFC protein.

ACKNOWLEDGMENTS

This work was supported by Grant CA53535 from the National Institutes of Health.

REFERENCES

1. Lucock M. Folic acid: nutritional biochemistry, molecular biology, and role in disease processes. Mol Genet Metab 2000;71:121–138.
2. Matherly LH, Goldman ID. Membrane transport of folates. Vitam Horm 2003;66: 403–456.
3. Sirotnak FM, Tolner B. Carrier-mediated membrane transport of folates in mammalian cells. Ann Rev Nutr 1999;19:91–122.
4. Goldman ID, Matherly LH. The cellular pharmacology of methotrexate. Pharmacol Ther 1985;28:77–100.
5. Matherly LH. Molecular and cellular biology of the human reduced folate carrier. In: Moldave K, ed. Progress in Nucleic Acid Research and Molecular Biology, Vol. 67. San Diego: Harcourt/Academic Press; 2001:131-161.
6. Jansen G. Receptor- and carrier-mediated transport systems for folates and antifolates. Exploitation for folate chemotherapy and immunotherapy. In: Jackman AL, ed. Anticancer Development Guide: Antifolate Drugs in Cancer Therapy. Totowa, NJ: Humana Press, 1999:293–321.
7. Goldman ID, Zhao R. Molecular, biochemical, and cellular pharmacology of pemetrexed. Semin Oncol 2002;29:3–17.

8. Schuetz JD, Matherly LH, Westin EH, Goldman ID. Evidence for a functional defect in the translocation of the methotrexate transport carrier in a methotrexate resistant murine L1210 leukemia cell line. J Biol Chem 1988;263:9840–9847.
9. Wong SC, McQuadeR, Proefke SA, Matherly LH. Human K562 transfectants expressing high levels of reduced folate carrier but exhibiting low transport activity. Biochem Pharmacol 1997;53:199–206.
10. Jansen G, Mauritz R, Drori S, et al. A structurally altered human reduced folate carrier with increased folic acid transport mediates a novel mechanism of antifolate resistance. J Biol Chem 1998;273:30189–30198.
11. Gong M, Yess J, Connolly T, et al. Molecular mechanism of antifolate transport deficiency in a methotrexate resistant MOLT-3 human leukemia cell line. Blood 1997;89:2494–2499.
12. Sadlish H, Williams FM, Flintoff WF. Cytoplasmic domains of the reduced folate carrier are essential for trafficking, but not function. Biochem J 2002;364:777–786.
13. Sirotnak FM, Moccio DM, Kelleher LE, Goutas LJ. Relative frequency and kinetic properties of transport-defective phenotypes among methotrexate resistant L1210 clonal cell lines derived in vivo. Cancer Res 1981;41:4442–4452.
14. Goldman ID, Lichtenstein NS, Oliverio VT. Carrier-mediated transport of the folic acid analogue methotrexate, in the L1210 leukemia cell. J Biol Chem 1968;243:5007–5017.
15. Sirotnak FM, Kurita S, Hutchison DJ. On the nature of a transport alteration determining resistance to amethopterin in the L1210 leukemia. Cancer Res 1968;28:75–80.
16. Dixon KH, Lanpher BC, Chiu J, Kelley K, Cowan KH. A novel cDNA restores reduced folate carrier activity and methotrexate sensitivity to transport deficient cells. J Biol Chem 1994;269:17–20.
17. Williams FMR, Murray RC, Underhill TM, Flintoff WF. Isolation of a hamster cDNA clone coding for a function involved in methotrexate uptake. J Biol Chem 1994;269:5810–5816.
18. Sirotnak FM. Correlates of folate analog transport, pharmacokinetics, and selective antitumor action. Pharmacol Ther 1980;8:71–103.
19. Sierra E E, Brigle KE, Spinella MJ, Goldman ID. pH dependence of methotrexate transport by the reduced folate carrier and the folate receptor in L1210 leukemia cells—further evidence for a third route mediated at low pH. Biochem Pharmacol 1997;53:223–231.
20. Kumar CK, Nguyen TT, Gonzales FB, Said HM. Comparison of intestinal folate carrier clone expressed in IEC-6 cells and in *Xenopus* oocytes. Am J Physiol 1998;274:C289–C294.
21. Chiao JH, Roy K, Tolner B, Yang CH, Sirotnak FM. RFC-1 gene expression regulates folate absorption in mouse small intestine. J Biol Chem 1997;273:11165–11170.
22. Horne DW, Reed KA. Transport of methotrexate into PC-3 human prostate cancer cells. Arch Biochem Biophys 2001;394:39–44.

Structure–Function of Reduced Folate Carrier

23. White JC, Bailey BD, Goldman ID. Lack of stereospecificity at carbon 6 of methyltetrahydrofolate transport in Ehrlich ascites tumor cells. J Biol Chem 1978; 253:242–245.
24. Sirotnak FM, Chello PL, Moccio DM, et al. Stereospecificity at carbon 6 of formyltetrahydrofolate as a competitive inhibitor of transport and cytotoxicity of methotrexate in vitro. Biochem Pharmacol 1979;28:2993–2997.
25. Smith GK, Bigley JW, Dev IK, Duch DS, Ferone R, Pendergast W. GW1843: a potent, noncompetitive thymidylate synthase inhibitor; preclinical and preliminary clinical studies. In: Jackman AL, ed. Anticancer Development Guide: Antifolate Drugs in Cancer Therapy. Totowa, NJ: Humana Press; 1999:203–227.
26. Henderson GB, Zevely EM. Use of non-physiological buffer systems in the analysis of methotrexate transport in L1210 cells. Biochem Int 1983;6:507–515.
27. Yang C-H, Sirotnak FM, Dembo M. Interaction between anions and the reduced folate/methotrexate transport system in L1210 cell plasma membrane vesicles: directional symmetry and anion specificity for differential mobility of loaded and unloaded carrier. J Membr Biol 1984;70:285–292.
28. Henderson GB, Zevely EM. Transport routes utilized by L1210 cells for the influx and efflux of methotrexate. J Biol Chem 1984;259:1526–1531.
29. Goldman ID. A model system for the study of heteroexchange diffusion: methotrexate-folate interactions in L1210 leukemia and Ehrlich ascites tumor cells. Biochim Biophys Acta 1971;233:624–634.
30. Goldman ID. The characteristics of the membrane transport of amethopterin and the naturally occurring folates. Ann NY Acad Sci 1971;186:400–422.
31. Henderson GB, Zevely EM. Anion exchange mechanism for transport of methotrexate in L1210 cells. Biochem Biophys Res Commun 1981;99:163–169.
32. Henderson GB, Zevely EM. Structural requirements for anion substrates of the methotrexate transport system of L1210 cells. Arch Biochem Biophys 1983;221: 438–446.
33. Henderson GB, Zevely EM. Transport of methotrexate in L1210 cells: effect of ions on the rate and extent of uptake. Arch Biochem Biophys 1980;200: 149–155.
34. Zhao R, Gao F, Wang Y, Diaz GA, Gelb BD, Goldman ID. Impact of the reduced folate carrier on the accumulation of active thiamin metabolites in murine leukemia cells. J Biol Chem 2001;276:1114–1118.
35. Sirotnak FM, Moccio DM, Yang CH. A novel class of genetic variants of the L1210 cell up-regulated for folate analogue transport inward. Isolation, characterization, and degree of metabolic instability of the system. J Biol Chem 1984;259: 13139–13144.
36. Jansen G, Westerhof GR, Jarmuszewski MJ, Kathmann I, Rijksen G, Schornagel JH. Methotrexate transport in variant human CCRF-CEM leukemia cells with elevated levels of the reduced folate carrier. Selective effect on carrier-mediated transport of physiological concentrations of reduced folates. J Biol Chem 1990; 265:18272–18277.

37. Matherly LH, Czajkowski CA, Angeles SM. Identification of a highly glycosylated methotrexate membrane carrier in K562 erythroleukemia cells up-regulated for tetrahydrofolate cofactor and methotrexate transport. Cancer Res 1991;51: 3420–3426.
38. Yang CH, Pain J, Sirotnak FM. Alteration of folate analogue transport inward after induced maturation of HL-60 leukemia cells. Molecular properties of the transporter in an overproducing variant and evidence for down-regulation of its synthesis in maturating cells. J Biol Chem 1992;267:6628–6634.
39. Henderson GB, Grzelakowska-Sztabert B, Zevely EM, Huennekens FM. Binding properties of the 5-methyltetrahydrofolate/methotrexate transport system in L1210 cells. Arch Biochem Biophys 1980;202:244–249.
40. Henderson GB, Zevely EM, Huennekens FM. Photoinactivation of the methotrexate transpoprt system of L1210 cells by 8-azidoadenosine-5′-monophosphate. J Biol Chem 1979;254:9973–9975.
41. Henderson GB, Zevely EM. Functional correlations between the methotrexate and general anion transport systems of L1210 cells. Biochem Int 1982;4:493–502.
42. Henderson GB, Zevely EM, Huennekens FM. Irreversible inactivation of the methotrexate transport systems in L1210 cells by carbodiimide activated substrates. J Biol Chem 1980;255:4826–4833.
43. Jansen G, Westerhof GR, Rijksen G, Schornagel JH. Interaction of N-hydroxy-(sulfo)succinimide active esters with the reduced folate/methotrexate transport system from human leukemic CCRF-CEM cells. Biochim Biophys Acta 1989;875: 266–270.
44. Henderson GB, Zevely EM. Affinity labeling of the 5-methyltetrahydrofolate/methotrexate transport protein of L1210 cells by treatment with an N-hydroxysuccinimide ester of [^{3}H]methotrexate. J Biol Chem 1984;259:4558–4562.
45. Freisheim JH, Ratnam M, McAlinden TP, et al. Molecular events in the membrane transport of methotrexate in human CCRF-CEM leukemia cell lines. Adv Enzyme Regul 1992;32:17–31.
46. Zhao R, Gao F, Liu L, Goldman ID. The reduced folate carrier in L1210 murine leukemia cells Is a 58 kDa protein. Biochim Biophys Acta 2000;1466:7–10.
47. Price EM, Sams L, Harpring KM, Kempton RJ, Freisheim JH. Photoaffinity analogues of methotrexate as probes for dihydrofolate reductase structure and function. Biochem Pharmacol 1986;35:4341–4343.
48. Underhill TM, Williams FMR, Murray RC, Flintoff WF. Molecular cloning of a gene involved in methotrexate uptake by DNA-mediated gene transfer. Somat Cell Mol Genet 1992;18,337–349.
49. Moscow JA, Gong MK, He R, et al. Isolation of a gene encoding a human reduced folate carrier (RFC1) and analysis of its expression in transport-deficient, methotrexate-resistant human breast cancer cells. Cancer Res 1995;55: 3790–3794.
50. Prasad PD, Ramamoorthy S, Leibach FH, Ganapathy V. Molecular cloning of the human placental folate transporter. Biochem Biophys Res Commun 1995;206; 681–687.

51. Williams FMR, Flintoff WF. Isolation of a human cDNA that complements a mutant hamster cell defective in methotrexate uptake. J Biol Chem 1995;270: 2987–2992.
52. Wong SC, Proefke SA, Bhushan A, Matherly LH. Isolation of human cDNAs that restore methotrexate sensitivity and reduced folate carrier activity in methotrexate transport-defective Chinese hamster ovary cells. J Biol Chem 1995;270: 17468–17475.
53. Nguyen TT, Dyer DL, Dunning DD, Rubin SA, Grant KE, Said HM. Human intestinal folate transport: cloning, expression, and distribution of complementary RNA. Gastroenterology 1997;112:783–791.
54. Brigle KE, Spinella MJ, Sierra EE, Goldman ID. Characterization of a mutation in the reduced folate carrier in a transport defective L1210 murine leukemia cell line. J Biol Chem 1995;270:22974–22979.
55. Wong SC, Zhang L, Proefke SA, Matherly LH. Effects of the loss of capacity for N-glycosylation on the transport activity and cellular localization of the human reduced folate carrier. Biochim Biophys Acta 1998;1375:6–12.
56. Kumar CK, Nguyen TT, Gonzales FB, Said HM. Comparison of intestinal folate carrier clone expressed in IEC-6 cells and in *Xenopus* oocytes. Am J Physiol 1998;274:C289–C294.
57. Rajgopal A, Sierra EE, Zhao R, Goldman ID. Expression of the reduced folate carrier SLC19A1 in IEC-6 cells results in two distinct transport activities. Am J Physiol Cell Physiol 2001;281:C1579–C1586.
58. Hoffman K, Stoffel W. TMBASE-A database of membrane spanning protein segments. Biol Chem Hoppe Seyler 1993;374:166.
59. Ferguson PL, Flintoff WF. Topological and functional analysis of the human reduced folate carrier by hemagglutinin epitope insertion. J Biol Chem 1999;274: 16269–18278.
60. Liu X, Matherly LH. Analysis of membrane topology of the human reduced folate carrier protein by hemagglutinin epitope insertion and scanning glycosylation insertion mutagenesis. Biochim Biophys Acta 2002;1564:333–342.
61. Popov M, Tam LY, Li J, Reithmeier RA. Mapping the ends of transmembrane segments in a polytopic membrane protein. Scanning N-glycosylation mutagenesis of extracytosolic loops in the anion exchanger, Band 3. J Biol Chem 1997;272: 18325–18332.
62. Wong SC, Zhang L, Witt TL, Proefke SA, Bhushan A, Matherly LH. Impaired membrane transport in methotrexate-resistant CCRF-CEM cells involves early translation termination and increased turnover of a mutant reduced folate carrier. J Biol Chem 1999;274:10388–10394.
63. Rothem L, Ifergan I, Kaufman Y, Priest DG, Jansen G, Assaraf YG. Resistance to multiple novel antifolates is mediated via defective drug transport resulting from clustered mutations in the reduced folate carrier gene in human leukemia cell lines. Biochem J 2002;367:741–750.
64. Zhao R, Assaraf YG, Goldman ID. A mutated murine reduced folate carrier (RFC1) with increased affinity for folic acid, decreased affinity for methotrexate,

and an obligatory anion requirement for transport function. J Biol Chem 1998;273: 19065–19071.
65. Gifford AJ, Haber M, Witt TL, et al. Role of the E45K reduced folate carrier gene mutation in methotrexate resistance in human leukemia cells. Leukemia 2002;16: 2379–2387.
66. Drori S, Jansen G, Mauritz R, Peters GJ, Assaraf YG. Clustering of mutations in the first transmembrane domain of the human reduced folate carrier in GW1843U89-resistant leukemia cells with impaired antifolate transport and augmented folate uptake. J Biol Chem 2000;275:30855–30863.
67. Zhao R, Gao F, Wang PJ, Goldman ID. Role of the amino acid 45 residue in reduced folate carrier function and ion-dependent transport as characterized by site-directed mutagenesis. Mol Pharmacol 2000;57:317–323.
68. Zhao R, Assaraf YG, Goldman ID. A reduced carrier mutation produces substrate-dependent alterations in carrier mobility in murine leukemia cells and methotrexate resistance with conservation of growth in 5-formyltetrahydrofolate. J Biol Chem 1998;273:7873–7879.
69. Yang R, Sowers R, Mazza B, et al. Sequence alterations in the reduced folate carrier are observed in osteosarcoma tumor samples. Clin Cancer Res 2003;9:837–844.
70. Tse A, Brigle K, Taylor SM, Moran RG. Mutations in the reduced folate carrier gene which confer dominant resistance to 5,10-dideazatetrahydrofolate. J Biol Chem 1998;273:25953–25960.
71. Zhao R, Gao F, Goldman ID. Discrimination among reduced folates and methotrexate as transport substrates by a phenylalanine substitution for serine within the predicted eighth transmembrane domain of the reduced folate carrier. Biochem Pharmacol 1999;58:1615–1624.
72. Roy K, Tolner B, Chiao JH, Sirotnak FM. A single amino acid difference within the folate transporter encoded by the murine RFC-1 gene selectively alters its interaction with folate analogues. implications for intrinsic antifolate resistance and directional orientation of the transporter within the plasma membrane of tumor cells. J Biol Chem 1998;273:2526–2531.
73. Zhao R, Gao F, Babani S, Goldman ID. Sensitivity of 5,10-dideazatetrahydrofolate is fully conserved in a murine leukemia cell line highly resistant to methotrexate due to impaired transport mediated by the reduced folate carrier. Clin Cancer Res 2000;6:3304–3311.
74. Liu XY, Matherly LH. Functional interactions between arginine-133 and aspartate-88 in the human reduced folate carrier: evidence for a charge-pair association. Biochem J 2001;358:511–516.
75. Sharina IG, Zhao R, Wang Y, Babani S, Goldman ID. Mutational analysis of the functional role of conserved arginine and lysine residues in transmembrane domains of the murine reduced folate carrier. Mol Pharmacol 2001;59:1022–1028.
76. Sadlish H, Williams FM, Flintoff WF. Functional role of arginine 373 in substrate translocation by the reduced folate carrier. J Biol Chem 2002;277: 42105–42112.

77. Witt TL, Matherly LH. Identification of lysine-411 in the human reduced folate carrier as an important determinant of substrate selectivity and carrier function by systematic site directed mutagenesis. Biochim Biophys Acta 2002;1567: 56–62.
78. Marchant JS, Subramanian VS, Parker I, Said HM. Intracellular trafficking and membrane targeting mechanisms of the human reduced folate carrier in mammalian epithelial cells. J Biol Chem 2002;277:33325–33333.
79. Sadlish H, Williams FM, Flintoff WF. Cytoplasmic domains of the reduced folate carrier are essential for trafficking, but not function. Biochem J 2002;364:777–786.
80. Sharina IG, Zhao R, Wang Y, Babani S, Goldman ID. Role of the C-terminus and the long cytoplasmic loop in reduced folate carrier expression and function. Biochem Pharmacol 2002;63:1717–1724.
81. Liu XY, Witt TL, Matherly LH. Restoration of high level transport activity by human reduced folate carrier/ThTr1 chimeric transporters: role of the transmembrane domain 6/7 linker region in reduced folate carrier function. Biochem J 2003;369:31–37.
82. Barril X, Aleman C, Orozco M, Luque FJ. Salt bridge interactions: stability of the ionic and neutral complexes in the gas phase, in solution, and in proteins. Proteins 1998;32:67–79.
83. Dunten RL, Sahin-Toth M, Kaback HR. Role of the charge pair aspartic acid-237-lysine-358 in the lactose permease of *Escherichia coli*. Biochemistry 1993;32: 3139–3145.
84. Merickel A, Kaback HR, Edwards RH. Charged residues in transmembrane domains II and XI of a vesicular monoamine transporter form a charge pair that promotes high affinity substrate recognition. J Biol Chem 1997;272:5403–5408.
85. Zhao R, Wang Y, Gao F, Goldman ID. Residues 45 and 404 in the murine reduced folate carrier may interact to alter carrier binding and mobility. Biochim Biophys Acta 2003;1613:49–56.
86. Karlin A, Akabas MH. Substituted-cysteine accessibility method. Methods Enzymol 1998;293:123–145.
87. Frillingos S, Sahin-Toth M, Wu J, Kaback HR. Cys-scanning mutagenesis: a novel approach to structure function relationships in polytopic membrane proteins. FASEB J 1998;12:1281–1299.
88. Loo TW, Clarke DM. Determining the structure and mechanism of the human multidrug resistance P-glycoprotein using cysteine-scanning mutagenesis and thiol modification techniques. Biochim Biophys Acta 1999;1461:315–325.
89. Loo TW, Clarke DM. Membrane topology of a cysteine-less mutant of human *P*-glycoprotein. J Biol Chem 1995;270:843–848.
90. Nicoll DA, Ottolia M, Lu L, Lu Y, Philipson KD. A new topological model of the cardiac sarcolemmal Na^+-Ca^{2+} exchanger. J Biol Chem 1999;274:910–917.
91. Hu YK, Kaplan JH. Site-directed chemical labeling of extracellular loops in a membrane protein. The topology of the Na,K-ATPase alpha-subunit. J Biol Chem 2000;275:19185–19191.

92. Dodd JR, Christie DL. Cysteine 144 in the third transmembrane domain of the creatine transporter is located close to a substrate-binding site. J Biol Chem 2001;276:46983–46988.
93. Loo TW, Clarke DM. Identification of residues within the drug-binding domain of the human multidrug resistance P-glycoprotein by cysteine-scanning mutagenesis and reaction with dibromobimane. J. Biol. Chem 2000;275:39272–39278.
94. Slotboom DJ, Konings WN, Lolkema JS. Cysteine-scanning mutagenesis reveals a highly amphipathic, pore-lining membrane-spanning helix in the glutamate transporter GltT. J Biol Chem 2001;276:10775–10781.
95. Kwaw I, Zen KC, Hu Y, Kaback HR. Site-directed sulfhydryl labeling of the lactose permease of *Escherichia coli:* helices IV and V that contain the major determinants for substrate binding. Biochemistry 2001;40:10491–10499.
96. Zeng FY, Hopp A, Soldner A, Wess J. Use of a disulfide cross-linking strategy to study muscarinic receptor structure and mechanisms of activation. J Biol Chem 1999;274:16629–16640.
97. Loo TW, Clarke DM. Determining the dimensions of the drug-binding domain of human P-glycoprotein using thiol cross-linking compounds as molecular rulers. J Biol Chem 2001;276:36877–36880.
98. Cao W, Matherly LH. Characterization of a cysteine-less human reduced folate carrier: localization of a substrate binding domain by cysteine scanning mutagenesis and cysteine accessibility methods. Biochem J 2003;374:27–36.
99. Saier MH Jr, Beatty JT, Goffeau A, et al. The major facilitator superfamily. J Mol Microbiol Biotechnol 1999;1:257–279.

13

Glutathione Transport in the Kidneys

Experimental Models, Mechanisms, and Methods

Lawrence H. Lash

Summary

Although investigators have often focused on the role of glutathione (GSH) in drug metabolism and protection from reactive oxygen species and toxic electrophiles, membrane transport processes also play a critical role in the overall homeostasis of GSH in the body. Although the liver is the primary source of extracellular GSH, the kidneys are relatively unique in possessing plasma membrane transport systems for both uptake and efflux of GSH and are the major sites for clearance of circulating GSH from the plasma. This chapter reviews the various aspects of how GSH is transported across the plasma and mitochondrial inner membranes in renal cells, with a focus on the appropriate choice of experimental model and considerations important in accurately quantifying transport. Model systems for measuring plasma membrane transport of GSH that are discussed include isolated cells and tubules and membrane vesicles. Model systems for measuring mitochondrial transport of GSH include isolated cells coupled with digitonin fractionation, isolated mitochondria and mitoplasts, purified and reconstituted carrier proteins, and bacterially expressed, purified and reconstituted recombinant carrier proteins. GSH is truly a "molecule on the move" and accomplishes this by highly regulated, carrier-mediated processes that can be exploited to modulate and characterize cellular and mitochondrial redox homeostasis.

Key Words

Apoptosis; basolateral plasma membrane; brush-border plasma membrane; *tert*-butylhydroperoxide; dibutylphthalate method; dicarboxylate carrier; digitonin fractionation; distal tubular cells; γ-glutamyltransferase; glutathione; glutathione disulfide; glutathione degradation; glutathione oxidation; interorgan metabolism; kidney; marker enzymes; membrane vesicles; mitochondria; mitoplasts; multidrug resistance proteins; NRK-52E cells; organic anion transporters; 2-oxoglutarate carrier; proximal tubular cells; sodium-dicarboxylate 2 cotransporter.

From: *Methods in Pharmacology and Toxicology,*
Drug Metabolism and Transport: Molecular Methods and Mechanisms
Edited by: L. Lash © Humana Press Inc., Totowa, NJ

1. INTRODUCTION

The purpose of this chapter is not to review the many cellular functions of glutathione (GSH) as a nucleophile and reductant. Rather, the goals are to review the various aspects of how GSH is transported across the plasma and mitochondrial inner membranes in renal cells, with a focus on the appropriate choice of experimental model and considerations important in accurately quantifying transport. Hence, although investigators have often focused on the role of GSH in drug metabolism and protection from reactive oxygen species and toxic electrophiles, membrane transport processes also play a critical role in the overall homeostasis of GSH in the body. The resistance of the γ-glutamyl peptide bond of the GSH molecule to hydrolysis by circulating proteases and the large efflux of GSH from the liver are thus responsible for micromolar concentrations of GSH in the plasma *(1)*. Accordingly, one function of this interorgan process has been ascribed to GSH acting as a relatively stable transport form for cysteine. This is likely to be one role for the interorgan process, as cysteine is relatively unstable, undergoing facile auto-oxidation at physiological pH, and is a limiting component for resynthesis of GSH or various proteins. Although most tissues have varying activity levels of the enzymes catalyzing synthesis of GSH, this interorgan process may also function to supply epithelial tissues, including the lungs, kidney, and small intestine, with exogenous GSH.

Selective tissue localization of membrane carriers for GSH and interorgan translocation are therefore major determinants of cellular GSH status *(1)*. Whereas hepatocytes are the primary source of plasma and other pools of extracellular GSH, possessing carriers on the sinusoidal and canalicular plasma membranes that mediate efflux of GSH *(2,3)*, the kidneys are relatively unique in possessing plasma membrane transport systems for both uptake and efflux of GSH and are the major sites for clearance of circulating GSH from the plasma *(1,4)* (Fig. 1). Moreover, the kidneys possess the highest activity of any tissue of γ-glutamyltransferase (GGT) *(5)*, which, along with dipeptidase activity, degrade GSH to its constituent amino acids in the tubular lumen. The constituent amino acids are reabsorbed into the proximal tubular (PT) cell by transport across the brush-border membrane (BBM), where they can serve as precursors for protein or for resynthesis of GSH. Hence, renal PT cells can obtain GSH from both the extracellular space, via transport across the basolateral membrane (BLM), or by intracellular synthesis from its precursors. Thus, processes on the BBM serve to provide renal cells with amino acid precursors for resynthesis of GSH or, via reabsorptive mechanisms, to supply extrarenal tissues with cysteine and the other amino acids for synthesis of GSH or proteins. Efflux from PT cells by transport

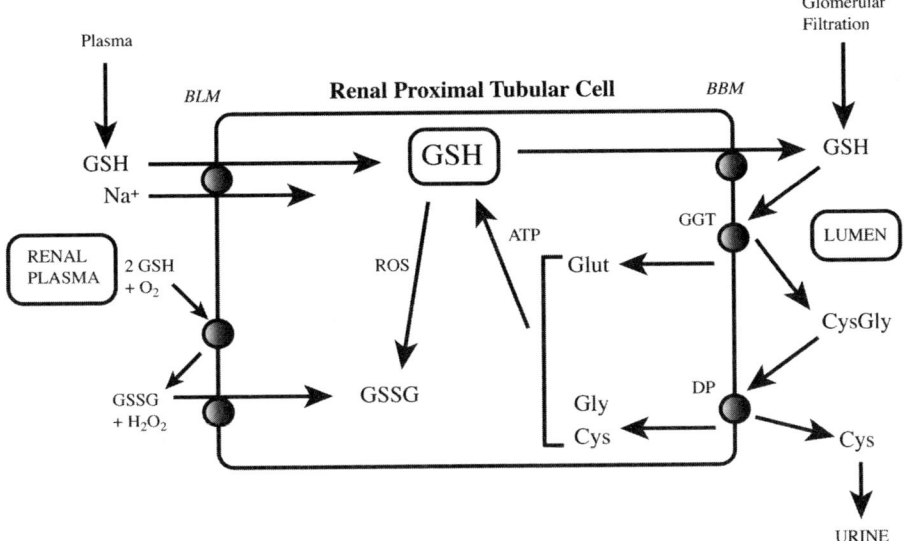

Fig. 1. Handling of GSH by renal PT cells. The scheme summarizes some of the major processes involved in GSH transport and metabolism in renal PT cells. These processes include uptake (coupled either directly or indirectly to Na$^+$ ions) across the BLM, efflux from the cell into the lumen by transport across the BBM, oxidation to GSSG at the BLM by a Cu-containing thiol oxidase, degradation at the BBM into the constituent amino acids by the γ-glutamyltransferase (GGT) and dipeptidase (DP), intracellular resynthesis of GSH from the constituent amino acids, and intracellular oxidation to GSSG to detoxify toxicants such as reactive oxygen species (ROS).

across the BBM and subsequent degradation by GGT account for turnover of renal GSH and for most of the turnover of GSH in the body. The physiological function of basolateral uptake of GSH is not completely understood, but the transport processes may be used pharmacologically to provide renal PT cells with exogenous GSH to protect against oxidant injury (6). Studies by Parks et al. (7) in isolated perfused PT segments from the S_1, S_2, and S_3 segments of rabbit proximal tubule also demonstrated cell-to-lumen and cell-to-bath secretion of GSH.

2. CARRIERS INVOLVED IN RENAL GSH TRANSPORT
2.1. Plasma Membrane Transport Processes

Observations in isolated, perfused kidneys from the rat and rabbit in the late-1970s through the mid-1980s (8–14) provided evidence that either endogenous or administered GSH was extracted from the plasma by both a basolateral and a luminal mechanism. Although the latter clearly involves glomerular filtration, degradation by BBM enzymes, and uptake of the constituent amino acids by renal PT cells *(1,9)*, there was controversy over whether a basolateral transport mechanism for the intact tripeptide of GSH actually existed or if the apparent basolateral extraction of plasma GSH was due to degradation of GSH by extraluminal GGT, renal cellular uptake of the constituent amino acids, and intracellular resynthesis of GSH *(11,15,16)*. This controversy was ultimately resolved by studies by Lash and Jones *(17,18)* and subsequent studies by Jones and colleagues *(6)*: these studies provide a biochemical description of an Na^+-dependent transport process for uptake of GSH in isolated BLM vesicles and isolated rat kidney cells. Additional studies *(19)* showed that GSH *S*-conjugates are transported across the BLM, at least in part, by the same process(es) that transport(s) GSH.

The process of GSH uptake across the BLM thus comprises at least two components, an Na^+-independent and an Na^+-dependent pathway. Measurement of the stoichiometry of the Na^+-dependent process showed coupling of GSH uptake to the uptake of at least two Na^+ ions with the net transfer across the membrane of at least one positive charge *(18)*. As such, the transport is electrogenic and is membrane potential sensitive. Because the intracellular milieu is negative relative to the extracellular space, transport under physiological conditions is predominantly uptake of GSH from renal plasma and interstitial space into the cell. GSH uptake is also inhibited by organic anions, such as *p*-aminohippurate and probenecid *(18)*. More recent studies of ours *(20)* showed that besides *p*-aminohippurate, which is transported across the renal BLM primarily by the organic anion transporter 1 (OAT1) but also by OAT3, transport of GSH across the BLM is also inhibited by dimethylsuccinate, which is a specific inhibitor of the sodium-dicarboxylate 2 (SDCT2) cotransporter. Besides the OAT proteins and SDCT2, multidrug resistance protein 5 (MRP5) is also localized on the renal BLM and may be an additional carrier that functions in GSH transport, although this possibility is yet to be investigated. Moreover, the nephron localization of MRP5 has not been established, so it is uncertain if this carrier is present in the proximal tubules. A schematic of the putative transporters for GSH across the BLM of renal PT cells is shown in Fig. 2.

Transport of GSH across the BBM of renal PT cells is not coupled to Na^+ or other ions, but is electrogenic, catalyzing transfer of one negative charge across the membrane and is driven by the membrane potential *(21)*. Because the intracellular milieu is negative relative to the luminal fluid, transport under physiological conditions is predominantly efflux of cellular GSH into the lumen. This process is the critical determinant in the renal cellular turnover of GSH, as the efflux of GSH into the lumen delivers GSH to the active site of GGT on the external surface of the BBM *(22,23)*. Furthermore, this process is critical to

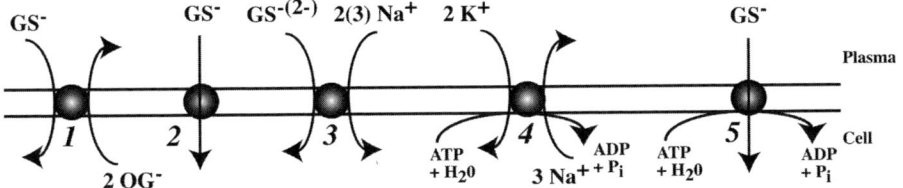

Fig. 2. Hypothesized mechanisms for transport of GSH across the BLM of renal PT cells. *1* = Oat1, *2* = Oat3, *3* = SDCT2, *4* = (Na$^+$ + K$^+$)-stimulated ATPase, *5* = Mrp5. GSH is suggested to be transported as either a monoanion or a dianion.

the turnover of whole body GSH because of the interorgan pathways and the predominant localization of GGT in the kidney.

No direct information is presently available about the potential function of any specific carrier on the BBM in GSH efflux. We can make certain suppositions, however, based on current knowledge; putative carriers are shown schematically in Fig. 3. There are three carriers on the BBM from the so-called multispecific organic anion carrier family that may be functional in GSH transport. Of these three, OATP1 is localized to the S_3 segment of rat PT cells and the form expressed in hepatic sinusoidal plasma membranes does transport GSH *(24)* and likely functions as an Na$^+$-independent, electroneutral exchanger of GSH with other organic anions (25). Besides OATP1, the two kidney-specific OAT proteins, OAT-K1 and OAT-K2, are also found in renal BBM and mediate Na$^+$-independent, facilitated efflux or exchange of organic anions. Relatively little is known about these two carriers. For example, it is not even certain whether the two carriers are separate proteins. Rather, OAT-K2 may be derived from the same gene product as OAT-K1. Rat OAT-K1 has a high degree of homology with rat and mouse OATP1 (72%). The substrate specificity of OAT-K1 appears to be rather narrow, with methotrexate and folates being the only identified substrates. Several other organic anions inhibit OAT-K1 but do not appear to be transported. Methotrexate efflux from Madin-Darby Canine Kidney (MDCK) cells overexpressing OAT-K1 was not enhanced by an inwardly directed gradient of GSH *(26)*, suggesting that OAT-K1 may not function in GSH transport across the BBM. It is important to note, however, that this absence of effect of GSH in MDCK cells may not occur in the in vivo rat proximal tubule. Despite being considered a homolog of OAT-K1, OAT-K2 transports taurocholate and prostaglandin E_2, which are not substrates for OAT-K1. MRP2 is found on the BBM of rat PT cells and does transport GSH conjugates *(27–29)* and GSH itself *(30–32)*. Hence, although its function in the renal PT cell has not been investigated directly, it will likely function in GSH efflux.

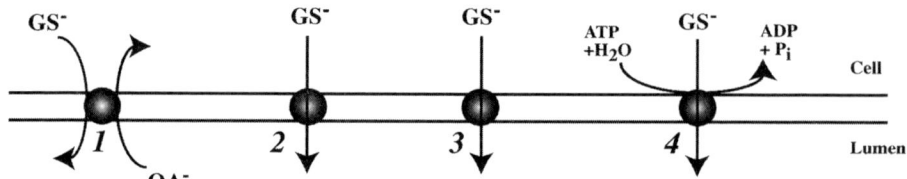

Fig. 3. Hypothesized mechanisms for transport of GSH across the BBM of renal PT cells. *1* = Oatp1, *2* = Oat-k1, *3* = Oat-k2, *4* = Mrp2.

2.2. Mitochondrial Membrane Transport Processes

GSH is compartmentalized within the renal PT cell. Turnover studies with radiolabeled GSH in both liver and kidney showed that there are at least two major pools of GSH, one with a relatively short half-life of 2 h and a smaller pool with a relatively long half-life of 30 h *(33,34)*. The long half-life pool was identified as being localized predominantly in the mitochondria *(34)*. Fractionation studies of rat renal proximal tubules showed that the mitochondrial pool comprises approx 15–30% of total cellular GSH *(35,36)*, which is the approximate volume fraction of mitochondria in the proximal tubules. Although there is no concentration gradient for GSH across the mitochondrial inner membrane, the net negative charge of the GSH molecule at physiological pH and the existence of a pH gradient and membrane potential across the mitochondrial inner membrane imply that the distribution of GSH between the cytoplasm and mitochondrial matrix cannot be regulated passively but must be regulated by some energy-dependent mechanism.

There are two possible sources of mitochondrial GSH, *de novo* synthesis from precursor amino acids or transport of intact GSH from the cytoplasm. As the enzymes for synthesis of GSH are localized predominantly, if not entirely, in the cytoplasm and little or no synthesis of GSH occurs within the mitochondria *(37,38)*, transport from the cytoplasm must be the mechanism by which mitochondria are supplied with their pool of GSH. The importance of understanding this mechanism lies in the predominance of GSH in the nonprotein thiol pool of mitochondria and its function to maintain redox status and activity of numerous sulfhydryl-dependent processes *(39–42)*. Moreover, selective depletion of mitochondrial GSH has been associated with enhanced susceptibility to several mechanisms of chemically induced injury, such as oxidative stress *(43–45)*.

Early studies on mitochondrial GSH transport *(46–48)* focused primarily on the relationship between mitochondrial respiratory state and transport activity. Although this provided insight into how transport activity varied with mitochondrial energetics, it did not address the critical issue of how GSH was translocated across the inner membrane and what source of energy was required to maintain this critical cellular pool of GSH.

Studies from Lash and colleagues in the 1990s in isolated mitochondria from rat kidney cortex *(38,49)* identified two of the anion carriers, the dicarboxylate carrier (DCC) and 2-oxoglutarate carrier (OGC), as being responsible for uptake of GSH from cytoplasm into the mitochondrial matrix. This conclusion was based on studies of substrate competition, inhibitor sensitivity, and energetics. Additional evidence for the function of these carriers was provided in studies where the carriers were partially purified from mitoplasts from rabbit kidney cortex and reconstituted into proteoliposomes *(50)*. More recent studies from Lash and colleagues *(51,52)* provided the most definitive evidence to date that the DCC is one carrier involved in mitochondrial GSH transport. The cDNA for rat DCC was amplified, expressed in bacteria, purified, and reconstituted into proteoliposomes; the reconstituted protein transported GSH and malonate with properties similar to what was observed previously in intact mitochondria or in a purified and reconstituted system. Furthermore, overexpression of the cDNA for rat DCC in a rat renal PT cell line (NRK-52E cells) enhanced cellular uptake and accumulation of GSH by 3- to 11-fold and markedly diminished sensitivity of the NRK-52E cells to apoptosis induced by either an oxidant (*tert*-butyl hydroperoxide [*t*-BH] or a mitochondrial toxicant (*S*-[1,2-dichlorovinyl]-L-cysteine; DCVC).

Similar studies to those described for the DCC were conducted, in which NRK-52E cells were transfected to overexpress mRNA for either the wild-type OGC or a mutant OGC that exhibits little GSH transport activity, and provided evidence for the critical role of this carrier in mitochondrial GSH transport *(53–55)*. Thus, cells that overexpressed the wild-type OGC, and thereby exhibited high activity of mitochondrial GSH transport, were protected from *t*-BH- or DCVC-induced apoptosis; in contrast, cells transfected to overexpress the mutant OGC and that exhibited very low mitochondrial GSH transport activity had a similar, high degree of sensitivity to *t*-BH- and DCVC-induced apoptosis.

3. EXPERIMENTAL MODEL SYSTEMS USED TO STUDY GSH TRANSPORT

This section will present a brief consideration of the different types of in vitro experimental model systems that one can use to directly quantify and characterize the various GSH transport processes. The choice of model system is guided by which process is being studied and the type of information that is desired. A critical issue regardless of the model system is that the GSH molecule is maintained intact so that transport can be measured accurately. For many transport studies, a limiting factor in accurately measuring transport is the ability to minimize intracellular metabolism of the transported substrate. In the case of GSH, however, metabolism, or more specifically, degradation, occurs at the brush-border membrane surface. Consequently, although one must be concerned about intracellular metabolism, metabolism at the membrane surface that competes directly with transport is the primary concern. Renal BBMs have extremely high activity levels of GGT. Consequently, when preparing subcellular fractions, even a very small amount of contamination (e.g., <5%) of the fraction of interest with BBMs can still produce significant degradation of GSH. In fact, in studies of GSH transport across the basolateral membrane (BLM) using BLM vesicles, it was estimated that contamination with brush-border membrane was <2% *(17,18)*. If GGT was not inhibited, the rate of GSH degradation was as high or higher than that of transport, thus making accurate measurements of transport difficult to achieve.

3.1. Model Systems for Measuring Plasma Membrane Transport

For any study of a renal plasma membrane transport process, an important concern is whether or not epithelial polarity is maintained so that processes occurring on one specific membrane can be distinguished from those occurring on the other membrane. This is even more important when transepithelial absorption or excretion are being determined. The choice of model also depends on the experimental goal. For example, if one wants to examine the role of the transport process in some cellular function or in a toxicological or pathological response, then an intact cellular model is needed. Although description of methods for the preparation of these intact cellular models is beyond the scope of this chapter, a few points are important as they relate to membrane transport. Nephron heterogeneity, or cell type purity, is critical as well, because available data indicate that most of the processes relating to GSH transport and metabolism are present predominantly in the PT region and are either absent or present at very low levels in the distal tubular (DT) region. Hence, most experiments will involve use of proximal tubules or PT cells or material (i.e., membrane vesicles) from PT cells, and a limiting factor will be the purity of these cells or subcellular fractions. Experimental approaches to purify PT cells from rat renal cortex have been described in depth, and the reader is referred to other publications for details *(56–58)*.

When performing studies of GSH transport across either the BLM or BBM of freshly isolated proximal tubules or PT cells, membrane polarity cannot be achieved because the biological material is usually used in suspension. However, primary cultures can readily be grown with the cells or tubule fragments plated on a semipermeable material, such as Millicell filter inserts (Fig. 4). In this case, cells or tubules are plated on the filters, which have usually been precoated with collagen or some collagen-derived material. The cells grow with

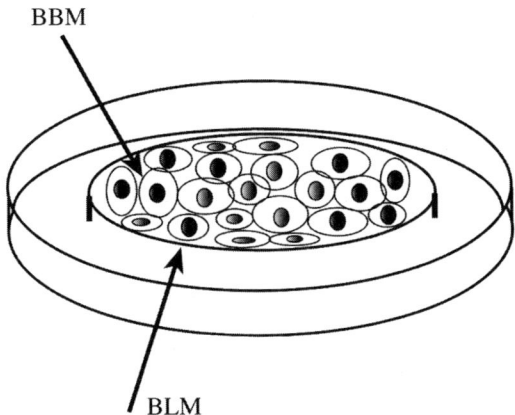

Fig. 4. Scheme showing model for measuring polarized flux across the BBM and BLM in primary cultures of renal PT cells.

their BBM facing up, so that substrate added to the upper compartment is in contact with only the BBM. Material can be added to the lower compartment so that substrate has contact with the BLM. Owing to the extremely high activity of GGT on the renal PT BBM, acivicin (L-[α,S,5S])-α-amino-3-chloro-4,5-dihydro-5-isoxazoleacetic acid) is usually used to irreversibly inhibit GGT activity. One typically pretreats cells or tubules with 0.25–0.5 mM acivicin for 15 min prior to conducting transport measurements. Acivicin is a glutamine analogue that was originally developed as an antitumor agent, but was shown to be a very selective inhibitor of GGT at relatively low concentrations *(59,60)*. It is important not to use too high a concentration of acivicin, because at higher concentrations acivicin becomes a relatively nonselective alkylating agent *(61)* and inhibits many other processes, including GSH transport *(17,18)*.

Another popular method to study plasma membrane transport processes has been the use of membrane vesicles. For most transport substrates, the primary rationale for using membrane vesicles is that the investigator isolates the subcellular fraction that contains the transporter and eliminates intracellular metabolism as a complicating factor in the measurement of intravesicular substrate content. As noted earlier, however, the situation is somewhat different for GSH because the enzymes that catalyze degradation of the GSH molecule (i.e., GGT and dipeptidase) are localized on the BBM with their active sites facing externally. Nonetheless, use of isolated BLM and BBM vesicles has distinct advantages for study of GSH transport. These advantages include the ease of preparation of membrane vesicles of high purity and homogeneity and the absence of intracellular metabolism.

3.2. Model Systems for Measuring Mitochondrial Transport

A variety of experimental models can be used to examine mitochondrial GSH transport. These various models and the methods used to quantify and characterize GSH transport have been discussed previously *(62)*. Models for measurement of mitochondrial GSH transport in the kidney include intact cells or tubules, isolated mitochondria, and mitoplasts. In all cases, it is important to inhibit GSH degradation by GGT with acivicin. Even with the isolated mitochondria and mitoplasts, it is estimated that contamination of the mitochondrial fraction with fragments of BBM can be as high as 2–5% *(38,49)*. The exceptionally high GGT activity on the renal PT BBM indicates that even such a small contamination can result in a significant capacity to degrade GSH.

To study GSH transport into renal mitochondria using intact cells or tubules as the experimental model, it is important to be able to efficiently and accurately separate the mitochondrial compartment from the cytoplasmic compartment. This is typically achieved by treatment of the cells or tubules with a material that can permeabilize the plasma membrane but not affect the mitochondrial inner membrane, followed by rapid centrifugation. We have used the detergent digitonin to achieve this *(35)*. As shown in Fig. 5, cells are rapidly mixed with a top layer containing buffer and 0.1 mg of digitonin/10^6 cells in a 2.9-mL polypropylene microcentrifuge tube. After a 30-s centrifugation of the cells through the digitonin and through a layer of silicone oil:mineral oil (6:1), cells are pelleted into a layer of 10% (w/v) perchloric acid. Material recovered in the top layer contains cytoplasm and extracellular medium whereas that recovered in the bottom layer contains predominantly the mitochondrial fraction. A paired sample is also run without digitonin in the top layer; in this case, material in the top layer contains that in the extracellular medium and that in the bottom layer contains the total cellular content. Comparison of values in the two sets of paired tubes allows determination of what is specifically in the cytoplasm and mitochondria.

Suspensions of isolated mitochondria are the most common model in which to study transport across the inner membrane. This subcellular fraction is relatively simple to prepare by differential centrifugation procedures and can be validated in terms of functionality and integrity by a large battery of established methods *(63)*. Common assessments of mitochondrial functional integrity include measurement of substrate- and ADP-dependent oxygen consumption with determination of respiratory control ratio, spectrophotometric monitoring of matrix swelling with polyethylene glycol or leakage of matrix enzymes, and measurement of membrane potential with various potential-sensitive dyes. An important aspect of the use of suspensions of isolated mitochondria is the buffer that is used to both prepare the mitochondria and in the final resuspension.

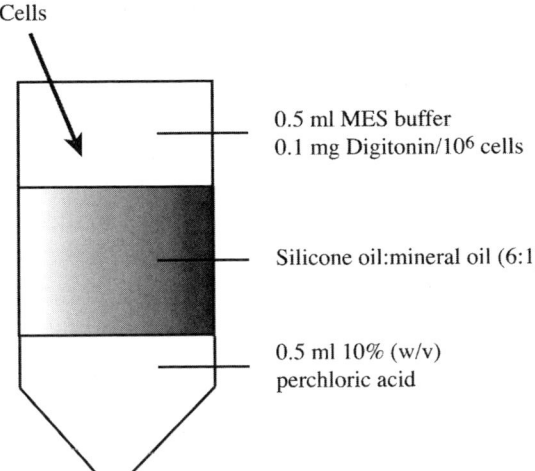

Fig. 5. Subcellular fractionation of renal PT cells with digitonin. To separate mitochondrial and cytoplasmic contents for analysis of GSH, other metabolites, or enzyme activities, renal PT cells can be centrifuged through a layer of buffer morpholinoethanesulfonic acid (MES) and digitonin, a layer of silicone oil : mineral oil (6 : 1), into a layer of perchloric acid.

Typically, preparations of isolated mitochondria use homogenization in buffers containing a high concentration of an impermeant solute, such as 225 mM sucrose, potassium phosphate, magnesium chloride, an organic buffer, such as Tris-HCl or triethanolamine HCl, and a divalent cation chelator such as ethylene glycol bis(β-aminoethyl ether)-N,N,N',N'-tetraacetic acid (EGTA). The final buffer that is used for resuspension of mitochondria and for assay of mitochondrial function and transport is the same as earlier but without EGTA. The buffer composition is critical because it enables isolation of mitochondria that maintain a high degree of structural integrity, selective permeability, and function.

Because mitochondria can adapt to their environment and assume an orthodox or condensed conformation, thereby changing the matrix volume, it is important to determine whether matrix volume changes during the course of transport incubations and measurements. Potential changes in matrix volume are often eliminated by inclusion of a metabolic inhibitor, such as antimycin A (49). This point is particularly important when measuring transport of substrates that undergo further metabolism in the matrix or by the mitochondrial electron transport chain.

A final experimental model that can be used to measure transport across the mitochondrial inner membrane is mitoplasts, which are mitochondria that have had their outer membrane and intermembrane space removed, leaving the matrix and inner membrane. Mitoplasts can be prepared by first isolating mitochondria by differential centrifugation and then applying a treatment to shear off or remove the outer membrane. Methods to remove the outer membrane include sonication or treatment with a nonionic detergent, such as Lubrol, that leaves the inner membrane intact (e.g., ref. 64). Functional integrity can be assessed in the same manner as is done with intact mitochondria. Advantages of using mitoplasts are that the outer membrane is missing and, therefore, cannot impede transport measurements. Functional integrity of mitoplasts is, however, more difficult to maintain than that of intact mitochondria.

3.3. Issues and Considerations in Measuring GSH Transport

This subheading briefly lists important considerations or cautions that are needed in the measurement of substrate transport in general and GSH transport in particular. Some considerations relate specifically to which experimental model is used while others are generic to all transport measurements, regardless of the model and substrate used. Regardless of the extent of contamination of the biological model with other subcellular fractions that can lead to oxidation or degradation of GSH, it is recommended that at least in pilot studies, transported GSH be quantified by a method that identifies the specific form of GSH. In other words, a method should be used that can specifically identify GSH, GSSG, and degradation products (i.e., L-glutamate and L-cysteine). An example of such a method would be high-performance liquid chromatography in which GSH and all the relevant metabolites are derivatized and can be identified by comparison with authentic standards (e.g., ref. 65). Once the form of GSH in the compartment of interest is determined, then other methods that would enable more rapid analysis of samples, such as scintillation counting of incubations with radiolabeled GSH, can be used with more precision and certainty.

3.3.1. General Considerations Related to the Experimental Model

The basic considerations and cautions that relate to measurement of transport of any metabolite, including GSH, include the following: (1) homogeneity or purity of the model; (2) viability of the model and the extent of leakiness of the membrane; (3) ability to distinguish transport from nonspecific binding or electrostatic association of the transport substrate with the membrane; and (4) ability to efficiently separate the interior and exterior compartments during the measurement of transport and to precisely quantify the extent of substrate carryover when separating compartments. Each of these points is discussed briefly in the paragraphs below.

(1) Homogeneity or purity of the experimental model is typically assessed by measurement of activities of marker enzymes. In the case of isolated renal PT

cells as the model, marker enzymes for PT cells, which are typically BBM enzymes such as GGT and alkaline phosphatase, should be high, whereas marker enzymes for other cell types, such as hexokinase for DT cells, should be low. When using BBM and BLM vesicles obtained from renal cortical homogenates, marker enzymes for each membrane are used, and include GGT and alkaline phosphatase for the BBM and the ($Na^+ + K^+$)-ATPase for the BLM. In addition, marker enzymes for other membrane-containing, subcellular fractions should also be measured and should be very low. These include markers for plasma membranes (BBM, BLM), lysosomes (e.g., acid phosphatase), endoplasmic reticulum (e.g., glucose 6-phosphatase), peroxisomes (e.g., catalase or glucose oxidase), and mitochondria (e.g., citrate synthase). When isolated mitochondria or mitoplasts are used, marker enzymes for other membrane-containing, subcellular fractions should be determined as described earlier.

(2) Assessments of viability of the models have been in the preceding above and elsewhere. As to assessment of the potential leakiness of the model, a typical approach is to use a radiolabeled, impermeant chemical, such as [^{3}H]inulin or [^{14}C]sucrose and compare its distribution to that of ^3H_2O. While the radiolabeled water should evenly distribute between the two compartments, the amount of radiolabeled inulin or sucrose that is recovered in the internal compartment (= apparent transport) provides a measure of leakiness. An example of the application of this method to determine leakiness and internal compartment volume for transport studies with isolated mitochondria is described in Subheading 5.

(3) The ability to distinguish transport from nonspecific binding or some electrostatic interaction when using charged substrates can be accomplished by washing steps after the transport process has been stopped and by performing incubations with boiled material. When performing transport measurements with membrane vesicles, a useful approach to quantify binding or nonspecific association is to measure equilibrium values of substrate that are retained with the membranes when the incubations are performed in a medium containing a very high concentration of sucrose (e.g., 1 M sucrose). This approach causes the intravesicular volume to shrink to essentially zero because of osmotic pressure so that transport should theoretically be zero.

(4) Efficient separation of compartments and quantitation of carryover is done essentially as described in point 2 earlier, using radiolabeled markers to quantify compartment volumes and leakiness or carryover.

3.3.2. Considerations Specific to GSH

The major considerations or cautions that are specific to measuring transport of GSH include maintenance or assessment of oxidation/reduction state and limiting or preventing degradation, as discussed above. Inclusion of an antioxidant, either in the form of a metal ion chelator (e.g., EDTA or bathophenanthroline disulfonate) or a thiol reductant (e.g., dithiothreitol), can ensure that little if any oxidation of GSH occurs. When measuring GSH uptake in intact PT cells, oxidation of GSH by the thiol oxidase on the BLM can also occur (66), leading to extracellular formation of glutathione disulfide (GSSG) (cf. Fig. 1). This complicates measurement of GSH transport because GSSG, while also transported across the BLM, is transported much more slowly than GSH (18). Because the thiol oxidase is a copper-containing protein, it can be inhibited by a metal ion chelator such as bathophenanthroline disulfonate (67). As discussed earlier, GSH degradation can be substantially (>98%) inhibited by brief pretreatment of acivicin.

4. MEASUREMENT OF GSH TRANSPORT ACROSS RENAL PLASMA MEMBRANES

GSH uptake across renal plasma membranes can be measured with various experimental models, including intact cells or tubules or membrane vesicles. With either type of model, similar constraints exist because the primary competing metabolic step is GGT-mediated degradation on the BBM. Another concern, which is particularly relevant to the intact cell models, is that of nephron heterogeneity. For example, we have shown previously that GSH transport is significantly faster in PT cells and has distinct kinetic properties and substrate specificity in PT and DT cells (20). Figure 6 illustrates rates for GSH uptake, oxidation, and degradation based on 30-min incubations of rat renal PT and DT cells with 5 mM GSH, both with and without acivicin and BSO pretreatment. Although acivicin is used to inhibit degradation of GSH, BSO is used to inhibit synthesis. This combination of inhibitors is often used in studies of GSH transport so that measured intracellular GSH can only be attributed to transport and not to a combination of degradation, uptake of the constituent amino acids, and intracellular resynthesis of GSH. The results clearly show the following: (1) GSH metabolism and transport are more rapid in PT cells; (2) oxidation is the predominant process regardless of the presence or absence of acivicin and BSO; and (3) uptake of intact GSH is minimally detectable in the absence of acivicin.

Accurate measurement of transport of GSH (or any substrate for that matter) in intact cells requires efficient and quantifiable separation of intracellular from extracellular material without postisolation artifacts. In other words, it is critical that procedures to terminate the transport process do not cause any additional changes in substrate distribution among the compartments or in substrate status (oxidation or degradation for GSH). This can be achieved with isolated cells or tubules by a number of methods. Two approaches that have been successful are to either filter cells under vacuum on 0.45-μm pore size nitrocellulose filters or

Renal Glutathione Transport

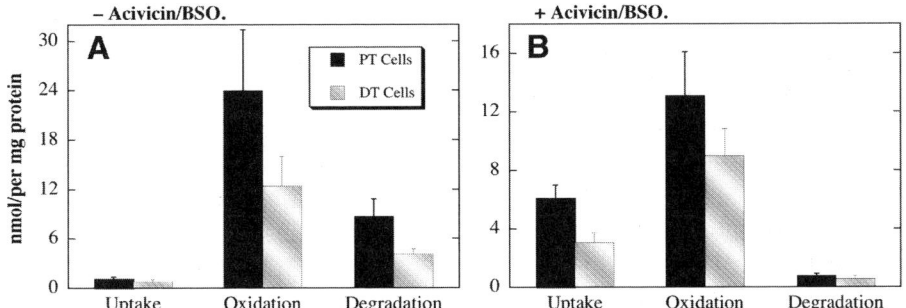

Fig. 6. Rates of GSH metabolism and loss in renal PT and DT cells. Rates of GSH uptake, oxidation, and degradation to the constituent amino acids are shown for cells preincubated with either buffer or 0.25 mM acivicin + 2 mM BSO (to inhibit GSH degradation and synthesis, respectively), and then incubated with 5 mM GSH at 37°C for 30 min. Values are means ± SEM of measurements from four separate cell preparations.

to rapidly centrifuge cells through a material that separates cells from the extracellular medium. One method is to layer cells (0.5 mL, 1–3 × 10⁶/mL) on 1 mL of 20% (v/v) Percoll in 1.5-mL polyethylene microcentrifuge tubes and centrifuge for 30 s at 13,000g. For studies with membrane vesicles, filtration under vacuum on 0.45-µm pore size filters is generally the method of choice. Although incubations of GSH with intact cells or tubules to quantify transport are usually performed at 37°C, incubations of GSH with membrane vesicles to quantify transport are usually performed at 25°C to extend the time period over which the vesicles retain their functional integrity and to enable measurement of very rapid processes. Incubation of membrane vesicles at 37°C would result in relatively rapid decrease in functional integrity and would exhibit rates of transport that would likely be too high to measure accurately.

5. MEASUREMENT OF GSH TRANSPORT ACROSS RENAL MITOCHONDRIAL INNER MEMBRANE

Similar to measurements of GSH transport in membrane vesicles, those in isolated mitochondria or mitoplasts are usually performed at reduced temperatures (25°C or 28°C are typically used). We have developed three methods for processing incubations of isolated mitochondria *(49,62)*. Each procedure gives virtually the same results once the appropriate corrections are made for nonspecific association/binding and extramitochondrial medium carryover.

Method 1: Single-step centrifugation. Aliquots (0.5 mL) of samples at various time points are placed in 1.5-mL polyethylene microcentrifuge tubes and are centrifuged at 13,000g for 30 s to separate extramitochondrial space (= supernatants) and mitochondria (= pellets).

Method 2: Centrifugation-resuspension. This method differs from method 1 in that pellets obtained after the first centrifugation step are resuspended in 0.5 mL of ice-cold buffer, centrifuged again, and then the final pellets are resuspended in 10% (v/v) perchloric acid.

Method 3: Dibutylphthalate method. Aliquots (0.5 mL) of samples at various time points are layered on top of a 0.5-mL dibutylphthalate layer and a 0.55-mL 10% (v/v) perchloric acid layer in 1.5-mL microcentrifuge tubes, tubes are immediately centrifuged at 13,000g for 30 s. Extramitochondrial material remains in the top (dibutylphthalate) layer, whereas intramitochondrial material is released into the bottom (perchloric acid) layer.

Determination of mitochondrial matrix volume. Mitochondrial suspensions are incubated with a buffer containing 0.1 µCi of [^{14}C]-sucrose and 1 µCi of ^{3}H$_2$O, either centrifuged through buffer *(single-step centrifugation method)* or centrifuged through dibutylphthalate into perchloric acid, and radioactivity determined in both pellet and supernatant, with separate counting in the ^{14}C and ^{3}H channels. The mitochondrial matrix volume is then calculated according to the following equation:

$$V_m = V_{H_2O} - V_{sucrose} = [(Net(^3H)_{pellet}/A^3H) - (Net(^{14}C)_{pellet}/A^{14}C)]$$

The matrix volume (V_m) is the volume of water in the pellet (V_{H_2O}), calculated by correcting net ^{3}H for specific ^{3}H counts (A^{3}H), minus the volume of sucrose in the pellet ($V_{sucrose}$), which is similarly calculated by correcting net ^{14}C counts for specific ^{14}C counts (A^{14}C). This value is then divided by mg protein in a 1-mL sample to give a volume in µL/mg.

By the *single-step centrifugation method*, pellet volume was approx 7 µL/mg of protein and matrix volume was 0.82–0.87 µL/mg of protein, or approx 11.5% of the total pellet volume. By the *dibutylphthalate method*, pellet volume was 4.2–4.8 µL/mg of protein and matrix volume was 0.95–1.1 µL/mg of protein, or 21–26% of the total pellet volume. Thus, a higher amount of carryover of substrate from the extramitochondrial space occurs with the first method.

6. SUMMARY AND CONCLUSIONS

This chapter has reviewed the current state of knowledge of renal GSH transport. The renal handling of GSH is truly unique in that the kidneys, primarily the proximal tubules, possess both enzymes to degrade GSH (principally if not exclusively on the BBM) and carrier proteins on the plasma membranes for uptake and efflux of GSH. In fact, although the liver plays a major role in producing GSH and mediating its efflux into bile and plasma, the kidneys are the primary organ that extracts circulating GSH. This chapter has reviewed several of the experimental models that are used to quantify and characterize GSH transport across the plasma membranes, focusing on validation of the models and cautions that are needed to optimize accurate measurement of GSH transport. Besides plasma membrane transport of GSH from outside the renal PT cell across the BLM or from inside the renal PT cell across the BBM into the lumen, intracellular GSH is compartmentalized into subcellular organelles with the mitochondria containing the major intracellular pool of GSH. Because the mitochondria catalyze little if any *de novo* synthesis of GSH, the intramitochondrial pool (primarily inside the matrix) must derive from transport across the inner membrane from the cytoplasm. Accordingly, different models for study of these transport processes were presented and the procedures to optimize accurate measurement of the transport process were presented. GSH is truly a "molecule on the move" and accomplishes this by highly regulated, carrier-mediated processes that can be exploited to modulate and characterize cellular and mitochondrial redox homeostasis.

ACKNOWLEDGMENT

Research from the author's laboratory was supported by a grant from the National Institute of Diabetes and Kidney Diseases (R01-DK40725), and is gratefully acknowledged.

REFERENCES

1. Lash LH, Jones DP, Anders MW. Glutathione homeostasis and glutathione S-conjugate toxicity in the kidney. Rev Biochem Toxicol 1988;9:29–67.
2. Ballatori N, Dutczak WJ. Identification and characterization of high and low affinity transport systems for reduced glutathione in liver cell canalicular membranes. J Biol Chem 1994;269:19731–19737.
3. Kaplowitz N, Aw TY, Ookhtens M. The regulation of hepatic glutathione. Annu Rev Pharmacol Toxicol 1985;25:715–744.
4. Lash LH. Glutathione and other antioxidant defense mechanisms. In: Goldstein RS, ed. Comprehensive Series in Toxicology, Vol. 7: Kidney Toxicology, Oxford: Elsevier; 1997:403–428.
5. Hinchman CA, Ballatori N. Glutathione-degrading capacities of liver and kidney in different species. Biochem Pharmacol 1990;40:1131–1135.
6. Hagen TM, Aw TY, Jones DP. Glutathione uptake and protection against oxidative injury in isolated kidney cells. Kidney Int 1988;34:74–81.
7. Parks LD, Zalups RK, Barfuss DW. Heterogeneity of glutathione synthesis and secretion in the proximal tubule of the rabbit. Am J Physiol 1998;274:F924–F931.
8. Fonteles MC, Pillio DJ, Jeske AH, Leibach FH. Extraction of glutathione by the isolated perfused rabbit kidney. J Surg Res 1976;21:169–174.
9. Griffith OW, Meister A. Glutathione: interorgan translocation, turnover, and metabolism. Proc Natl Acad Sci USA 1979;76:5606–5610.
10. Häberle D, Wahlländer A, Sies H. Assessment of the kidney function in maintenance of plasma glutathione concentration and redox state in anesthetized rats. FEBS Lett 1979;108:335–340.

11. Anderson ME, Bridges RJ, Meister A. Direct evidence for inter-organ transport of glutathione and that the non-filtration mechanism for glutathione utilization involves γ-glutamyl transpeptidase. Biochem Biophys Res Commun 1980;96: 848–853.
12. Ormstad K, Låstbom T, Orrenius S. Evidence for different localization of glutathione oxidase and γ-glutamyltransferase activities during extracellular glutathione metabolism in isolated perfused kidney. Biochim Biophys Acta 1982;700:148–153.
13. Rankin BB, Curthoys NP. Evidence for renal paratubular transport of glutathione. FEBS Lett 1982;147:193–196.
14. Rankin BB, Wells W, Curthoys NP Rat renal peritubular transport and metabolism of plasma [^{35}S]glutathione. Am J Physiol 1985;249:F198–F204.
15. Abbott WA, Bridges RJ, Meister A. Extracellular metabolism of glutathione accounts for its disappearance from the basolateral circulation of the kidneys. J Biol Chem 1984;259:15393–15400.
16. Inoue M, Shinozuka S, Morino Y. Mechanism of peritubular extraction of plasma glutathione: the catalytic activity of contralumenal γ-glutamyltransferase is prerequisite to the apparent peritubular extraction of plasma glutathione. Eur J Biochem 1986;157:605–609.
17. Lash LH, Jones DP. Transport of glutathione by renal basal-lateral membrane vesicles. Biochem Biophys Res Commun 1983;112:55–60.
18. Lash LH, Jones DP. Renal glutathione transport: characteristics of the sodium-dependent system in the basal-lateral membrane. J Biol Chem 1984;259: 14508–14514.
19. Lash LH, Jones DP. Uptake of the glutathione conjugate S-(1,2-dichlorovinyl) glutathione by renal basal-lateral membrane vesicles and isolated kidney cells. Mol Pharmacol 1985;28:278–282.
20. Lash LH, Putt DA. Renal cellular transport of exogenous glutathione: heterogeneity at physiological and pharmacological concentrations. Biochem Pharmacol 1999;58:897–907.
21. Inou M, Morino Y. Direct evidence for the role of the membrane potential in glutathione transport by renal brush-border membranes. J Biol Chem 1985;260: 326–331.
22. Griffith OW, Meister A. Translocation of intracellular glutathione to membrane-bound γ-glutamyl transpeptidase as a discrete step in the γ-glutamyl cycle: glutathionuria after inhibition of transpeptidase. Proc Natl Acad Sci USA 1979;76: 268–272.
23. Scott RD, Curthoys NP. Renal clearance of glutathione measured in rats pretreated with inhibitors of glutathione metabolism. Am J Physiol 1987;252:F877–F882.
24. Mittur A, Wolkoff AW, Kaplowitz N. The thiol sensitivity of glutathione transport in sidedness-sorted basolateral liver plasma membrane and in Oatp1-expressing HeLa cell membrane. Mol Pharmacol 2002;61:425–435.
25. Li L, Lee TK, Meier PJ, Ballatori N. Identification of glutathione as a driving force and leukotriene C_4 as a substrate for oatp1, the hepatic sinusoidal organic solute transporter. J Biol Chem 1998;273:16184–16191.

26. Takeuchi A, Masuda S, Saito H, Hashimoto Y, Inui K. Trans-stimulation effects of folic acid derivatives on methotrexate transport by rat renal organic anion transporter, OAT-K1. J Pharmacol Exp Ther 2000;293:1034–1039.
27. Keppler D, Leier I, Jedlitschky G. Transport of glutathione conjugates and glucuronides by the multidrug resistance proteins MRP1 and MRP2. Biol Chem 1997; 378:787–791.
28. Gerk PM, Vore M. Regulation of expression of the multidrug resistance-associated protein 2 (MRP2) and its role in drug disposition. J Pharmacol Exp Ther 2002; 302:407–415.
29. Terlouw S, Masereeuw R, van den Broek PHH, Notenboom S, Russel FGM. Role of multidrug resistance protein 2 (MRP2) in glutathione-bimane efflux from Caco-2 and rat renal proximal tubule cells. Br J Pharmacol 2001;134:931–938.
30. Evers R, de Haas M, Sparidans R, et al. Vinblastine and sulfinpyrazone export by the multidrug resistance protein MRP2 is associated with glutathione export. Br J Cancer 2000;83:375–383.
31. Paulusma CC, van Geer MA, Evers R, et al. Canalicular multispecific organic anion transporter/multidrug resistance protein 2 mediates low-affinity transport of reduced glutathione. Biochem J 1999;338:393–401.
32. Rebbeor JF, Connolly GC, Ballatori N. Inhibition of Mrp2- and Ycf1p-mediated transport by reducing agents: evidence for GSH transport on rat Mrp2. Biochim Biophys Acta 2002;1559:171–178.
33. Moldéus P, Ormstad K, Reed DJ. Turnover of cellular glutathione in isolated rat kidney cells: role of cystine and methionine. Eur J Biochem 1981;116:13–16.
34. Meredith MJ, Reed DJ. Status of the mitochondrial pool of glutathione in the isolated hepatocyte. J Biol Chem 1982;257:3747–3753.
35. Lash LH, Visarius TM, Sall JW, Qian W, Tokarz JJ. Cellular and subcellular heterogeneity of glutathione metabolism and transport in rat kidney cells. Toxicology 1998;130:1–15.
36. Schnellmann RG, Gilchrist SM, Mandel LJ. Intracellular distribution and depletion of glutathione in rabbit renal proximal tubules. Kidney Int 1988;34:229–233.
37. Griffith OW, Meister A. Origin and turnover of mitochondrial glutathione. Proc Natl Acad Sci USA 1985;82:4668–4672.
38. McKernan TB, Woods EB, Lash LH. Uptake of glutathione by renal cortical mitochondria. Arch Biochem Biophys 1991;288:653–663.
39. Yagi T, Hatefi Y. Thiols in oxidative phosphorylation: inhibition and energy-potentiated uncoupling by monothiol and dithiol modifiers. Biochemistry 1984;23: 2449–2455.
40. Beatrice MC, Stiers DL, Pfeiffer DR. The role of glutathione in the retention of Ca^{2+} by liver mitochondria. J Biol Chem 1984;259:1279–1287.
41. Lê-Quôc K, Lê-Quôc D. Crucial role of sulfhydryl groups in the mitochondrial inner membrane structure. J Biol Chem 1985;260:7422–7428.
42. Lê-Quôc D, Lê-Quôc K. Relationships between the NAD(P) redox state, fatty acid oxidation, and inner membrane permeability in rat liver mitochondria. Arch Biochem Biophys 1989;273:466–478.

43. Martensson J, Meister A. Mitochondrial damage in muscle occurs after marked depletion of glutathione and is prevented by giving glutathione monoester. Proc Natl Acad Sci USA 1989;86:471–475.
44. Shan X, Jones DP, Hashmi M, Anders MW. Selective depletion of mitochondrial glutathione concentrations by (*R,S*)-3-hydroxy-4-pentenoate potentiates oxidative cell death. Chem Res Toxicol 1993;6:75–81.
45. Hashmi M, Gräf S, Braun M, Anders MW. Enantioselective depletion of mitochondrial glutathione concentrations by *(S)*- and *(R)*-3-hydroxy-4-pentenoate. Chem Res Toxicol 1996;9:361–364.
46. Kurosawa K, Hayashi N, Sato N, Kamada T, Tagawa K Transport of glutathione across the mitochondrial membranes. Biochem Biophys Res Commun 1990;167: 367–372.
47. Martensson J, Lai JCK, Meister A. High-affinity transport of glutathione is part of a multicomponent system essential for mitochondrial function. Proc Natl Acad Sci USA 1990;87:7185–7189.
48. Schnellmann RG. Renal mitochondrial glutathione transport. Life Sci 1991;49: 393–398.
49. Chen Z, Lash LH. Evidence for mitochondrial uptake of glutathione by dicarboxylate and 2-oxoglutarate carriers. J Pharmacol Exp Ther 1998;285:608–618.
50. Chen Z, Putt DA, Lash LH. Enrichment and functional reconstitution of glutathione transport activity from rabbit kidney mitochondria: further evidence for the role of the dicarboxylate and 2-oxoglutarate carriers in mitochondrial glutathione transport. Arch Biochem Biophys 2000;373:193–202.
51. Lash LH, Putt DA, Hueni SE, et al. Cellular energetics and glutathione status in NRK-52E cells: toxicological implications. Biochem Pharmacol 2002;64:1533–1546.
52. Lash LH, Putt DA, Matherly LH. Protection of NRK-52E cells, a rat renal proximal tubular cell line, from chemical induced apoptosis by overexpression of a mitochondrial glutathione transporter. J Pharmacol Exp Ther 2002;303:476–486.
53. Xu F, Lash LH, Putt DA, Sun B, Matherly LH. Expression and stable transfection in NRK-52E cells of the mitochondrial 2-oxoglutarate carrier (OGC), a glutathione transporter. Toxicol Sci 2003;72(1-S):351.
54. Lash LH, Xu F, Putt DA, Sun B, Matherly LH. Expression and stable transfection in NRK-52E cells of the mitochondrial 2-oxoglutarate carrier (OGC), a glutathione transporter. FASEB J 2003;17:A1046.
55. Lash LH, Putt DA, Xu F, et al. Modulation of mitochondrial glutathione (GSH) transport in NRK-52E cells alters susceptibility to oxidative injury. J Am Soc Nephrol 2003;14:355A.
56. Lash LH, Tokarz JJ. Isolation of two distinct populations of cells from rat kidney cortex and their use in the study of chemical-induced toxicity. Anal Biochem 1989; 182:271–279.
57. Lash LH. In vitro methods of assessing renal damage. Toxicol Pathol 1998;26:33–42.
58. Lash LH. Use of freshly isolated and primary cultures of proximal tubular and distal tubular cells from rat kidneys. In: Zalups RK, Lash LH, eds. Methods in Renal Toxicology. Boca Raton, FL: CRC Press; 1996:189–215.

59. Jayaram HN, Cooney DA, Ryan JA, Neil G, Dion RL, Bono VH. L-[αS,5S]-α-Amino-3-chloro-4,5-dihydro-5-isoxazoleacetic acid (NSC-163501): a new amino acid antibiotic with the properties of an antagonist of L-glutamine. Cancer Chemother Rep 1975;59:481–491.
60. Reed DJ, Ellis WW, Meck RA. The inhibition of γ-glutamyl transpeptidase and glutathione metabolism of isolated rat kidney cells by L-(αS,5S)-α-amino-3-chloro-4,5-dihydro-5-isoxazoleacetic acid (AT-125; NSC-163501). Biochem Biophys Res Commun 1980;94:1273–1277.
61. Schasteen CS, Curthoys NP, Reed DJ. The binding mechanism of glutathione and the anti-tumor drug L-(αS,5S)-α-amino-3-chloro-4,5-dihydro-5-isoxazoleacetic acid (AT-125; NSC-163501) to γ-glutamyltransferase. Biochem Biophys Res Commun 1981;112:564–570.
62. Lash LH. Intracellular distribution of thiols and disulfides: assay of mitochondrial glutathione transport. Methods Enzymol 1995;252:14–26.
63. Lash LH, Sall JM. Mitochondrial isolation from liver and kidney: strategy, techniques, and criteria for purity. In: Lash LH, Jones DP, eds. Methods in Toxicology, Vol. 2; Mitochondrial Dysfunction, San Diego: Academic Press; 1993; 8–28.
64. Greenawalt JW. The isolation of outer and inner mitochondrial membranes. Methods Enzymol 1974;31:310–323.
65. Fariss MW, Reed DJ. High-performance liquid chromatography of thiols and disulfides: dinitrophenyl derivatives. Methods Enzymol 1987;143:101–109.
66. Lash LH, Jones DP. Localization of the membrane-associated thiol oxidase of rat kidney to the basal-lateral plasma membrane. Biochem J 1982;203:371–376.
67. Lash LH, Jones DP. Purification and properties of thiol oxidase from porcine kidney. Arch Biochem Biophys 1986;247:120–130.

14

Human Cytosolic Sulfotransferases

Properties, Physiological Functions, and Toxicology

Charles N. Falany

Summary

Sulfation is a major reaction in phase II drug and xenobiotic metabolism. It is catalyzed by a family of enzymes, the sulfotransferases (SULTs), and involves the enzymatic transfer of a sulfonate group from a donor molecule (known as 3′-phosphoadenosine 5′-phosphosulfate [PAPS]) to either an hydroxyl moiety or an amine group. Although sulfation often results in enhanced excretion of xenobiotics, there is an increasing appreciation for examples whereby sulfation results in bioactivation and hence increased toxicity. This chapter provides background on the current state of knowledge of the SULT enzymes in humans, focusing on both those that metabolize endogenous substrates such as androgens and estrogens, and those that metabolize drugs and other xenobiotics. Insight into techniques for the expression and purification of human SULTs is also presented, highlighting difficulties that have arisen and approaches that have circumvented these problems. The chapter then describes procedures for the enzymatic assay of SULT activity, again highlighting some of the unexpected problems that have arisen and approaches that have circumvented some of these difficulties. Finally, the last two sections summarizes approaches that have been used to detect SULTs and immunohistochemistry approaches that have been used to localize these enzymes.

Key Words

Allozymes; estrogen metabolism; phenol metabolism; sulfotranferases; SULTs; SULT1A subfamily; SULT2 subfamily.

1. INTRODUCTION

Sulfation is a major reaction in phase II drug and xenobiotic metabolism initially identified in the mid-19th century *(1)*. The reaction involves the enzymatic transfer of a sulfonate group from 3′-phosphoadenosine 5′-phosphosulfate

From: *Methods in Pharmacology and Toxicology,*
Drug Metabolism and Transport: Molecular Methods and Mechanisms
Edited by: L. Lash © Humana Press Inc., Totowa, NJ

(PAPS) to either a hydroxyl moiety to form a sulfate or to an amine group to form a sulfamate *(2,3)*. Sulfate conjugation is generally an inactivation reaction since the conjugates are biologically inactive owing to the presence of the bulky charged sulfonate group. The sulfonate group has a pK_a of approx 2 and is ionized at physiological pHs resulting in rapid excretion of the sulfonates by the kidneys and liver. Figure 1 shows the sulfation of the classical substrates 4-nitrophenol (PNP) and β-estradiol (E2). The ability of human tissues to conjugate a broad variety of small phenols and aliphatic hydroxyl-containing compounds with sulfate has emphasized the role of sulfation in xenobiotic and drug metabolism. However, sulfation of small endogenous compounds in tissues by members of the cytosolic sulfotransferase (SULT) family is also important in hormone and monoamine neurotransmitter metabolism *(4)*. Steroid sulfation in human tissues has unique properties that distinguish it from sulfation in most laboratory animals. Synthesis and secretion of dehydroepiandrosterone (DHEA) sulfate from the reticular layer of the adrenal cortex results in plasma levels of DHEA-sulfate that are several hundredfold higher than in most research animals *(5,6)*. DHEA that is released from DHEA-sulfate by sulfatase activity can be converted into both androgens and estrogens in peripheral tissues *(7)*. During pregnancy, humans also have micromolar levels of estrogen sulfates in plasma that are synthesized from DHEA-sulfate secreted by both the fetal adrenal and maternal adrenal cortex. The significance of the high levels of estrogen sulfates during pregnancy is not well understood. Sulfation is also a major reaction in dopamine metabolism in humans *(4,8)*.

2. GENERATION OF REACTIVE INTERMEDIATES

The role of conjugation reactions in drug metabolism is generally related to decreases in the biological activity of the acceptor compound and an associated increase in water solubility resulting in enhanced excretion. As with most biological processes, there are important exceptions to these rules. Conjugation of small drugs and xenobiotics has been associated with both increases in biological activity as well as the generation of reactive electrophilic compounds capable of covalently binding DNA and eliciting mutagenic effects on DNA structure.

Minoxidil represents a second generation of compounds originally synthesized for the treatment of hypertensive disease and used for resistant hypertension *(9,10)*. During long-term treatment with minoxidil, both men and women developed hypertrichosis or excessive hair growth *(11)*. Subsequently, minoxidil became popular as a topical agent for the treatment of alopecia androgenetica or male pattern baldness. Analysis of the mechanism of minoxidil in

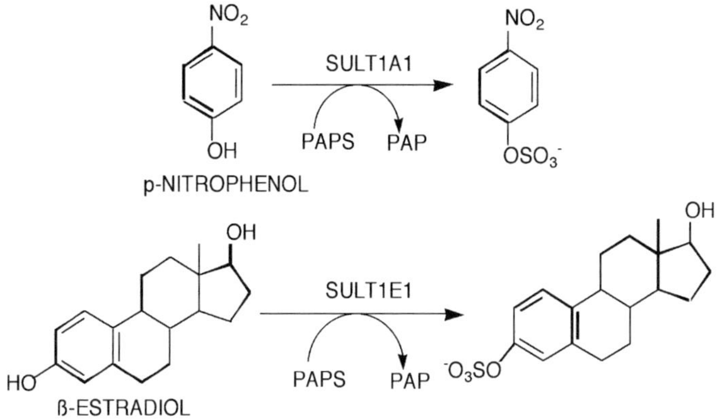

Fig. 1. Sulfonation of the prototypical substrates 4-nitrophenol (PNP) and β-estradiol. 3′-Phosphoadenosine 5′-phosphosulfate (PAPS) is the sulfonate donor for all sulfation reactions. PNP is a widely used substrate for assaying phenol SULT activity. β-Estradiol is a high-affinity substrate for assaying SULT1E1 activity.

hair growth established that minoxidil sulfate was the active agent in this process *(10)* and possibly also in cardiac tissue *(12,13)*. Minoxidil is a pyrimidine *N*-oxide that is sulfated to form the *N,O*-sulfate ester. Sulfation of the *N*-oxide moiety of minoxidil is unique in that the minoxidil *N,O*-sulfate is more hydrophobic than unconjugated minoxidil owing to intramolecular hydrogen bonding *(10)*. In cardiac tissue, minoxidil sulfate acts as a K^+ channel agonist whereby the hydrophobicity of this compound increases its accessibility to its binding site in the K^+ channel *(13)*. The mechanism for the stimulation of hair growth remains unclear although the major sulfotransferase (SULT) isoform involved with the sulfation of minoxidil is localized in the outer root sheath of the rat hair follicle *(14)*.

Sulfation is also important in the generation of reactive electrophilic metabolites of a variety of compounds. The role of sulfation in the bioactivation of promutagens was initially characterized by James and Elizabeth Miller at the McArdle Laboratory for Cancer Research, University of Wisconsin. The Millers were involved in the initial studies establishing the function of biotransformation reactions in the generation of mutagenic and carcinogenic metabolites. These investigators established that sulfation of the procarcinogens, 1′-hydroxysafrole and *N*-hydroxy-acetylaminofluorene (N-OH-AAF), was necessary for the generation of their carcinogenic activity. Safrole is a constituent of the natural flavoring sassafras and cinnamon oils that may be hydroxylated by the cytochromes P450 mixed function oxidation (MFO) system to generate 1′-hydroxysafrole

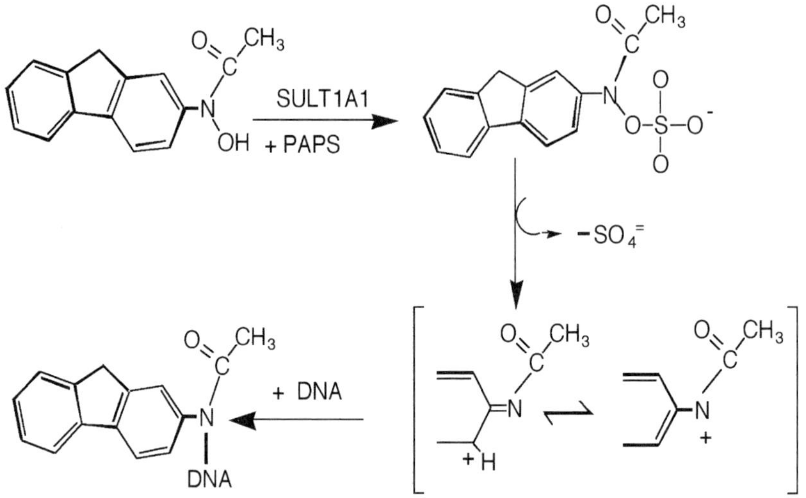

Fig. 2. Bioactivation of N-hydroxyacetylaminofluorene (NOH-AAF) by SULT1A1. NOH-AAF is conjugated by SULT1A1 to form the sulfoxy derivative. The sulfoxy derivative is unstable and spontaneously degrades to generate the nitrenium ion. The charge may be stabilized by the conjugated ring system to also form a carbocation. The reactive electrophilic group can covalently react with cellular nucleophiles including DNA, RNA and proteins.

(15,16). Sulfation activity results in the formation of 1′-sulfoxysafrole that undergoes spontaneous heterolytic cleavage to generate a carbocation. Treatment of mice with radiolabeled safrole resulted in the formation of DNA adducts and the production of hepatic tumors. Similar studies were carried out using AAF that was also demonstrated to be a potent hepatic carcinogen (17). N-OH AAF formed by the MFO system can be bioactivated by either sulfation or acetylation. As shown in Fig. 2, sulfation of N-OH AAF may lead to the heterocyclic cleavage of the sulfate ester generating the reactive nitrenium ion. Resonance stabilization of the charged AAF molecule can result in translocalization of the charge to the benzene ring resulting in the formation of a carbocation. Procarcinogen activation via sulfation is now recognized as a common property of SULTs although the types and rates at which individual compounds are activated can vary greatly (18,19).

3. HUMAN SULTs

In humans, there are two SULT families that are distinguished by their subcellular localization. One family consists of the membrane-associated SULTs involved with the sulfation of glycosaminoglycans, glycoproteins, and proteins in the Golgi apparatus (20–23). These enzymes are not involved in the conjugation of xenobiotics or drugs. The cytosolic SULT gene family is responsible for the sulfation of drugs and xenobiotics *(2,24)* and, to date, consists of 10 genes encoding 11 SULT isoforms. In addition, Freimuth et al. *(25)* recently identified a novel human SULT isoform termed SULT6B1 by data mining of the human genome. This isoform is expressed in testis and is very similar to the gorilla and chimpanzee orthologs. Further characterization of this putative SULT6B1 will likely result in its inclusion in the cytosolic SULT family. Although it is possible that more novel human SULT isoforms will be identified, it is anticipated that this number would be low.

Naming the human SULTs has generated a confusing quagmire that has not been sufficiently clarified. Table 1 contains the most commonly used nomenclature for the human SULTs as well as several of the more frequently used common names. Initial attempts to refer to the individual SULTs based on substrate reactivities or physical properties has proven confusing following the identification and cloning of isoforms with crossreacting substrate specificities as well as identification of major allelic variants with different physical properties *(26–29)*.

Novel SULT cDNAs that are not expressed in humans have been identified in nonhuman mammals. A unique canine *SULT1D1* cDNA has been isolated and expressed by Tsoi et al. *(30)*. This cDNA is similar to that of the *SULT1A* and *SULT1B* family members, suggesting that it is a novel member of the *SULT1* family. Although dopamine is a superior substrate, the canine *SULT1D1* is also capable of sulfating PNP and has no activity toward the prototypical steroid substrates, E2 and DHEA. Meinl and Glatt *(31)* subsequently identified a *SULT1D1* pseudogene in the gene cluster containing the human *SULT1E1* and *SULT1B1* genes on chromosome 4.

3.1. SULT1A Subfamily

The identification and analysis of phenol sulfation activity in human blood platelets initiated the investigation of phenol and monoamine sulfation in humans *(32)*. Human platelet cytosol was demonstrated to possess two significant phenol sulfation activities. Numerous studies established the presence of two separate phenol SULT activities in platelets based on differences in substrate reactivities, thermal stability, response to inhibitors, and physical separation by anion-exchange chromatography *(33–36)*. The phenol SULT activities in platelet cytosol were initially named phenol-sulfating phenol SULT (P-PST) and monoamine-sulfating phenol SULT (M-PST) to reflect their preference for phenol and dopamine sulfation, respectively *(37)*. Purification of MPST *(SULT1A3)* and PPST *(SULT1A1)* from platelet and liver, respectively, was instrumental in providing the background for the cloning and expression of the phenol SULT gene subfamily. Currently, the phenol SULT family consists of

Table 1
Human Cytosolic SULTs

Current nomenclature	Previously used names
SULT1A1	Phenol-sulfating phenol sulfotransferase (P-PST, P-PST-1) (40,130) Thermostable phenol sulfotransferase (TS-PST, TS-PST-1) (47) Human aryl sulfotransferase 1 (HAST1) (53)
SULT1A2	Phenol-sulfating phenol sulfotransferase-2 (P-PST-2) (STP2) (131) Thermostable phenol sulfotransferase-2 (TS-PST-2) (132) HAST4 (53) ST1A2 (54)
SULT1A3	Monoamine-sulfating phenol sulfotransferase (M-PST) (60,130,133) Thermolabile phenol sulfotransferase (TL-PST)(STM) (51) HAST3 (134) ST1A5 (135) Placental estrogen sulfotransferase (114)
SULT1B1	Thyroid hormone sulfotransferase (ST1B2) (63,64)
SULT1C1	SULT 1C sulfotransferase 1 (70) SULT1C2 (69)
SULT1C2	SULT 1C sulfotransferase 2 (70) SULT1C3 (69)
SULT1E1	Estrogen sulfotransferase (EST) (72,74)
SULT2A1	Dehydroepiandrosterone sulfotransferase (DHEA-ST) (88,136) Hydroxysteroid sulfotransferase (HST) (85) Alcohol/hydroxysteroid sulfotransferase (hSTa) (137)
SULT2B1a	Hydroxysteroid sulfotransferase (92)
SULT2B1b	Hydroxysteroid sulfotransferase (92)
SULT4A1	Brain sulfotransferase-like cDNA (BR-STL) (100)

eight members encoded by separate genes that are arranged in clusters on separate chromosomes *(25,29,38)*.

3.1.1. SULT1A1: Phenol-Sulfating Phenol SULT-1

SULT1A1 is arguably the major xenobiotic and drug conjugating SULT in human tissues. Subsequent to purification to homogeneity from human liver cytosol *(39)*, the cDNA was cloned from a human liver cDNA library *(40)*. SULT1A1 has proven to be easily expressed in a variety of systems with great stability. The expressed native enzyme possesses kinetic properties similar to those of the purified liver enzyme *(40,41)*. Analysis of SULT1A1 substrate reactivity indicates that it is capable of sulfating a wide variety of small phenolic compounds, including estrogens, phytoestrogens, small phenols, minoxidil, and iodothyronines. SULT1A1 also conjugates amines to generate sulfamates *(42)* and activates promutagens such as 1-hydroxymethylpyrene (HMP) and N-OH AAF to mutagenic reactive electrophiles *(18,43,44)*. The importance of SULT1A1 in xenobiotic metabolism is emphasized by its high levels of expression in the liver and GI tract. SULT1A1 immunoreactive protein and/or message has been detected in many human tissues including endometrium, breast, brain, platelets, kidney, skin, and prostate.

The early detection and characterization of *SULT1A1* in human blood platelets demonstrated the variability of activity and established the likely genetic basis for this variability *(45,46)*. Subsequent molecular characterization of *SULT1A1* resulted in the identification of multiple allelic variants in human tissues. Several of these variants generate allozymes with different kinetic properties including procarcinogen activation *(18,47,48)*.

At least 17 allelic variants of human *SULT1A1* have been reported encoding six different amino acid changes *(19)*. The expression of several of these alleles is significant and variable in different human populations. Carlini et al. *(28)* reported the allelic frequencies for *SULT1A1* in Caucasian, Chinese, and African-American populations. The frequencies for *SULT1A1*1, 1A1*2* and *1A1*3* in Caucasians were 0.656, 0.332, and 0.012 respectively. In the Chinese population, these frequencies were 0.914, 0.080 and 0.006, whereas in African-Americans the frequencies were 0.477, 0.294 and 0.229. Expression of the SULT1A1*2 allozyme is associated with the level of thermal sensitivity of PNP sulfation activity in human liver cytosol. The sensitivity of PNP sulfation has been extensively used to characterize genetic differences in phenol SULT activity *(19,37,47)*. The expressed SULT1A1*2 allozyme shows decreased thermostability compared to the wild-type allozyme and SULT1A1*3, and is apparently responsible for the thermostability differences described in Caucasian platelet PPST activities *(48)*.

The structural genes for the *SULT1A* family are located on chromosome 16q12.1–11.2 *(49–51)*. This locus contains the genes for *SULT1A1*, *SULT1A2*, and *SULT1A3* that are greater than 92% identical in sequence, indicating that these genes arose by duplication of a single ancestral gene. The proximity of the structural genes is also responsible for the linkage in the expression of allelic variants of the *SULT1A* genes *(52)*. Structural analysis of the *SULT1A* gene family demonstrates considerable conservation of exonic structure between the human SULT as well as the rodent SULT genes *(38)*.

3.1.2. SULT1A2

SULT1A2 was identified at the molecular level before the protein or activity was observed or recognized *(53)*. SULT1A2 is approx 96% similar to SULT1A1 and SULT1A3 and the gene for SULT1A2 is at the *SULT1A* loci (Fig. 3). Although SULT1A2 has been expressed and characterized, expression of the SULT1A2 enzyme in human tissues has been difficult to detect *(48,54)*. Because of its sequence similarity to the other SULT1As, SULT1A2 is detectable by immunoblotting with polyclonal anti-SULT1A antibodies. Expressed SULT1A2 migrates slightly differently from SULT1A1 and SULT1A3 during sodium dodecyl sulfate-polyacrylamide gel electrophoresis (SDS-PAGE). SULT1A2 protein is usually not detectable in human tissue specimens, suggesting its impact on sulfation is small.

Characterization of SULT1A2 activity was carried out with the enzyme activity expressed in mammalian COS-1 cells *(48)*. Kinetically, SULT1A2 displays properties intermediate between those of SULT1A1 and SULT1A3. The wild-type SULT1A2 isoform has a K_m for the sulfation of the prototypical phenolic substrate, PNP, approx 10-fold higher than that of SULT1A1 *(48,53)*. Sulfation of dopamine is low or negligible, suggesting a greater similarity to SULT1A1 than to SULT1A3. As observed with most of the SULT isoforms, SULT1A2 bioactivates several promutagens to reactive electrophilic forms *(19)*. SULT1A2 expressed in *S. typhimurium* was capable of efficiently activating N-OH-AAF and 2-hydroxylamino-5-phenylpyridine (OH-APP) to mutagens. Glatt et al. *(19)* compared the ability of the human SULT isoforms to activate a set of 11 promutagens in the *S. typhimurium* mutagenesis assay. The pattern of activation of these compounds by SULT1A1 and SULT1A2 is similar except for the greater activity of SULT1A1 with 1-hydroxymethylpyrene (HMP). Interpretation of the importance or role of SULT1A2 in both xenobiotic sulfation and promutagen activation is hindered because its expression in human tissues has not been delineated. Compared to SULT1A1 and SULT1A3, the expression of SULT1A2 in human tissues is low or absent; however, a thorough evaluation of the expression of SULT1A2 activity or protein in human tissues has not been reported.

	1A1	1A2	1A3	1B1	1C1	1C2	1E1	2A1	2B1a	2B1b	4A1
1A1											
1A2	96										
1A3	93	90									
1B1	53	55	52								
1C1	52	52	51	53							
1C2	53	54	53	53	63						
1E1	50	49	49	56	48	44					
2A1	35	36	35	36	36	36	36				
2B1a	36	36	37	39	35	33	35	48			
2B1b	37	37	38	38	36	35	36	48	99		
4A1	34	33	36	33	33	36	34	30	34	33	

Fig. 3. Sequence identities of the SULT isoforms. The sequences of the SULTs were determined using the ClustalW program. The percent identity for each individual pair is presented. The SULT sequences and accession numbers used in this analysis were: 1A1, L19999; 1A2, U28169; 1A3, U08032; 1B1, U95726; 1C1, U66036; 1C2, AF055584; 1E1, S77383; 2A1, L20000; 2B1a, U92314; 2B1b, U92315; 4A1, AF188698.

3.1.3. SULT1A3

SULT1A3 (M-PST) was initially described as one of the platelet phenol SULT activities *(34,37)* that, along with SULT1A1, was extensively studied in platelet cytosol. Initial studies demonstrated that human platelet cytosol contained a high-affinity dopamine sulfating activity that was physically distinct from the smaller phenol sulfating activity *(34–37)*. The dopamine sulfating activity was initially termed monoamine-sulfating phenol SULT or M-PST. Because of its sensitivity to thermal inactivation compared to SULT1A1, the enzyme activity was also termed thermostable PST *(34)*. Characterization and physical separation of the phenol and dopamine sulfating activities in platelet cytosol established that these were separate enzymes *(34,35,37,55)*. Heroux and Roth *(36)* purified SULT1A3 from human platelets, confirming that it was distinct from SULT1A1. Although SULT1A1 has not been purified form platelet cytosol, Falany et al. *(39)* purified this SULT from human liver and established that it was kinetically and physically identical to the platelet enzyme. Molecular characterization of the SULT1A1 and SULT1A3 cDNAs established that the sequences of the proteins were approximately 93% identical. Multiple allelic variants of SULT1A1 and 1A2 have been reported but no allelic variants resulting in multiple allozymes of SULT1A3 have been reported in Caucasians *(56)*. However, earlier studies of SULT1A3 activity in platelets suggested a genetic basis for the observed variability in activity *(57)*. One allelic variant encoding a sequence change has been reported in African-Americans *(56)*.

Despite their similarity in structure, SULT1A3 and SULT1A1 have distinct substrate reactivities. SULT1A1 has a high affinity for the sulfation of small neutral phenols including phenol and PNP. In contrast, SULT1A3 has a high affinity for the sulfation of monoamine neurotransmitters. High-affinity dopamine sulfation is limited to higher primates and is characterized by the observation that greater than 95% of circulating dopamine is sulfated. Eisenhofer et al. *(58)* suggested that the majority of the dopamine sulfate is generated in the GI tract that is the site of a novel dopamine autocrine/paracrine system that produces approx 50% of the dopamine in human tissues. In concordance with this theory, SULT1A3 is highly expressed in the human GI tract. In addition, dopamine sulfate is found in cerebrospinal fluid, suggesting synthesis in the brain. Both SULT1A1 and 1A3 are expressed in brain and have been immunolocalized in neurons of the CNS *(59)*. It is estimated that SULT1A3 is responsible for 15% of dopamine metabolism in brain *(8)*.

SULT1A3 has a K_m for dopamine sulfation of approx 4 μM whereas the K_m for PNP sulfation is 100-fold higher *(35,60)*. It is also capable of sulfating epinephrine, norepinephrine, levodopa, fenoterol, acetaminophen, and triiodothyronine. Taskinen et al. *(61)* determined the sulfation rates for 53 catechol compounds by six expressed human SULT isoforms and found the highest activity and broadest reactivity with SULT1A3. SULT1A3 sulfated 47 of the catechols tested; SAR analysis suggested that additional hydroxyls on the catechol or the presence of a carboxylate ion significantly inhibited the rate of sulfation. Mutagenesis studies and analysis of the crystal structure of SULT1A3 indicate that Glu146 is primarily responsible for the differences in the substrate specificity of SULT1A3 compared to SULT1A1 *(62)*. The presence of the Glu146 is also proposed to interact with the Tyr240 residue to enhance hydrogen bonding with catechols *(61)*. The Tyr240 residue apparently is nonreactive; however, high-affinity catechol substrates for SULT1A3 are stabilized by hydrogen bonding to the Tyr240 residue. SULT1C2, which does not possess the Tyr240 residue, was the only SULT tested with only trace levels of catechol sulfation activity.

3.2. SULT1B1

SULT1B1 was initially cloned and identified at the molecular level using the orthologous rat cDNA sequence as a probe *(63)*. It represents the first human SULT cDNA to be identified at the molecular level prior to characterization of its enzymatic activity. Sequence alignment as well as substrate reactivity have placed *SULT1B1* in the *SULT1* gene family *(64)*. The *SULT1B1* gene has been localized to human chromosome 4q13.1 at the same loci as the *SULT1E1* gene and the *SULT1D1* pseudogene. Association of these genes at the same loci would suggest that they arose by gene duplication. The SULT1B1 amino acid sequence is 52–56% identical to that of the other members of the SULT1 family (Fig. 3); however, rabbit antibodies raised to either SULT1B1 or SULT1E1 tend to show crossreactivity on immunoblot analysis *(64)*. This suggests a greater structural similarity between these SULT isoforms than is apparent from sequence analysis.

SULT1B1 was initially referred to as a thyroid hormone-sulfating SULT because of its ability to sulfate thyroid hormones including T3 and T4 *(64)*. Subsequently, it has been established that it is not the most efficient human SULT involved in thyroid hormone sulfation *(65,66)*. SULT1B1 has properties suggesting that it is primarily a xenobiotic sulfating enzyme. The substrate reactivity of SULT1B1 is representative of a phenol SULT with selectivity for smaller phenolic structures. Expressed SULT1B1 efficiently conjugates several prototypical phenolic substrates such as 1-naphthol and PNP, although its kinetic parameters are somewhat different from those of the SULT1A family *(64,67)*. In contrast to SULT1E1, SULT1B1 does not sulfate E2, estrone, or dihydroequilenin. As reported for many of the SULTs, SULT1B1 is capable of efficiently bioactivating several procarcinogens including 6-hydroxymethylbenzo(a)pyrene (HMBP) and 4-hydroxycyclopenta[def]chrysene (OH-CPC) *(19)*. In contrast, SULT1A1 and SULT1A2 do not react with these compounds but rapidly activate N-OH-AAF, which is a poor substrate for SULT1B1. The enzyme is highly expressed in the small intestine and colon as well as in white blood cells and spleen *(64)*. SULT1B1 is detectable in liver but is not detected in other tissues including breast, endometrium, kidney, and lung.

3.3. SULT1C1 and SULT1C2

SULT1C1 and SULT1C2 are recently described, related SULT isoforms belonging to the SULT1 family. Her et al. *(68)* reported the initial cloning of the human SULT1C1 cDNA using an expressed sequence database screening procedure. A highly conserved SULT signature sequence from the carboxy-region of the proteins (RKxxGDWKNxFT) was used to screen expressed sequence tag databases. The cDNA was isolated from a human fetal liver-spleen cDNA library. SULT1C2 was subsequently identified by a database search for sequences related to the SULT1C1 sequence *(69,70)*. The SULT1C isoforms are 63% identical in amino acid sequence and display approx 50% amino acid sequence identity with the human SULT1 isoforms resulting in inclusion in the SULT1 subfamily. The chromosomal localization of both

SULT1C structural genes is 2q11.2, distinct from the site of the *SULT1A* and *SULT1B/1E* chromosomal loci.

Both SULT1C1 and SULT1C2 messages were detected in fetal kidney and fetal liver by dot-blot analysis of human tissue mRNAs. A SULT1C1 message was also detected in adult kidney, thyroid and stomach while a SULT1C2 message was found in adult human heart, kidney, and ovarian tissues (69). To date, the substrate reactivities of the SULT1C isoforms are not well characterized. In a study of several typical SULT substrates and environmental estrogens, Suiko et al. (71) report that both SULT1C1 and 1C2 enzymes were capable of sulfating the prototypical phenol substrate PNP but with different kinetic properties. SULT1C1 had little activity even at high PNP concentrations (50 µM) whereas SULT1C2 had significant activity. SULT1C2 also had activity towards several environmental estrogens but not 17α-EE2, DHEA, or dopamine. Both SULT1C isoforms sulfate N-OH-AAF at high concentrations; however, the enzymes are not mutagenic in the *S. typhimurium* mutagenesis assay, in all likelihood because the N-OH-AAF levels required for mutagenesis are toxic (19). The high substrate concentrations required for activity with the SULT1C isoforms leaves their physiological substrates and function in question.

3.4. SULT1E1: Estrogen SULT

The sulfation of estrogens in human tissues is an important mechanism for the regulation of estrogenic activity. The local formation, metabolism, and action of steroid hormones occurs in peripheral target tissues and thus the activity of the SULTs in these specific target tissues is critical in regulation of intracellular estrogen levels. In humans, this process is also closely linked to the ability to synthesize estrogens from the high levels of circulating DHEA (6,7). The major SULT involved in the sulfation of physiological levels of E2 and estrone is SULT1E1 (72,73).

Aksoy et al. (74) initially cloned SULT1E1 from a human liver cDNA library. The expressed enzyme in COS-1 cells catalyzed E2, estrone, and DHEA. SULT1E1 is responsible for the high-affinity sulfation of E2, estrone, and 17α-EE2 (72,73). Detailed kinetic characterization of expressed pure SULT1E1 indicates that the K_ms for E2 and PAPS are 5 nM and 59 nM, respectively (73). The expressed enzyme is also capable of sulfating a number of other phenolic compounds and steroids including DHEA, pregnenolone, diethylstilbestrol, and equilenin, with affinities in the micromolar range (72). SULT1E1 also displays substrate inhibition with increasing E2 and estrone concentrations (72,73). Maximal E2 sulfation is observed at concentrations of 15–20 nM. This is a result of the combination of ternary (dead-end) complex formation as well as allosteric inhibition of SULT1E1 by E2 (73). The physiological function of the allosteric modulation of SULT1E1 may be a moot point because the K_i of 80 nM is not in the physiological range of E2 concentrations. SULT1E1 is also very active in thyroid hormone sulfation *(66)* and bioactivates several mutagens in *S. typhimurium* mutagenesis assays *(19,75)*.

SULT1E1 is expressed in liver, intestinal tract, testes, breast, and endometrium *(76–78)*. In human endometrium, SULT1E1 is selectively expressed during the secretory phase of the menstrual cycle *(76)*. In contrast, no SULT1E1 message RNA or protein is detected during the proliferative phase of the cycle. SULT1E1 expression is inducible by progestins in human Ishikawa endometrial adenocarcinoma cells *(79)*, suggesting that the increase in progesterone level that occurs after ovulation induces SULT1E1 expression. It is proposed that the elevated SULT1E1 activity in secretory endometrium has a role in regulating E2 activity in the endometrial tissues after ovulation.

3.5. SULT2 Subfamily

3.5.1. SULT2A1

One unique aspect of human endocrinology is the high level of DHEA-sulfate synthesized by the human fetal adrenal and the reticular layer of the adult adrenal *(80)*. SULT2A1 is the SULT isoform responsible for DHEA sulfation in the adrenal *(81,82)* and is highly expressed in the reticular layer of the adult human adrenal *(83)* as well as in the fetal adrenal *(84,85)*. The enzyme is also highly expressed in liver, where it is proposed to have a role in bile acid sulfation *(86)* and in the intestinal tract *(78)*, including the lining of the stomach *(87)*. Expression in the GI tract may be associated with xenobiotic sulfation because the expressed enzyme has a broad substrate reactivity.

SULT2A1 was the first human SULT cloned *(88)*, although the enzyme had been previously purified to homogeneity from human liver cytosol *(81)*. The structural gene is localized to chromosome 19q13.3 at the same locus as the *SULT2B* gene *(89)*. SULT2A1 sulfates 3α, 3β, and 3-phenolic hydroxysteroids and similar compounds as well as many aliphatic alcohols *(81,83,90)*. It has been reported that purified SULT2A1 is responsible for bile acid sulfation in human liver *(86)*. Consistent with the protective effects of sulfation on bile acid toxicity during cholestasis, *SULT2A1* expression is regulated by bile acids via the FXR *(91)*.

3.5.2. Human SULT2B1 Isoforms

Currently, the SULT2 family consists of two genes encoding three SULT isoforms. Two isoforms of SULT2B1 are transcribed from the same gene utilizing different transcriptional start sites so that different first exons are incorporated (Fig. 4). Her et al. *(92)* initially identified the two messages and termed them SULT2B1a and SULT2B1b. SULT2B1b is 365 amino acids in length whereas SULT2B1a is 350 amino acids in length due to different lengths of the

```
hSULT2B1a    1                      MASPPPFHSQKLPGEYFRYKGVPFPVGLYSLESIS   35
hSULT2B1b    1  MDGPAEPQIPGLWDTYEDDISEISQKLPGEYFRYKGVPFPVGLYSLESIS   50
hSULT2A1     1                     MSDDFLWFEGIAFPTMGFRSETLR              24
                                  .  ..  . *. **   .  *..

hSULT2B1a   36  LAENTQDVRDDDIFIITYPKSGTTWMIEIICLILKEGDPSWIRSVPIWER   85
hSULT2B1b   51  LAENTQDVRDDDIFIITYPKSGTTWMIEIICLILKEGDPSWIRSVPIWER  100
hSULT2A1    25  KVRDEFVIRDEDVIILTYPKSGTNWLAEILCLMHSKGDAKWIQSVPIWER   74
                .**.*. *.*******.*. **.**.    ** **.*******

hSULT2B1a   86  APWCETIVGAFSLPDQYSPRLMSSHLPIQIFTKAFFSSKAKVIYMGRNPR  135
hSULT2B1b  101  APWCETIVGAFSLPDQYSPRLMSSHLPIQIFTKAFFSSKAKVIYMGRNPR  150
hSULT2A1    75  SPWVESEIGYTALSESESPRLFSSHLPIQLFPKSFFSSKAKVIYLMRNPR  124
                .** *. .*  .*   **** *******.*  *.*********. ****

hSULT2B1a  136  DVVVSLYHYSKIAGQLKDPGTPDQFLRDFLKGEVQFGSWFDHIKGWLRMK  185
hSULT2B1b  151  DVVVSLYHYSKIAGQLKDPGTPDQFLRDFLKGEVQFGSWFDHIKGWLRMK  200
hSULT2A1   125  DVLVSGYFFWKNMKFIKKPKSWEEYFEWFCQGTVLYGSWFDHIHGWMPMR  174
                **.** *  .*    .*  .... *   * .* *.*******.**. *.

hSULT2B1a  186  GKDNFLFITYEELQQDLQGSVERICGFLGRPLGKEALGSVVAHSTFSAMK  235
hSULT2B1b  201  GKDNFLFITYEELQQDLQGSVERICGFLGRPLGKEALGSVVAHSTFSAMK  250
hSULT2A1   175  EEKNFLLLSYEELKQDTGRTIEKICQFLGKTLEPEELNLILKNSSFQSMK  224
                 ***  .. ****.**    ..*.**  ***. *    *.  .*.* **

hSULT2B1a  236  ANTMSNYTLLPPSLLDHRRGAFLRKGVCGDWKNHFTVAQSEAFDRAYRKQ  285
hSULT2B1b  251  ANTMSNYTLLPPSLLDHRRGAFLRKGVCGDWKNHFTVAQSEAFDRAYRKQ  300
hSULT2A1   225  ENKMSNYSLLSVDYVVDK-AQLLRKGVSGDWKNHFTVAQAEDFDKLFQEK  273
                 * ****.**     .    . *****.***********.* **. ...  .

hSULT2B1a  286  MRGMP--TFPWDEDPEEDGSPDPEPSPEPEPKPSLEPNTSLEREPRPNSS  333
hSULT2B1b  301  MRGMP--TFPWDEDPEEDGSPDPEPSPEPEPKPSLEPNTSLEREPRPNSS  348
hSULT2A1   274  MADLPRELFPWE*                                       286
                *  .* ***.

hSULT2B1a  334  PSPSPGQASETPHPRPS  350
hSULT2B1b  349  PSPSPGQASETPHPRPS  365
```

Fig. 4. Sequence alignment of the human SULT2 family. Sequences were compared using the ClustalW program. The accession numbers are SULT2A1, L20000; 2B1a, U92314; 2B1b, U92315. An asterisk denotes an identical amino acid and a dot denotes a conserved amino acid substitution. Gaps are inserted to optimize the alignment.

first exon. The final 341 amino acids of both sequences are identical. These investigators expressed both isoforms in COS-1 cells utilizing the pCR3.1 vector. Subsequent expression studies of the histidine (His)-tagged and native forms of the SULT2B1 cDNAs in *E. coli* demonstrated difficulty in the expression of the native form of SULT2B1b *(93)*. However, SULT2B1b can be expressed in bacteria with histidine or GST-tag sequences *(93,94)* and the active native enzyme can then be obtained by cleavage of the tag. The presence of a histidine tag significantly alters the kinetic activities of both SULT2B1a and SULTB1b compared to the native enzymes *(93)*. The native expressed form of

SULT2B1b obtained after removal of the tag is unstable and is inactivated by freeze-thawing.

Her et al. *(92)* initially identified both SULT2B1 messages in a placental cDNA library and isolated the clones from Marathon-ready cDNA prepared from placenta/prostate tissues by RACE analysis. Subsequent immunoblot analysis of multiple human tissues detected the presence of only SULT2B1b protein *(95)*. In addition, Northern blot analysis of RNA from human tissues using isoform-selective oligonucleotides detected only SULT2B1b message whereas both messages were detected by RT-PCR *(96,97)*. These results suggest that only SULT2B1b is significantly expressed in most human tissues.

The enzymatic activity of the SULT2B1 isoforms has been characterized using expressed enzymes *(93,96,97)*. To date, active SULT2B1b has not been isolated from human tissues or cells, although immunoreactive protein is present in these preparations. DHEA sulfation activity and immunoreactive SULT2B1b protein have been demonstrated in intact cultured MCF-7 breast cancer cells *(98)* and isolated placental nuclei *(95)*; however, following preparation of lysate or cytosol, no DHEA sulfation activity could be detected. Apparently, disruption of cells or nuclei during lysate or cytosol preparation results in inactivation of the enzyme.

Both expressed SULT2B1 isoforms are selective for the sulfation of the 3β-OH position of hydroxysteroids such as DHEA and pregnenolone. No activity was observed using 3α-OH steroids or 3-phenolic steroids *(93)*; however, both expressed isoforms were capable of sulfating dihydrotestosterone *(96)*. Fuda et al. *(99)* report that expressed SULT2B1b selectively sulfates cholesterol whereas both isoforms are active in pregnenolone sulfation. The unique 23-amino-acid terminus of SULT2B1b was necessary for cholesterol sulfation but not for pregnenolone sulfation.

3.6. SULT4A1

Falany et al. *(100)* initially reported the cloning and expression of novel SULT-related sequences from human and rat brain. These cDNAs have been termed SULT4A based on their sequence similarity to the human SULTs. The SULT4A family is notable in the high degree of sequence conservation between mammalian species. The sequences of the human, rat, and rabbit sequences are 98% identical and the mouse sequence is identical to the rat sequence. The human SULT4A1 sequence is also 96.7% identical to a 270-amino-acid fragment of the chicken SULT4A1 protein, suggesting a high degree of conservation even in nonmammalian species *(98)*. SULT4A1 message expression is detected primarily in human and rat brain cytosol *(100)*. Liyou et al. *(101)* immunolocalized SULT4A1 in neurons in multiple brain tissues. Several investigators expressed SULT4A1 in a variety of expression systems, yet only marginal levels of activity using high substrate concentrations have been reported *(102)*. The high level of sequence conservation for SULT4A1 from different mammalian species combined with selective expression in brain tissues, suggest an important function for this enzyme; however, the marginal activity and the inactivity of the expressed protein has limited the investigation of the physiological properties of SULT4A1.

4. EXPRESSION AND PURIFICATION OF HUMAN SULTS

The multiplicity of the SULTs was first established using differences in substrate reactivity and in responses of the SULT activities to inhibition and thermal inactivation, as well as physical separation of PNP and dopamine sulfation activities in human platelet cytosol by anion-exchange chromatography *(37)*. The initial purification of a human SULT to apparent homogeneity was accomplished by Heroux and Roth *(36)*, who isolated SULT1A3 (M-PST) from platelet cytosol utilizing DEAE-cellulose chromatography, Sephacryl S-200 size-exclusion chromatography, and PAP-agarose affinity chromatography. The combination of anion-exchange chromatography with affinity chromatography provided the basic procedures for the purification of the human SULTs prior to the advent of molecular cloning and expression systems. Combinations of anion-exchange chromatography and PAP-agarose affinity chromatography were utilized to purify both SULT1A1 (P-PST) *(39)* and SULT2A1 (DHEA-ST) *(81)* from human liver cytosol. Preparation of these pure SULT isoforms permitted the generation of widely applicable polyclonal antibodies in rabbits. These antibodies were important in comparing and identifying the SULTs in different human tissues. Comer et al. *(82)* demonstrated that DHEA-ST purified from human liver cytosol was structurally and functionally similar to the adrenal enzyme. However, studies on the purification of the human SULTs were limited by the availability of high-quality human tissues and the appearance of HIV in the blood supply.

The advent of molecular cloning of the SULTs not only identified several new isoforms of human SULT but also led to the expression and purification of large amounts of the SULT enzymes, generally utilizing tag sequences to facilitate purification. Several new problems resulted from these advances in technology. Native forms of the SULTs can be expressed in bacteria including *E. coli* and *S. typhimurium*, or in cultured mammalian or insect cells. The value of each system depends on whether the SULT activity will be isolated for characterization or will be used in intact cells. Also, the SULTs can be expressed with tags such as 6xHis or GST to facilitate purification.

Most human SULTs are readily expressed in *E. coli* in an active native form, and must be isolated from bacterial cell lysates or cytosol for further applications, particularly because bacterial cytosol possesses several phosphatase or sulfatase activities that rapid degrade PAPS and interfere with quantitative activity assays. One of the initial bacterial systems involved expression of the native SULT form using the pKK233-3 vector. SULT activity was isolated from bacterial cytosol by DEAE-Sepharose column chromatography with NaCl gradient elution. This procedure generates an active preparation of partially purified SULT activity useful for kinetic and activity studies and has been applied to SULT1A1, 1A3, 1B1, 1C2, 1E1 2A1, and SULT2B1a *(41,60,64,72,93)*. The SULTs could be further purified by PAP-agarose affinity chromatography analogous to the protocol for purification from liver cytosol; however, the commercial sources of the affinity resin are of varying quality and binding capacity. There are some concerns that although the pKK233-2 vector generates active enzyme, it is a relatively low level expression system *(103)*. Djani et al. *(104)* compared the properties of SULT1A3 expressed in *E. coli* with those of the enzyme expressed in *S. cerevisiae*, COS-7, and V79 cells as well as the platelet enzyme. The investigators concluded that the enzyme and kinetic properties were essentially the same in all expression systems. Although most SULTs are readily expressed in *E. coli*, SULT4A1 and SULT2B1b are exceptions. SULT4A1 has not been expressed in any system with a high level of activity. Native SULT2B1b protein can be expressed in *E. coli* using different expression vectors including pKK233-2; however, the enzyme is not enzymatically active following preparation of lysate or cytosol *(93)*. The active SULT2B1b isoform can be expressed with a cleavable His- or GST-tag, with the active form then generated by removal of the tag *(93,99)*.

Extensive bioactivation studies have been carried out with the individual SULT isoforms expressed in *S. typhimurium*. Expression of the individual native forms of the human SULTs in *S. typhimurium* has allowed evaluation of their activity in the Ames assay *(18,44)*. His⁻ *S. typhimurium* cells are transformed with expression vectors containing the individual SULT cDNAs then intact cells are treated with the procarcinogen. These studies generally utilize native SULT proteins. The cells undergoing mutagenesis demonstrate the ability to grow on His-depleted agar. Several of the SULTs have been coexpressed with cytochromes P450 to investigate the sequential activity of these enzymes in activating polyaromatic hydrocarbons and aromatic amines *(105,106)*. With the exceptions of SULT4A1 and the SULT2B1s, all SULTs demonstrate the ability to bioactive procarcinogens and are positive in the *S. typhimurium* mutagenesis assay *(19)*.

The native SULTs have also been expressed in mammalian COS monkey kidney fibroblasts for characterization of activity. Sufficient levels of activity for enzymatic analysis are generated in cytosolic preparations of the cells with only negligible background levels of sulfation activity. The system has the advantage of being a mammalian expression system and enables comparison of expression levels and stability of SULT haplotypes *(27–29)*. The use of mammalian cells for expression studies also allows posttranslational modification and processing of the SULTs. To date, however, no posttranslational modifications of any of the human SULTs have been reported. Expression in COS cells has been used by Weinshilboum's group at the Mayo Clinic for the analysis of the kinetic properties and differences in expression of genetic haplotypes for SULT1A1, SULT2A1, and SULT1E1 *(26,27,56)*. Stable expression of human SULTs in Chinese hamster ovary (CHO) cells has proven useful in studies investigating the bioactivation of 2-amino-1-methyl-6-phenylimidazo[4,5-β]pyridine (PhiP) *(107)*.

Several cultured mammalian cell lines have been stably transformed with individual SULTs. These cells lines are used to evaluate SULT activities in intact cells as well as the possible physiological roles of sulfation. Chinese hamster V79 cells have been used for stable expression of the SULTs and for characterization of their properties in mammalian cell mutagenesis *(106)*. V79 cells have also been used as a source of specific SULT activity expressed in mammalian cells for comparison with bacterially expressed SULT activity *(104)*.

Stable expression of SULT isoforms in mammalian cells is used as a tool to analyze the effect of either overexpression of a SULT activity that occurs naturally in a cell, or the effect of introducing a SULT activity into a cell where it does not occur naturally. Most native SULTs are efficiently expressed using mammalian expression vectors such as pcDNA3.1 that confer geneticin resistance *(108–110)*. SULT1A1 and SULT1E1 have been stably expressed in human MCF-7 cells to investigate their roles in E2 sulfation. Although SULT1A1 is naturally expressed in MCF-7 cells, a 10-fold higher activity level of SULT1A1 was achieved in cells subsequent to selection by geneticin resistance. SULT1E1 expression in hormone-responsive breast cancer cells, including MCF-7 cells, achieves activity levels similar to those found in primary breast epithelial cells. The high-affinity E2 sulfation activity of SULT1E1 may limit the growth of the cells owing to inactivation of estrogens required for growth, making it difficult to obtain cells with extremely high SULT1E1 activity by geneticin selection. Figure 5 shows the comparison of 20 n*M* E2 sulfation by MCF-7 cells expressing SULT1E1 and SULT1A1. SULT1E1 is responsible for the high-affinity sulfation of E2; sulfation by SULT1A1 becomes significant only when E2 concentrations approach nonphysiological levels.

The expression of SULTs with tags such as 6xHis or GST is utilized to facilitate isolation of the enzymes for characterization and/or structural analysis. Typically, expression is carried out with either a tag that is not removed or with a cleavable tag, depending on whether it is anticipated that the tag will affect SULT activity. The addition of a His-tag appears to have no significant effect on the activity of most of the human SULTs, whereas a few may be greatly

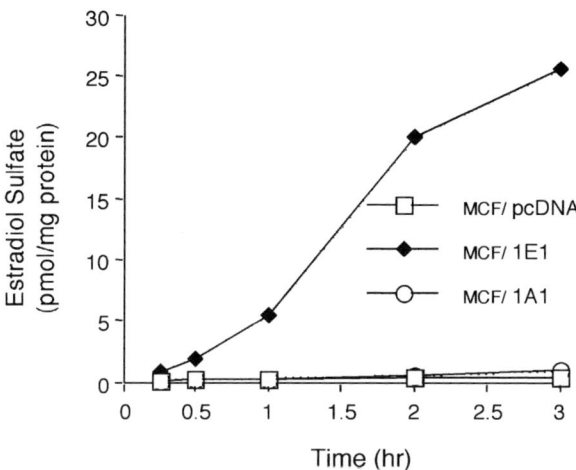

Fig. 5. Sulfation of increasing concentrations of β-estradiol by MCF-7 cells expressing SULT1E1 or SULT1A1. MCF-7 cells were stably transfected with the pcDNA3.1 vector expressing SULT1A1. The MCF-7/1A1 cells possessed 10-fold higher rates of PNP sulfation than the control pcDNA3.1 cells and MCF-7/1E1 cells. The three cell lines were grown to 70% confluency, washed with serum-free medium and 20 nM tritiated E2 added to the cells in serum-free medium. Aliquots of the medium were sampled at different times, extracted with chloroform, and the tritiated E2-sulfate determined by scintillation counting.

affected. SULT1A1 and SULT1B1 activity and kinetic properties appear to be relatively unaffected by the presence of N-terminal His tags (64). In contrast, the presence of an N-terminal His-tag significantly alters the activity and properties of the SULT2B1 isoforms (93). To avoid possible differences in substrate reactivity, the use of cleavable tags is generally advisable for kinetic or functional studies.

The pMAL fusion protein system (New England Biolabs) has proven very useful for the generation of highly purified human SULT1E1 (72). This system generates a maltose binding protein (MBP)–SULT fusion protein where the initial methionine of the enzyme is cloned immediately 3' to a factor X protease cleavage site. The fusion protein can be grown in E. coli and purified from bacterial cytosol by amylose affinity chromatography. The fusion protein is cleaved with activated factor X protease generating the native SULT protein. Uncut fusion protein and MBP can be removed by a second amylose affinity procedure then the factor X is removed by DEAE-Sepharose chromatography. The isolated enzyme is highly purified and useful for detailed mechanistic studies (73).

5. SULT ENZYMATIC ASSAYS

The identification of SULT activities depends in part on the assay of their enzymatic activities. Early studies routinely identified three to four isoforms of human SULT via the use of selective substrates. The platelet phenol SULTs were identified by the specificity of PNP sulfation by SULT1A1, and dopamine sulfation by SULT1A3 *(34)*. High-affinity E2 sulfation in endometrium was associated with estrogen SULT (1E1) and DHEA sulfation in the adrenal with DHEA SULT (SULT2A1) *(111,112)*. Identification of additional isoforms of SULT, primarily through molecular approaches, has led to the realization that, as with many other drug metabolizing enzyme families, the individual SULT isoforms show broad overlapping substrate reactivities. Substrate inhibition is also a common feature of SULT kinetics. Figure 6 shows the increase in DHEA sulfation catalyzed by expressed SULT2A1 followed by a decrease in activity as substrate concentrations are increased further. E2 sulfation by SULT1E1 also displays substrate inhibition with maximal activity observed at a concentration of 15–20 nM *(72)*. Analysis of SULT1E1 kinetics indicates that the enzyme has a random order bi bi reaction mechanism allowing for the formation of enzyme-PAP-E2 and enzyme-E2-sulfate-PAPS dead-end products. Zhang et al. *(73)* reported that SULT1E1 displays a K_m of 60 nM for PAPS and a K_i of 40 nM for PAP during the E2 sulfation reaction, suggesting the formation of SULT1E1-PAP-E2. These authors have also demonstrated that each SULT1E1 monomer is capable of binding two E2 molecules. One molecule binds at the active site and the second molecule at an inhibitory allosteric site. Substrate inhibition during the sulfation of E2 by SULT1E1 is the result of product inhibition as well as allosteric inhibition. Gamage et al. *(113)* reported the presence of two molecules of PNP at the active site of SULT1A1 during analysis of its crystal structure, suggesting that allosteric modulation of this enzyme may also be occurring. Potent substrate inhibition must be taken into account in the kinetic analysis of the SULTs. In general, very low substrate concentrations are used to avoid substrate inhibition when determining kinetic constants.

A complication that arises in characterizing SULT activity in tissue samples involves the ability of several SULTs to conjugate the same substrates. The classic example involves E2 sulfation. Falany et al. *(41,72)* reported that SULT1E1, SULT1A1, and SULT2A1 are capable of sulfating E2 with very different kinetic properties. Bernier et al. *(114)* reported that SULT1A3 is also capable of sulfating E2 and Faucher et al. *(115)* demonstrated that expressed SULT1A3 (hEST-1) is capable of sulfating E2, but not estrone, at micromolar substrate concentrations. In addition, it has been reported that SULT1A3 does not sulfate E2 at a significant rate at physiological low nanomolar concentrations *(60)*. SULT1A1 and SULT2A1 also conjugate E2 and estrone at micromolar

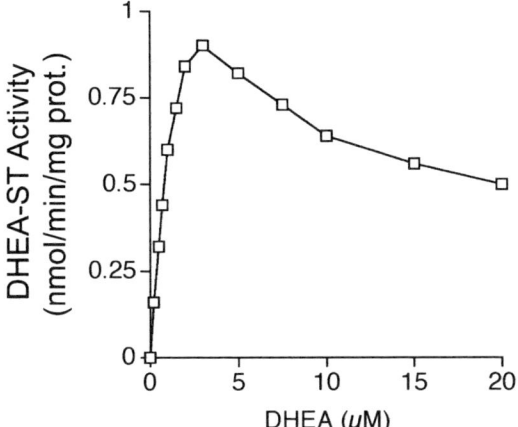

Fig. 6. Substrate inhibition of DHEA sulfation catalyzed by SULT2A1.

concentrations while little sulfation occurs at nanomolar concentrations. Figure 5 shows the disparity of E2 sulfation by human breast cancer MCF-7 cells. MCF-7 cells do not express SULT1E1 but express both SULT1A1 and SULT1A3 *(77)*. Thus, MCF-7 cells do not significantly sulfate E2 at a concentration of 20 nM because they lack SULT1E1. The stable expression of physiological levels of SULT1E1 in MCF-7 cells results in rapid E2 sulfation at low nanomolar concentrations. Even the stable expression of SULT1A1 activity in MCF-7 cells at 10-fold normal levels does not result in a significant increase in 20 nM E2 sulfation. However, increasing the E2 substrate concentration results in the detection of E2 sulfation by SULT1A1 (Fig. 7). Similar differences are observed in the sulfation of small phenols by several SULTs. PNP is frequently used to assay phenol sulfation activity. SULT1A1 is the primary SULT involved with PNP sulfation in human liver but SULT1B1 also sulfates PNP with a somewhat lower affinity. SULT1B1 is not highly expressed in liver but is well expressed in intestine and colon. Thus, PNP sulfation in different tissues can be attributed to different SULTs. SULT1C2 has also been reported to sulfate PNP but at significantly higher concentrations *(71)*. Therefore, PNP sulfation potentially involves the combined activity of at least two and possibly three separate SULTs. Some distinction between the contributions of the different isoforms can be made by careful attention to substrate concentrations and kinetic properties of the reactions.

Another consideration when assaying SULT activity is the promiscuity of most of the isoforms. The SULTs are drug metabolizing enzymes and several of the isoforms have evolved to conjugate a variety of substrates. SULT1A1 is

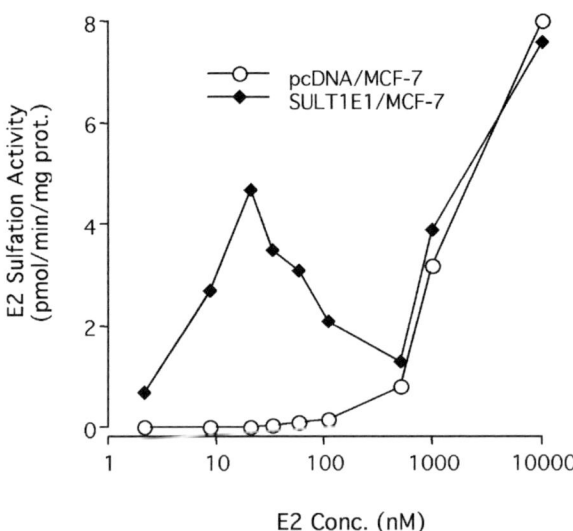

Fig. 7. Sulfation of β-estradiol by MCF-7 cells and MCF-7 cells stably expressing SULT1E1. MCF-7 human breast cancer cells were stably transfected with the pcDNA3.1 mammalian expression vector or with SULT1E1 inserted in the vector. The levels of SULT1E1 activity were very similar to the levels assayed in human primary mammary epithelial cells (77). The ability of the MCF-7 cells to sulfate increasing concentrations of β-estradiol added to the medium was assayed. The cells were grown to 70% confluency, washed with serum-free medium and the appropriate concentration of tritiated E2 added to the medium. After incubation, the medium was removed and extracted with chloroform to separate the E2 and the E2-sulfate, then counted in a scintillation counter.

generally considered the major xenobiotic phenol SULT in human tissues. SULT1A1 is highly expressed in liver and the GI tract and is present in many other tissues. Characterization of the substrate reactivity of SULT1A1 shows that it is able to sulfate a wide variety of chemical structures (39,41,116). Gamage et al. (113) analyzed the crystal structure of SULT1A1 and suggested that the broad substrate reactivity may be related to the flexibility of the substrate binding site. This broad substrate reactivity must be taken into account in assaying the activity of SULT1A1 and is a factor that must be considered in assaying most of the SULTs.

Several assays have been used to determine of SULT activity. The barium precipitation assay originally described by Foldes and Meek (117) has been widely used to assay SULT activity. This assay utilizes [^{35}S]PAPS and measures the formation of ^{35}S-conjugated substrates. Barium precipitation is utilized to remove the [^{35}S]PAPS from the reaction mixture allowing determination of the

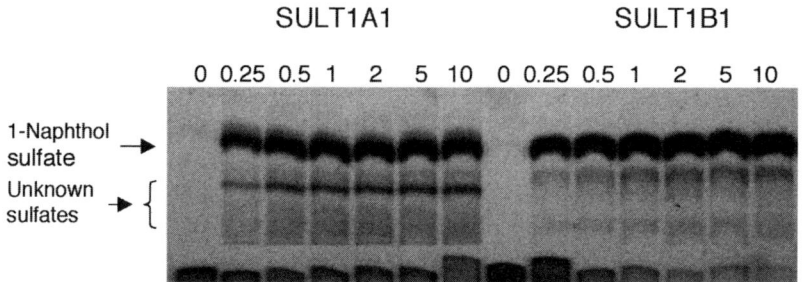

Fig. 8. Thin-layer chromatographic analysis of 1-naphthol sulfation products. Increasing concentrations of 1-naphthol were sulfated using [^{35}S]PAPS and SULT1A1 and SULT1B1 expressed in *E. coli* and purified by DEAE-Sepharose chromatography. The reactions were stopped by application to the loading zone of a silica gel F-250 TLC plate, dried and developed in a methylene chloride–MeOH–ammonium hydroxide (81:15:5) system. The plates were air-dried and exposed to autoradiograph film.

^{35}S-products via scintillation counting. The procedure works well with small phenols where greater than 95% recovery of ^{35}S-labeled phenols can be obtained. The procedure is less efficient with larger, hydrophobic substrates such as steroids. The recovery of sulfated steroids is variable depending on the steroid and is as low as 60% for DHEA sulfate. In general, the barium precipitation assay is not reliable for steroids and similar hydrophobic compounds. Another problem with the use of the barium precipitation assay is the sulfation of buffer components, substrate contaminants, and tissue preparations, largely because the assay does not distinguish between sulfated products. Figure 8 is an autoradiograph of a thin-layer chromatography plate demonstrating the sulfation of 1-naphthol by SULT1A1 expressed in *E. coli*. Despite the fact that a single substrate was provided for the reaction, multiple products are formed as indicated by the multiple bands. With the barium precipitation assay, these multiple products are not separated but rather are quantified with the specific reaction products. Thus, high background rates are a problem with the barium precipitation assay and sufficient controls must be included. Also, product identification needs to be carried out during assay validation. Previous investigators have reported that SULT1A1 is capable of sulfating contaminants in substrate preparations. Hernandez et al. *(42)* noted that β-naphthylamine was contaminated with low levels of β-naphthol and the initial detection of high levels of sulfation with β-naphthylamine were a result of β-naphthol sulfation. SULT1A1 does form naphthylamine sulfamate but at a much lower rate than for β-naphthol. Some Tris buffers contain a low level of phenol contamination that is readily sulfated by SULT1A1 *(unpublished observation)*. Sakakibara et al. *(118)* demonstrated that SULT1A3 sulfates small peptides containing tyrosines as well as free tyrosine, indicating that peptide sulfation may be involved in the high backgrounds generated with cytosol and lysate preparations. Platelet cytosol also possesses tyrosines containing peptide sulfation activity that is most likely associated with SULT1A1 *(119)*. Duffel *(120)* has reported the ability of rat aryl sulfotransferase IV to sulfate several tyrosine containing peptides. The high backgrounds cause problems in kinetic studies, especially when low substrate concentrations are used to avoid substrate inhibition. The barium precipitation assay is more reliable when used to assay purified preparations of the phenolic SULTs with appropriate controls and product identification. The use of [^{35}S]PAPS to assay SULT activity is advantageous because unradiolabeled acceptor substrates can be utilized. Because of the problems with the barium precipitation assay, thin-layer chromatography (TLC) or high-performance liquid chromatography (HPLC) assays are commonly used at present to isolate specific products and for more reliable quantitation and kinetic analyses. Zhang et al. *(73)* used TLC in a very thorough analysis of the reaction mechanism and kinetics of SULT1E1. Product analysis is sometimes beneficial because multiple products may be identified. Tibolone disulfate has been identified in human plasma; subsequent characterization of tibolone sulfation demonstrated that SULT2A1 is responsible for the formation of this tibolone disulfate. SULT1E1 and SULT2B1b also sulfate tibolone but form only monosulfates *(121)*.

Although it limits the array of substrates that can be utilized, the use of specific radiolabeled substrates with nonradiolabeled PAPS avoids several of the problems associated with using [^{35}S]PAPS. The use of tritium-labeled steroids combined with organic solvent extraction provides a simple and rapid assay for steroid sulfation. This assay is exemplified by the use of [^{3}H]DHEA to assay SULT2A1 activity *(81)*. Reactions are run with [^{3}H]DHEA and PAPS for a specified time, then stopped with the addition of chloroform, followed by low-speed centrifugation to separate the organic and aqueous phases. Greater than 98% of the [^{3}H]DHEA is in the organic phase, whereas greater than 99% of the [^{3}H]DHEA-sulfate is in the aqueous phase. This assay can be used for most steroids and many hydrophobic substrates such as 1-naphthol. Limitations of the assay are the requirement of specific radiolabeled substrates that can be expensive or that are not commercially available. Also, the substrates must be highly soluble in the organic solvent in order to obtain low backgrounds. Some substrates, such as [^{3}H]E2, will develop relatively high backgrounds over time, apparently due to degradation or to tritium exchange with the storage solvent.

6. DETECTION OF SULTs

One problem with the activity analyses of the individual SULTs in human tissues is the lack of well-defined substrates for most of the isoforms. The

Table 2
Crossreactivity of Polyclonal Antibodies Raised Against SULT Isoforms

SULT isoform/immunogen	Crossreactive isoforms
SULT1A1	SULT1A2, SULT1A3
SULT1B1	SULT1E1
SULT1C1	SULT1C2
SULT1E1	SULT1B1
SULT2A1	Not detected
SULT2B1a	SULT2B1b
SULT4A1	Not detected

All antisera are raised in rabbits except the anti-SULT4A1 antibody which raised in chickens. Crossreactivity was determined by immunoblot analysis *(39,82)*.

expression of SULT isoforms in a tissue should be confirmed by the detection of specific RNA message or immunoreactive protein. Identification of SULT expression by immunoblot analysis is preferred, although Northern blot and RT-PCR analysis of specific SULT messages is widely used.

Antibodies to the individual SULTs have been developed in rabbits as well as in chickens and have proven very useful in the identification of the individual SULTs in human tissues during immunoblot analysis. Appropriate application of the antibodies with known SULT standards allows the quantitation of SULT expression in a given tissue. Table 2 shows the general crossreactivity of rabbit antibodies raised to a pure SULT. Polyclonal antibodies raised in rabbits to any of the SULT1A isoforms crossreact strongly with all three isoforms. The individual SULT1A1 and SULT1A3 isoforms can be readily distinguished during immunoblot analysis owing to differences in their mobility during SDS-PAGE *(39)*. SULT1A3 migrates with an apparent mass approx 2000 Da larger than SULT1A1, although its estimated mass from its translation is actually slightly less than that of SULT1A1. Expressed SULT1A2 migrates between the positions of SULT1A1 and SULT1A3, although SULT1A2 is either not expressed or not present at levels detectable by immunoblot analysis in most human tissues. The development of selective SULT1A1 and SULT1A3 antibodies using peptides synthesized from one of the few regions of difference in the sequences of the proteins has been reported *(122)*; however, these antibodies have not been used extensively. In many instances, the polyclonal antibodies raised in rabbits to a purified and expressed SULT crossreact with related forms. This is the case with the rabbit polyclonal antibody raised to bacterially expressed SULT1B1 that also displays a low level of reactivity with SULT1E1. SULT1B1 is most similar to SULT1E1 when the SULT amino acid sequences are compared *(64,98)*. In antibody preparations where the crossreactivity is low, immunoabsorption against expressed SULT1E1 covalently bound to Sepharose can be utilized to remove most of the crossreacting antibodies *(64)*.

Northern blot analysis is a valuable tool for identification and quantitation of individual SULTs; however, there are limitations. The high similarity in sequence between the SULT1A isoforms prohibits the use of cDNA probes in Northern blotting experiments. The individual SULT1A mRNAs can be probed using specific oligonucleotide probes, although this results in a distinct loss of sensitivity. Also, the similarity between the sequences limits the positions at which the oligonucleotides can be synthesized within the coding regions. The design and use of primers to the 5′-region of SULT1A1 and SULT1A3 must take into account that multiple start sites of transcription are utilized by these isoforms *(38)*. Our understanding of the transcriptional regulation of these genes is limited and is an area for further investigation.

Several of the SULTs express mRNA forms in human tissues that apparently do not translate into functional SULT proteins. SULT2B1a and SULT2B1b represent two separate isoforms that are transcribed from the same gene but utilize different transcriptional start sites, resulting in the incorporation of different first exons *(92)*. Several investigators have reported the presence of specific RNA message for SULT2B1a in human tissues by reverse transcriptase-polymerase chain reaction (RT-PCR) or RACE analysis: however, to date only SULT2B1b immunoreactive protein has been detected in the human tissues analyzed *(95,98)*. SULT2B1a expression may be below the detection limits of immunoblot analysis; however, this would suggest that the levels of SULT2B1a expression may not be physiologically relevant when compared to SULT2B1b. Another possibility is that SULT2B1a is specifically in only a few tissues or cell types *(96)*. SULT4A1 is a recently described SULT isoform that was initially detected in a screening and sequencing of messages expressed in human pancreatic islet cells *(100)*. The apparently full-length message was identified in human brain and translation of the cDNA results in a SULT-like protein. To date, expression of the SULT4A1 in heterologous bacterial and mammalian expression systems has not resulted in the detection of convincing enzymatic activity *(100,102)*. SULT4A1 mRNA has been detected by RT-PCR in several human tissues, including liver and pancreas. Analysis of the SULT4A1 mRNA in these tissues indicates the presence of unspliced introns compared to the exonic structure of the other human SULTs *(100)*. To date, appropriately spliced message generating the assumed functional form of SULT4A1 has been identified only in brain and testes.

RT-PCR is a selective and sensitive method for the detection of SULT mRNA in preparations of tissue RNA. The use of specific primers permits detection of message for the specific SULTs as well as for the detection of allelic variants. However, as with Northern blot analysis, care must be taken to ensure that the SULT isoform being examined is present in the tissue specimen by either enzymatic activity or immunoblotting. RT-PCR is capable of detecting low levels of SULT mRNA, such as SULT2B1a, in tissue preparations where protein expression is not detectable by immunoblotting.

7. IMMUNOHISTOCHEMISTRY

The application of immunohistochemical techniques to investigation of the localization and function of the human SULTs has been underutilized. Early studies were limited by difficulty in purifying the enzyme to the homogeneity required for quality antibody preparation as well as by the inability to generate antibodies that distinguished between members of the SULT1A family. Using a rabbit antibody developed to purified human platelet SULT1A3, Zou et al. *(59)* reported that the SULT1A family was localized in neurons in the CNS. These studies were supported by purification studies and by chemical deletion studies in rodents *(123)*; however, owing to crossreactivity of the antibody with all SULT1A forms, differences in isoform distribution could not be discerned. Hume and Coughtrie have collaborated on the immunolocalization of the SULT1A and SULT2A families in multiple adult and fetal human tissues *(85,124,125)*, providing us with our most complete insight into SULT localization in human tissues.

Rabbit antibodies to SULT2A1 were used to localize expression in the reticular layer of the adrenal cortex *(83,126,127)* and in the fetal adrenal *(84)*. Although SULT2A1 immunoreactivity was also reported in human breast cancer tissue *(128)*, subsequent investigators have failed to detect SULT2A1 by immunoblot analysis in human breast cancer *(77)*. Thus, interpretation of immunohistochemical results must be cautious and, optimally, confirmed by immunoblot analysis. Nonspecific binding or crossreactivity of the antibody could result in positive immunohistochemical staining but would not be confirmed by immunoblot analysis that distinguishes proteins by molecular weight. Another example of this occurs with a commercial rabbit anti-SULT1E1 peptide antibody that was raised to the initial 13 amino acids of SULT1E1 linked to keyhole limpet hemocyanin. The antibody has been used in immunohistochemical studies of human breast cancer *(129)* and, as shown in Fig. 9, reacts with SULT1E1 in liver cytosol during immunoblot analysis; however, no detectable SULT1E1 is observed in breast cancer tissues. Strong crossreactivity is observed with a larger protein in breast cancer cytosol during immunoblotting, suggesting

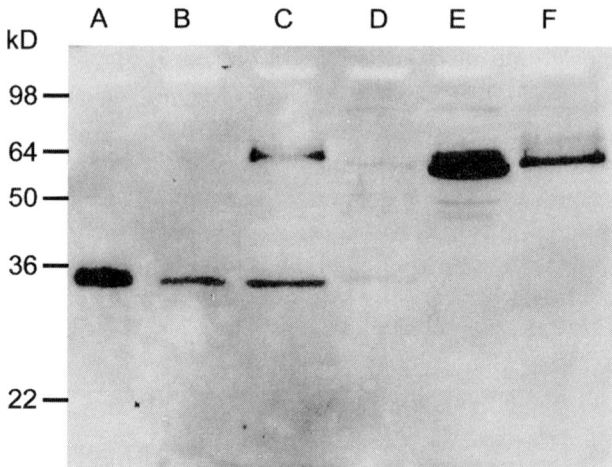

Fig. 9. Immunoblot analysis of SULT1E1 expression. The tissue samples were resolved in a 12% SDS-polyacrylmide gel and transferred to a nitrocellulose membrane. The membrane was incubated with rabbit anti-SULT1E1 peptide antiserum (1/5000 dil.) purchased from Medical Biological Laboratory (Nagoya, Japan). The secondary antibody was goat antirabbit IgG HRP-conjugate (Southern Biotech, Birmingham, AL). The signal was visualized with West Pico reagent (Pierce, Chicago, IL) and autoradiography. *Lane A* contained expressed SULT1E1 (200 ng); *lanes B, C,* normal human liver cytosol (200 µg); *lane D,* normal small intestine lysate (200 µg); and *lanes E, F,* breast tumor lysate (200 µg).

that the reactivity in immunohistochemical breast cancer sections is an artifact. Once again, this confirms that immunohistochemical localization studies of SULT expression should be supported by alternative procedures.

Recently, He et al. *(95)* reported the immunohistochemical localization of SULT2B1b in nuclei of term human placental synchiotrophoblasts. This was the first report of a cytosolic SULT expressed in nuclei. The localization was confirmed by isolation of nuclei using an Optiprep gradient with subsequent detection of DHEA sulfation activity and SULT2B1b protein in these isolated nuclei. In contrast, SULT2B1b was detectable only in cytosol of human LnCaP prostate adenocarcinoma cells and sections of normal and cancerous human prostate. Immunohistochemical analysis of SULT expression is a research area that has been largely ignored and, in the future, will generate novel insights into the properties and functions of the human SULTs.

8. SUMMARY

Our understanding of the role of cytosolic SULTs in human drug metabolism and toxicology has progressed rapidly as our understanding of the genetic character of the family has expanded. Sulfation has an important role in the inactivation and excretion of a large number of drugs and xenobiotic compounds. However, sulfate conjugation is also a mechanism for the activation of many aromatic amines, polycyclic aromatic amines and hydroxymethyl polyaromatic hydrocarbons to potent mutagens. Analysis of the kinetic, biochemical, genetic, and regulatory properties of each of the SULTs is necessary to understand their physiological functions and properties. Because of the role of sulfation in steroid synthesis and metabolism, SULT expression and function in hormone responsive cancers has been especially interesting. Although often overlooked, sulfation is still a major aspect of the metabolism and inactivation of therapeutic drugs and xenobiotics. Detailed studies of substrate reactivity and structures of the individual SULT isoforms are needed to further understand and account for sulfation in drug pharmacokinetics and efficacy. Developing and characterizing the molecular, analytical, and immunological tools required to pursue these studies is essential.

REFERENCES

1. Baumann E. Ueber sulfosauren im harn. Ber Dtsch Chem Ges 1876;54.
2. Mulder GJ. Sulfation. In: Bridges JW, Chasseaud LF, eds. Progress in Drug Metabolism. London: Taylor & Francis; 1984;35–100.
3. Jakoby WB, Sekura RD, Lyon ES, Marcus CJ, Wang J-L. Sulfotransferases. In: Jakoby WB, ed. Enzymatic Basis of Detoxication, New York: Academic Press; 1980;199–227.
4. Roth JA. Sulfoconjugation: role in neurotransmitter and secretory protein activity. Trends Pharmacol Sci 1986;7:404–407.
5. Casey ML, MacDonald PC, Simpson ER. Endocrinological changes of pregnancy. In: Wilson JD, Foster DW, eds. Williams Textbook of Endocrinology. Philadelphia: W.B. Saunders; 1987;422–437.
6. Kalimi M, Regelson W. The Biologic Role for Dehydroepiandrosterone. New York: Walter de Gruyter; 1990.
7. Labrie F, Luu-The V, Labrie C, Simard J. DHEA and its transformation into androgens and estrogens in peripheral target tissues: intracrinology. Front Neuroendocrinol 2001;22:185–212.
8. Roth JA, Rivett AJ. Does sulfate conjugation contribute to the metabolic inactivation of catecholamines in humans? Biochem Pharmacol 1982;31:3017–3021.
9. DuCharme DW, Freyburger WA, Graham BE, Carlson RG. Pharmacologic properties of minoxidil: a new hypotensive agent. J Pharmacol Exp Ther 1973;184:662–670.
10. McCall JM, Aiken JW, Chidester CG, DuCharme DW, Wendling MG. Pyrimidine and triazine 3-oxide sulfates: a new family of vasodilators. J Med Chem 1983;26: 1791–1793.
11. Clissold SP, Heel RC. Topical minoxidil. A preliminary review of its pharmacodynamic properties and therapeutic efficacy in alopecia areata and alopecia androgenetica. Drugs 1987;33:107–122.

12. Meisheri KD, Cipkus LA. Biochemical mechanisms by which minoxidil sulfate influences mammalian cells. Dermatologica 1987;175 (Suppl 2):3–11.
13. Meisheri KD, Cipkus LA, Taylor CJ. Mechanism of action of minoxidil sulfate-induced vasodilation: a role for increased K^+ permeability. J Pharmacol Exp Ther 1988;245:751–760.
14. Dooley TP, Walker CJ, Hirshey SJ, Falany CN, Diani AR. Localization of minoxidil sulfotransferase in the liver and outer root sheath of rat anagen pelage and vibrissa follicles. J Invest Dermatol 1991;96:65–70.
15. Boberg EW, Miller EC, Miller JA, Poland A, Liem A. Strong evidence from studies with brachymorphic mice and pentachlorophenol that 1′-sulfooxysafrole is the major ultimate electrophilic and carcinogenic metabolite of 1′-hydroxysafrole in mouse liver. Cancer Res 1983;43:5163–5173.
16. Miller EC, Miller JA, Boberg EW, et al. Sulfuric acid esters as ultimate electrophilic and carcinogenic metabolites of some alkenylbenzenes and aromatic amines in mouse liver. Carcinogenesis 1985;11:93–107.
17. Miller JA, Miller EC. Electrophilic sulfuric acid ester metabolites as ultimate carcinogens. Adv Exp Med Biol 1986;197:583–595.
18. Glatt H. Sulfotransferases in the bioactivation of xenobiotics. Chem Biol Interact 2000;129;141–170.
19. Glatt H, Boeing H, Engelke CE, et al. Human cytosolic sulphotransferases: genetics, characteristics, toxicological aspects. Mutat Res 2001;482:27–40.
20. Grunwell JR, Bertozzi CR. Carbohydrate sulfotransferases of the GalNAc/Gal/GlcNAc6ST family. Biochemistry 2002;41:13117–13126.
21. Honke K, Taniguchi N. Sulfotransferases and sulfated oligosaccharides. Med Res Rev 2002;22:637–654.
22. Ouyang Y, Lane WS, Moore KL. Tyrosylprotein sulfotransferase: purification and molecular cloning of an enzyme that catalyzes tyrosine O-sulfation, a common posttranslational modification of eukaryotic proteins. Proc Natl Acad Sci USA 1998;95:2896–2901.
23. Mandon E, Kempner ES, Ishihara M, Hirschberg CB. A monomeric protein in the Golgi membrane catalyzes both N-deacetylation and N-sulfation of heparan sulfate. J Biol Chem 1994;269:11729–11733.
24. Falany CN. Enzymology of human cytosolic sulfotransferases. FASEB J 1997;11:206–216.
25. Freimuth RR, Wiepert M, Chute CG, Wieben ED, Weinshilboum RM. Human cytosolic sulfotransferase database mining: identification of seven novel genes and pseudogenes. Pharmacogenomics J 2003;4:54–65.
26. Adjei AA, Thomae BA, Prondzinski JL, Eckloff BW, Wieben ED, Weinshilboum RM. Human estrogen sulfotransferase (SULT1E1) pharmacogenomics: gene resequencing and functional genomics. Br J Pharmacol 2003;139:1373–1382.
27. Thomae BA, Eckloff BW, Freimuth RR, Wieben ED, Weinshilboum RM. Human sulfotransferase SULT2A1 pharmacogenetics: genotype-to-phenotype studies. Pharmacogenomics J 2002;2:48–56.

28. Carlini EJ, Raftogianis RB, Wood TC, et al. Sulfation pharmacogenetics: SULT1A1 and SULT1A2 allele frequencies in Caucasian, Chinese and African-American subjects. Pharmacogenetics 2001;11:57–68.
29. Freimuth RR, Eckloff B, Wieben ED, Weinshilboum RM. Human sulfotransferase SULT1C1 pharmacogenetics: gene resequencing and functional genomic studies. Pharmacogenetics 2001;11:747–756.
30. Tsoi C, Falany CN, Morgenstern R, Swedmark S. Identification of a new subfamily of sulphotransferases: cloning and characterization of canine SULT1D1. Biochem J 2001;356 891–897.
31. Meinl W, Glatt H. Structure and localization of the human SULT1B1 gene: neighborhood to SULT1E1 and a SULT1D pseudogene. Biochem Biophys Res Commun 2001;288:855–862.
32. Hart RF, Renskers KJ, Nelson EB, Roth JA. Localization and characterization of phenol sulfotransferase in human platelets. Life Sci 1979;24:125–130.
33. Anderson RJ, Weinshilboum RM, Phillips SF, Broughton DD. Human platelet phenol sulphotransferase: assay procedure, substrate and tissue correlations Clin Chim Acta 1981;110:157–167.
34. Reiter C, Mwaluko G, Dunnette J, Van Loon J, Weinshilboum R. Thermolabile and thermostable human platelet phenol sulfotransferase: substrate specificity and physical separation. Naunyn Schmiedebergs Arch Pharmacol 1983;324:140–147.
35. Whittemore RM, Pearce LB, Roth JA. Purification and characterization of a dopamine-sulfating form of phenol sulfotransferase from human brain. Biochemistry 1985;24:2477–2482.
36. Heroux JA, Roth JA. Physical characterization of a monoamine-sulfating form of phenol sulfotransferase from human platelets. Mol Pharmacol 1988;34:29–33.
37. Weinshilboum RM. Phenol sulfotransferase in humans: properties, regulation, and function. Fed Proc 1986;45:2223–2228.
38. Weinshilboum R, Otterness D, Aksoy I, Wood T, Her C, Raftogianis R. Sulfotransferase molecular biology: cDNAs and genes. FASEB J 1997;11:3–14.
39. Falany CN, Vazquez ME, Heroux JA, Roth JA. Purification and characterization of human liver phenol-sulfating phenol sulfotransferase. Arch Biochem Biophys 1990;278:312–318.
40. Wilborn TW, Comer KA, Dooley TP, Reardon IM, Heinrikson RL, Falany CN. Sequence analysis and expression of the cDNA for the phenol-sulfating form of human liver phenol sulfotransferase. Mol Pharmacol 1993;43:70–77.
41. Falany CN, Wheeler J, Oh TS, Falany JL. Steroid sulfation by expressed human cytosolic sulfotransferases. J Steroid Biochem Mol Biol 1994;48:369–375.
42. Hernandez JS, Powers SP, Weinshilboum RM. Human liver arylamine N-sulfotransferase activity. Thermostable phenol sulfotransferase catalyzes the N-sulfation of 2-naphthylamine. Drug Metab Dispos 1991;19:1071–1079.
43. Glatt H, Pauly K, Czich A, Falany JL, Falany CN. Activation of benzylic alcohols to mutagens by rat and human sulfotransferases expressed in *Escherichia coli*. Eur J Pharmacol 1995;293:173–181.

44. Glatt H. Sulfation and sulfotransferases 4: bioactivation of mutagens via sulfation. FASEB J 1997;11:314–321.
45. Price RA, Cox NJ, Spielman RS, Van Loon JA, Maidak BL, Weinshilboum RM. Inheritance of human platelet thermolabile phenol sulfotransferase (TL PST) activity. Genet Epidemiol 1988;5:1–15.
46. Weinshilboum R. Phenol sulfotransferase inheritance. Cell Mol Neurobiol 1988; 8:27–34.
47. Raftogianis RB, Wood TC, Otterness DM, Van Loon JA, Weinshilboum RM. Phenol sulfotransferase pharmacogenetics in humans: association of common SULT1A1 alleles with TS PST phenotype. Biochem Biophys Res Commun 1997; 239:298–304.
48. Raftogianis RB, Wood TC, Weinshilboum RM. Human phenol sulfotransferases SULT1A2 and SULT1A1: genetic polymorphisms, allozyme properties, and human liver genotype–phenotype correlations. Biochem Pharmacol 1999;58:605–616.
49. Dooley TP, Probst P, Obermoeller RD, et al. Mapping of the phenol sulfotransferase gene (STP) to human chromosome 16p12.1-p11.2 and to mouse chromosome 7. Genomics 1993;18:440–443.
50. Dooley TP, Mitchison HM, Munroe PB, et al. Mapping of two phenol sulphotransferase genes, STP and STM, to 16p: candidate genes for Batten disease. Biochem Biophys Res Commun 1994;205:482–489.
51. Aksoy IA, Callen DF, Apostolou S, Her C, Weinshilboum RM. Thermolabile phenol sulfotransferase gene (STM): localization to human chromosome 16p11.2. Genomics 1994;23:275–277.
52. Engelke CE, Meinl W, Boeing H, Glatt H. Association between functional genetic polymorphisms of human sulfotransferases 1A1 and 1A2. Pharmacogenetics 2000; 10:163–169.
53. Zhu X, Veronese ME, Iocco P, McManus ME. cDNA cloning and expression of a new form of human aryl sulfotransferase Int J Biochem Cell Biol 1996;28: 565–571.
54. Ozawa SH, Nagata K, Shimada M, et al. Primary structures and properties of two related forms of aryl sulfotransferase in human liver. Pharmacogenetics 1995;5: S135–S140.
55. Campbell NR, Van Loon JA, Weinshilboum RM. Human liver phenol sulfotransferase: assay conditions, biochemical properties and partial purification of isozymes of the thermostable form. Biochem Pharmacol 1987;36:1435–1446.
56. Thomae BA, Rifki OF, Theobald MA, Eckloff BW, Wieben ED, Weinshilboum RM. Human catecholamine sulfotransferase (SULT1A3) pharmacogenetics: functional genetic polymorphism. J Neurochem 2003;87:809–819.
57. Price RA, Spielman RS, Lucena AL, Van Loon JA, Maidak BL, Weinshilboum RM. Genetic polymorphism for human platelet thermostable phenol sulfotransferase (TS PST) activity. Genetics 1989;122:905–914.
58. Eisenhofer G, Coughtrie MW, Goldstein DS. Dopamine sulphate: an enigma resolved. Clin Exp Pharmacol Physiol Suppl 1999;26:S41–S53.

59. Zou J, Pentney R, Roth JA. Immunohistochemical detection of phenol sulfotransferase-containing neurons in human brain. J Neurochem 1990;55:1154–1158.
60. Ganguly TC, Krasnykh V, Falany CN. Bacterial expression and kinetic characterization of the human monoamine-sulfating form of phenol sulfotransferase. Drug Metab Dispos 1995;23:945–950.
61. Taskinen J, Ethell BT, Pihlavisto P, Hood AM, Burchell B, Coughtrie MW. Conjugation of catechols by recombinant human sulfotransferases, UDP-glucuronosyltransferases, and soluble catechol O-methyltransferase: structure–conjugation relationships and predictive models. Drug Metab Dispos 2003;31:1187–1197.
62. Dajani R, Hood AM, Coughtrie MW. A single amino acid, glu146, governs the substrate specificity of a human dopamine sulfotransferase, SULT1A3. Mol Pharmacol 1998;54:942–948.
63. Fujita K, Nagata K, Ozawa S, Sasano H, Yamazoe Y. Molecular cloning and characterization of rat ST1B1 and human ST1B2 cDNAs, encoding thyroid hormone sulfotransferases. J Biochem (Tokyo) 1997;122:1052–1061.
64. Wang J, Falany JL, Falany CN. Expression and characterization of a novel thyroid hormone-sulfating form of cytosolic sulfotransferase from human liver. Mol Pharmacol 1998;53:274–282.
65. Kester MH, Kaptein E, Roest TJ, et al. Characterization of human iodothyronine sulfotransferases. J Clin Endocrinol Metab 1999;84:1357–1364.
66. Kester MH, van Dijk CH, Tibboel D, et al. Sulfation of thyroid hormone by estrogen sulfotransferase. J Clin Endocrinol Metab 1999;84:2577–2580.
67. Fujita K, Nagata K, Yamazaki T, Watanabe E, Shimada M, Yamazoe Y. Enzymatic characterization of human cytosolic sulfotransferases; identification of ST1B2 as a thyroid hormone sulfotransferase. Biol Pharm Bull 1999;22:446–452.
68. Her C, Kaur GP, Athwal RS, Weinshilboum RM. Human sulfotransferase SULT1C1: cDNA cloning, tissue-specific expression, and chromosomal localization. Genomics 1997;41:467–470.
69. Yoshinari K, Nagata K, Shimada M, Yamazoe Y. Molecular characterization of ST1C1-related human sulfotransferase. Carcinogenesis 1998;19:951–953.
70. Sakakibara Y, Yanagisawa K, Katafuchi J, et al. Molecular cloning, expression, characterization of novel SULT1C sulfotransferases that catalyze the sulfonation of N-hydroxy-2-acetylaminofluorene. J Biol Chem 1998;273:33929–33935.
71. Suiko M, Sakakibara Y, Liu MC. Sulfation of environmental estrogen-like chemicals by human cytosolic sulfotransferases. Biochem Biophys Res Commun 2000;267:80–84.
72. Falany CN, Krasnykh V, Falany JL. Bacterial expression and characterization of a cDNA for human liver estrogen sulfotransferase. J Steroid Biochem Mol Biol 1995;52:529–539.
73. Zhang H, Varmalova O, Vargas FM, Falany CN, Leyh TS. Sulfuryl transfer: the catalytic mechanism of human estrogen sulfotransferase. J Biol Chem 1998;273:10888–10892.

74. Aksoy IA, Wood TC, Weinshilboum R. Human liver estrogen sulfotransferase: identification by cDNA cloning and expresion. Biochem Biophys Res Commun 1994;200:1621–1629.
75. Hagen M, Pabel U, Landsiedel R, Bartsch I, Falany CN, Glatt H. Expression of human estrogen sulfotransferase in Salmonella typhimurium: differences between hHST and hEST in the enantioselective activation of 1-hydroxyethylpyrene to a mutagen. Chem Biol Interact 1998;109:249–253.
76. Falany JL, Azziz R, Falany CN. Identification and characterization of the cytosolic sulfotransferases in normal human endometrium. Chem Biol Interact 1998; 109:329–339.
77. Falany JL, Falany CN. Expression of cytosolic sulfotransferases in normal mammary epithelial cells and breast cancer cell lines. Cancer Res 1996;56:1551–1555.
78. Her C, Szumlanski C, Aksoy I, Weinshilboum R. Human jejunal estrogen sulfotransferase and dehydroepiandrosterone sulfotransferase: immunological characterization of individual variation. Drug Metab Dispos 1996;24:1328–1335.
79. Falany JL, Falany CN. Regulation of estrogen sulfotransferase in human endometrial adenocarcinoma cells by progesterone. Endocrinology 1996;137:1395–1401.
80. Baxter JD, Tyrrell JB. The Adrenal Cortex. In Felig P, et al. Endocrinology and Metabolism. New York: McGraw-Hill; 1987;511–632.
81. Falany CN, Vazquez ME, Kalb JM. Purification and characterization of human liver dehydroepiandrosterone sulfotransferase. Arch Biochem Biophys 1989;260:641–646.
82. Comer KA, Falany CN. Immunological characterization of dehydroepiandrosterone sulfotransferase from human liver and adrenals. Mol Pharmacol 1992;41:645–651.
83. Falany CN, Comer KA, Dooley TP, Glatt H. Human dehydroepiandrosterone sulfotransferase: purification, molecular cloning, and characterization. Ann NY Acad Sci 1995;774:59–72.
84. Parker CR, Falany CN, Stockard CR, Stankovic AK, Grizzle WE. Immunohistochemical localization of dehydroepiandrosterone sulfotransferase in human fetal tissues. J Clin Endocrinol Metab 1993;78:234–236.
85. Forbes KJ, Hagen M, Glatt H, Hume R, Coughtrie MWH. Human fetal adrenal hydroxysteroid sulphotransferase: cDNA cloning, stable expression in V79 cells and functional characterization of the expressed enzyme. Mol Cell Endocrinol 1995;112:53–60.
86. Radominska A, Comer KA, Ziminak P, Falany J, Iscan M, Falany CN. Human liver steroid sulfotransferase sulphates bile acids. Biochem J 1991;273:597–604.
87. Tashiro A, Sasano H, Nishikawa T, et al. Expression and activity of dehydroepiandrosterone sulfotransferase in human gastric mucosa. J Steroid Biochem Mol Biol 2000;72:149–154.
88. Otterness DM, Wieben ED, Wood TC, et al. Human liver dehydroepiandrosterone sulfotransferase: molecular cloning and expression of the cDNA. Mol Pharmacol 1992;41:865–872.
89. Otterness D, Mohrenweiser HW, Brandiff BF, Weinshilboum RM. Dehydroepiandrosterone sulfotransferase gene (STD): Localization to human chromosome 19q13.3. Cytogenet Cell Genet 1995;70:45–52.

90. Meloche CA, Sharma V, Swedmark S, Andersson P, Falany CN. Sulfation of budesonide by human cytosolic sulfotransferase, dehydroepiandrosterone-sulfotransferase (DHEA-ST), Drug Metab Dispos 2002;30:582–585.
91. Kitada H, Miyata M, Nakamura T, et al. Protective role of hydroxysteroid sulfotransferase in lithocholic acid-induced liver toxicity. J Biol Chem 2003;278: 17838–17844.
92. Her C, Wood TC, Eichler EE, et al. Human hydroxysteroid sulfotransferase SULT2B1: two enzymes encoded by a single chromosome 19 gene. Genomics 1998;53:284–295.
93. Meloche CA, Falany CN. Cloning and expression of the human 3β-hydroxysteroid sulfotransferases (SULT 2B1a and SULT 2B1b). J Steroid Biochem Mol Biol 2001;77:261–269.
94. Pai TG, Sugahara T, Suiko M, Sakakibara Y, Xu F, Liu MC. Differential xenoestrogen-sulfating activities of the human cytosolic sulfotransferases: molecular cloning, expression, and purification of human SULT2B1a and SULT2B1b sulfotransferases. Biochim Biophys Acta 2002;1573:165–170.
95. He D, Meloche CA, Dumas NA, Frost AR, Falany CN. Different subcellular localization of sulfotransferase 2B1b (SULT2B1b) in human placenta and prostate. Biochem J 2004;379:533–540.
96. Geese WJ, Raftogianis R. Biochemical characterization and tissue distribution of human SULT2B1. Biochem Biophys Res Commun 2001;288:280–289.
97. Javitt NB, Lee YC, Shimizu C, Fuda H, Strott CA. Cholesterol and hydroxycholesterol sulfotransferases: identification, distinction from dehydroepiandrosterone sulfotransferase, and differential tissue expression. Endocrinology 2001;142: 2978–2984.
98. Falany CN, Meloche CA, He D, Falany JL. Molecular cloning of the human cytosolic sulfotransferases. In Pacifici GM, Coughtrie MWH, eds. Human Cytosolic Sulfotransferases. London: Taylor and Francis; 2004;in press.
99. Fuda H, Lee YC, Shimizu C, Javitt NB, Strott CA. Mutational analysis of human hydroxysteroid sulfotransferase SULT2B1 isoforms reveals that exon 1B of the SULT2B1 gene produces cholesterol sulfotransferase, whereas exon 1A yields pregnenolone sulfotransferase. J Biol Chem 2002;277:36161–36168.
100. Falany CN, Xie X, Wang J, Ferrer J, Falany JL. Molecular cloning and expression of novel sulfotransferase-Like cDNAs from human and rat brain. Biochem J 2000; 346:857–864.
101. Liyou NE, Buller KM, Tresillian MJ, et al. Localization of a brain sulfotransferase, SULT4A1, in the human and rat brain: an immunohistochemical study. J Histochem Cytochem 2003;51:1655–1664.
102. Sakakibara Y, Suiko M, Pai TG, et al. Highly conserved mouse and human brain sulfotransferases: molecular cloning, expression, and functional characterization. Gene 2002;285:39–47.
103. Bidwell LM, Gillam EM, Gaedigk A, Zhu X, Grant D, McManus ME. Bacterial expression of two human aryl sulfotransferases. Chem Biol Interact 1998;109: 137–141.

104. Dajani R, Sharp S, Graham S, et al. Kinetic properties of human dopamine sulfotransferase (SULT1A3) expressed in prokaryotic and eukaryotic systems: comparison with the recombinant enzyme purified from *Escherichia coli*. Protein Express Purif 1999;16:11–18.
105. Glatt H, Bartsch I, Christoph S, et al. Sulfotransferase-mediated activation of mutagens studied using heterologous expression systems. Chem Biol Interact 1998;109:195–219.
106. Arlt VM, Glatt H, Muckel E, et al. Activation of 3-nitrobenzanthrone and its metabolites by human acetyltransferases, sulfotransferases and cytochrome P450 expressed in Chinese hamster V79 cells. Int J Cancer 2003;105:583–592.
107. Wu RW, Panteleakos FN, Kadkhodayan S, Bolton-Grob R, McManus ME, Felton JS. Genetically modified Chinese hamster ovary cells for investigating sulfotransferase-mediated cytotoxicity and mutation by 2-amino-1-methyl-6-phenylimidazo[4,5-b]pyridine. Environ Mol Mutagen 2000;35:57–65.
108. Kotov A, Falany JL, Wang J, Falany CN. Regulation of estrogen activity by sulfation in human Ishikawa endometrial adenocarcinoma cells. J Steroid Biochem Mol Biol 1999;68:137–144.
109. Falany JL, Falany CN. Regulation of estrogen activity by sulfation in human MCF-7 breast cancer cells. Oncol Res 1998;9:589–596.
110. Falany JL, Macrina N, Falany CN. Regulation of MCF-7 breast cancer cell growth by beta-estradiol sulfation. Breast Cancer Res Treat 2002;74:167–176.
111. Adams JB, McDonald D. Enzymatic synthesis of steroid sulphates. XII. Isolation of Dehydroepiandrosterone sulphotransferase from human adrenals by affinity chromatography. Biochim Biophys Acta 1979;567:144–153.
112. Liu H-C, Tseng L. Estradiol metabolism in isolated human endometrial epithelial glands and stromal cells. Endocrinology 1979;104:1674–1694.
113. Gamage NU, Duggleby RG, Barnett AC, et al. Structure of a human carcinogen-converting enzyme, SULT1A1. Structural and kinetic implications of substrate inhibition. J Biol Chem 2003;278:7655–7662.
114. Bernier F, Lopez Solache I, Labrie F, Luu-The V. Cloning and expression of cDNA encoding human placental estrogen sulfotransferase. Mol Cell Endocrinol 1994;99:R11–R15.
115. Faucher F, Lacoste L, Dufort I, Luu-The V. High metabolization of catechole-strogens by type 1 estrogen sulfotransferase (hEST1). J Steroid Biochem Mol Biol 2001;77:83–86.
116. Campbell NR, Van Loon JA, Sundaram RS, Ames MM, Hansch C, Weinshilboum R. Human and rat liver phenol sulfotransferase: structure–activity relationships for phenolic substrates. Mol Pharmacol 1987;32:813–819.
117. Foldes A, Meek JS. Rat brain phenol sulfotransferase. Biochim Biophys Acta 1973;327:365–374.
118. Sakakibara Y, Katafuchi J, Takami Y, et al. Manganese-dependent Dopa/tyrosine sulfation in HepG2 human hepatoma cells: novel Dopa/tyrosine sulfotransferase activities associated with the human monoamine-form phenol sulfotransferase. Biochim Biophys Acta 1997;1355:102–106.

119. Sane DC, Baker MS. Human platelets possess tyrosylprotein sulfotransferase (TPST) activity. Thromb Haemost 1993;69:272–275.
120. Duffel MW. Molecular specificity of aryl sulfotransferase IV (tyrosine-ester sulfotransferase) for xenobiotic substrates and inhibitors. Chem Biol Interact 1994;92: 3–14.
121. Falany JL, Macrina N, Falany CN. Sulfation of tibolone and tibolone metabolites by expressed human cytosolic sulfotransferases. J Steroid Biochem Mol Biol 2004;88:383–391.
122. Sharp S, Coughtrie MW, Forbes KJ, Hume R. Preparation and characterization of anti-peptide antibodies directed against human phenol and hydroxysteroid sulphotransferases. J Pharmacol Toxicol Methods 1995;34:89–95.
123. Rivett AJ, Francis A, Whittemore R, Roth JA. Sulfate conjugation of dopamine in rat brain: regional distribution of activity and evidence for neuronal localization. J Neurochem 1984;42:1444–1449.
124. Hume R, Barker EV, Coughtrie MW. Differential expression and immunohistochemical localisation of the phenol and hydroxysteroid sulphotransferase enzyme families in the developing lung. Histochem Cell Biol 1996;105:147–152.
125. Hume R, Richard K, Kaptein E, Stanley EL, Visser TJ, Coughtrie MW. Thyroid hormone metabolism and the developing human lung. Biol Neonate 2001;80 (Suppl 1):18–21.
126. Kennerson AR, McDonald DA, Adams JB. Dehydroepiandrosterone sulfotransferase localization in human adrenal glands: a light and electron microscopic study. J Clin Endocrinol Metab 1983;56:786–790.
127. Sasano H, Sato F, Shizawa S, Nagura H, Coughtrie MW. Immunolocalization of dehydroepiandrosterone sulfotransferase in normal and pathologic human adrenal gland. Mod Pathol 1995;8:891–896.
128. Sharp S, Anderson JM, Coughtrie MW. Immunohistochemical localisation of hydroxysteroid sulphotransferase in human breast carcinoma tissue: a preliminary study. Eur J Cancer 1994;30A:1654–1659.
129. Suzuki T, Nakata T, Miki Y, et al. Estrogen sulfotransferase and steroid sulfatase in human breast carcinoma. Cancer Res 2003;63:2762–2770.
130. Jones AL, Hagen M, Coughtrie MW, Roberts RC, Glatt H. Human platelet phenolsulfotransferases: cDNA cloning, stable expression in V79 cells and identification of a novel allelic variant of the phenol-sulfating form. Biochem Biophys Res Commun 1995;208:855–862.
131. Dooley TP, Huang Z. Genomic organization and DNA sequences of two human phenol sulfotransferase genes (STP1 and STP2) on the short arm of chromosome 16. Biochem Biophys Res Commun 1996;228:134–140.
132. Her C, Raftogianis R, Weinshilboum RM. Human phenol sulfotransferase STP2 gene: Molecular cloning, structural characterization and chromosomal localization. Genomics 1996;33:409–420.
133. Dooley TP, Probst P, Munroe PB, Mole SE, Liu Z, Doggett NA. Genomic organization and DNA sequence of the human catecholamine-sulfating phenol sulfotransferase gene (STM). Biochem Biophys Res Commun 1994;205:1325–1332.

134. Zhu X, Veronese ME, Sansom LN, McManus ME. Molecular characterisation of a human aryl sulfotransferase cDNA. Biochem Biophys Res Commun 1993;192: 671–676.
135. Honma W, Kamiyama Y, Yoshinari K, et al. Enzymatic characterization and interspecies difference of phenol sulfotransferases, ST1A forms. Drug Metab Dispos 2001;29:274–281.
136. Comer KA, Falany JL, Falany CN. Cloning and expression of human liver dehydroepiandrosterone sulfotransferase. Biochem J 1993;289:233–240.
137. Kong A-NT, Yang L, Ma M, Tao D, Bjornsson TD. Molecular cloning of the alcohol/hydroxysteroid form (hSTa) of sulfotransferase from human liver. Biochem Biophys Res Commun 1992;187:448–454.

Index

AA, *see* Arachidonic acid
Acetaminophen
  bioactivation, 201, 202
  metabolism, 199, 201
  safety, 197, 198
  toxicity
    N-acetylcysteine management, 199
    acute liver failure epidemiology, 198
    cytochrome P450 transgenic mouse studies, 216–218
    DNA microarray studies of gene upregulation, 219, 220
    glutathione depletion, 255–257
    glutathione *S*-transferase transgenic mouse studies, 217, 218
    hepatocyte extrinsic death
      cytokine and chemokine roles, 208, 209
      nitric oxide and reactive nitrogen species role, 209, 213, 264, 265
      nuclear factor-κB role, 213, 214
      transgenic animal studies, 211, 212
    hepatocyte intrinsic death
      apoptosis, 202, 207
      mitochondria role, 202–205, 207
      protein targets, 203
      stress gene upregulation, 205
      transgenic animal studies, 210, 211
    lipid peroxidation, 257–260
    phases, 198, 199
    prospects for study, 221, 222
    small interfering RNA studies, 218, 219
N-Acetylcysteine (NAC), acetaminophen overdose management, 199
N-Acetyltransferase (NAT)
  isoforms and homology, 176
  polymorphisms
    allele types
      NAT1, 177–179
      NAT2, 179–183
    discovery, 173–176
    genotyping, 187
    phenotype determination
      deduced versus measured phenotype concordance, 188, 189
      NAT1 phenotype, 187
      NAT2 phenotype, 183, 185, 186
    single nucleotide polymorphism functional effects in NAT2, 182, 183
  substrates, 175, 176
Akt
  chemical inhibitors, 65
  insulin and growth factor signaling, 54, 55
p-Aminosalicylate (PAS), *N*-acetylation phenotype determination, 187
Antiviral therapy, *see* Interferons; Protease inhibitors, human immunodeficiency virus; Reverse transcriptase inhibitors; *specific drugs*; Viral fusion inhibitors

Apoptosis, hepatocytes in acetaminophen toxicity, 202, 207
Arachidonic acid (AA)
  glucuronidation of metabolites, see Fatty acid glucuronidation
  metabolism, 110

Baculovirus–Sf9 cell expression system, see Multidrug resistance proteins
BD, see 1,2-Butadiene
Bile flow
  bile acid-dependent, 274, 276
  bile acid-independent, 274, 276
Bilirubin, UDP-glucuronosyltransferase in clearance, 163
1,2-Butadiene (BD)
  carcinogenicity, 2
  metabolic oxidation products, 2, 3
  renal metabolism, 2, 3

Caffeine, N-acetylation phenotype determination, 183, 185, 186
ChIP, see Chromatin immunoprecipitation
Chromatin immunoprecipitation (ChIP), protein–DNA interaction analysis, 33, 34
CYP1A1
  discrimination between transcriptional versus posttranscriptional regulation
    inhibitors of transcription or translation, 20–22
    nuclear runoff assay, 22
  promoter
    analysis and reporter assays, 23, 25
    protein–DNA interaction analysis
      chromatin immunoprecipitation, 33, 34
      DNA footprinting, 29, 30, 34–36
      electrophoretic mobility shift assay, 30–33
      site affinity amplification binding, 33
      Southwestern blot, 26, 27
      ultraviolet crosslinking, 25
      yeast one-hybrid screening, 27–29
  transcription factor modulation studies
    inhibition, 40, 41
    overexpression
      stable cell line generation, 37, 39
      transient transfection, 36, 37
      viral transduction, 39, 40
CYP2A5, 1,2-butadiene metabolism, 3
CYP2E1
  acetaminophen bioactivation, 201
  1,2-butadiene metabolism, 3, 11
  suppression by insulin, 47, 49
CYP3A4, P-glycoprotein interactions, 240, 241
CYP4B1, 1,2-butadiene metabolism, 3, 10
Cytochrome P450, see also specific CYPs
  acetaminophen toxicity, transgenic mouse studies, 216–218
  diabetes effects on expression, 46–48
  gene expression regulation, see CYP1A1; specific hormone and growth factor signal transduction components
  human immunodeficiency virus antiviral drug metabolism, 235–240
  interferon therapy effects, 242
  pharmacokinetic boosting with drug–drug interactions, 233–235, 242–244
  regulation overview, 20

Index

DHA, *see* Docosahexaenoic acid
Diabetes, drug-metabolizing enzyme effects, 46–48
DNA footprinting
  protein–DNA interaction analysis
    in vitro, 29, 30
    in vivo, 34–36
  UDP-glucuronosyltransferase promoter analysis, 152, 153
DNA microarray, gene upregulation in acetaminophen toxicity, 219, 220
Docosahexaenoic acid (DHA), signaling pathway modulation, 110, 113

EGFR, *see* Epidermal growth factor receptor
Electrophoretic mobility shift assay (EMSA)
  protein–DNA interaction analysis, 30–33
  UDP-glucuronosyltransferase promoter analysis, 153–155
EMSA, *see* Electrophoretic mobility shift assay
Epidermal growth factor receptor (EGFR), signaling, 53

Fatty acid glucuronidation
  assays
    kinetic analysis, 121, 122
    mass spectrometry analysis of glucuronides, 124–126
    thin-layer chromatography, 120, 121
    UDP-glucuronosyltransferase incubation conditions, 119, 120
  hydrolysis conditions, 120
  kinetic parameters of UGT2B7, 123, 128

oxidized fatty acid glucuronidation
  biological significance, 114
  preparative synthesis of glucuronides, 122, 124
  prospects for study, 126, 128
  substrates
    commercial availability, 115
    gas chromatography-mass spectrometry analysis, 118, 119
    high-performance liquid chromatography purification, 118, 119
    13(S)-hydroxyoctadecadienoic acid synthesis, 116
    13-hydroxyperoxy-(z, e)-9,11-octadecadienoic acid synthesis, 115, 116
    linoleic acid epoxide and diol synthesis, 117, 118
    13-oxooctadecadienoic acid synthesis, 116, 117
Flavin-containing monooxygenases (FMOs)
  isoforms and renal expression, 13, 14
  tetrachloroethylene metabolism, 11, 13–15
  trichloroethylene metabolism, 11, 13–15
FMOs, *see* Flavin-containing monooxygenases
Folate, functions, 291, 292

Gene regulation
  discrimination between transcriptional versus posttranscriptional regulation
    inhibitors of transcription or translation, 20–22
    nuclear runoff assay, 22
    promoter analysis and reporter assays, 23, 25

protein–promoter interaction
    analysis
    DNA footprinting
        in vitro, 29, 30
        in vivo, 34–36
    electrophoretic mobility shift
        assay, 30–33
    site affinity amplification binding,
        33
    Southwestern blot, 26, 27
    ultraviolet crosslinking, 25
    yeast one-hybrid screening, 27–29
transcription factor modulation
    studies
    inhibition, 40, 41
    overexpression
        stable cell line generation, 37,
            39
        transient transfection, 36, 37
        viral transduction, 39, 40
UDP-glucuronosyltransferase, see
    UDP-
    glucuronosyltransferase
Glutathione
    acetaminophen depletion and
        metabolite interactions,
        255–257
    drug oxidative stress and depletion,
        261, 262
    functions, 262
    liver synthesis, 320
    renal transport
        assay
            general considerations, 330–
                332
            mitochondrial inner membrane
                transport, 333, 334
            plasma membrane transport,
                332, 333
        experimental model systems for
            study
            mitochondrial transport, 328–
                330
            overview, 325, 326

plasma membrane transport,
    326, 328
mitochondrial membrane
    transporters, 324, 325
overview, 320, 321
plasma membrane transporters,
    321–323
prospects for study, 334, 335
Glutathione reductase (GR)
    drug inhibition, 263, 265, 266
    functions, 262, 263
Glutathione S-transferase (GST)
    acetaminophen toxicity, transgenic
        mouse studies, 217, 218
    1,2-butadiene metabolism, 3
    classification, 85, 86
    diabetes effects on expression, 46–48
    functional overview, 86, 87
    tetrachloroethylene metabolism, 6,
        8
    trichloroethylene metabolism, 6, 8
    zeta isoform
        activity of variants, 92, 93
        antiserum generation, 94
        catalytic activities and assays
            α-halo acids as substrates, 95–
                97
            maleylacetoacetate isomerase,
                94, 95
        catalytic mechanism, 97–99
        crystal structure, 92, 94
        deficiency
            gene knockout studies, 100,
                101
            human disease, 100
            inhibitor studies, 101, 102
        discovery, 87, 88
        inactivation by α-halo acids, 99,
            100
        polymorphism detection by
            bioinformatics, 88–90
        recombinant protein expression in
            Escherichia coli, 91, 92
GR, see Glutathione reductase

Index

GST, *see* Glutathione S-transferase
13-HODE, *see* Fatty acid glucuronidation
31-HPODE, *see* Fatty acid glucuronidation
Human immunodeficiency virus antiviral therapy, *see* Protease inhibitors, human immunodeficiency virus; Reverse transcriptase inhibitors; *specific drugs*

Immunohistochemistry, sulfotransferases, 367, 368
Insulin
 CYP2E1 suppression, 47, 49
 receptor, 51, 52
Interferons
 antiviral therapy, 242
 cytochrome P450 interactions, 242
 drug–drug interactions, 242

Kinases, *see also specific kinases*
 assays
  activity assays, 62
  immunoblot, 61
 chemical inhibitors, 62–65
 dominant-negative protein kinase constructs, 65, 69
 small interfering RNA inhibition, 69–71

Linoleic acid (LA)
 glucuronidation of metabolites, *see* Fatty acid glucuronidation
 oxidative metabolites and biological activities, 109–112
Lipid peroxidation
 acetaminophen toxicity, 257–260
 thiobarbituric acid-reactive substances assay, 258, 260

MAPK, *see* Mitogen-activated protein kinase

Minoxidil, hair growth mechanisms, 342, 343
Mitochondria
 acetaminophen toxicity role, 202–205, 207
 glutathione transporter, 324, 325, 328–330, 333, 334
 nucleoside analog impairment of function, 237
Mitogen-activated protein kinase (MAPK)
 chemical inhibitors, 63, 64
 insulin and growth factor signaling, 51
 phosphatases, 59, 60
 phosphatidylinositol 3-kinase crosstalk, 57, 58
 signaling cascades, 55–57
 types, 55
MRPs, *see* Multidrug resistance proteins
Multidrug resistance proteins (MRPs)
 assays
  ATPase activity, 280–282
  liver tissue preparation for study, 277, 278
  membrane vesicle uptake, 279, 280
  transmonolayer flux, 280
 ATP requirement, 274
 MRP2
  baculovirus–Sf9 cell expression system, 278, 279, 283
  crude vesicle preparation, 285, 286
  freezing and thawing of Sf9 cells, 283, 284
  subculture, 283, 284
  sucrose-fractionated vesicle preparation, 284, 285
 expression modulators, 277
 hepatocyte function, 277
 reverse transcriptase inhibitor transport by MRP4, 235
 types and substrates, 276, 277

NAC, *see* N-Acetylcysteine
NAT, *see* N-Acetyltransferase
NF-κB, *see* Nuclear factor-κB
Nitric oxide (NO), acetaminophen toxicity role, 209, 213, 264, 265
NO, *see* Nitric oxide
Northern blot
   sulfotransferases, 366
   UDP-glucuronosyltransferase expression analysis, 141, 145
Nuclear factor-κB (NF-κB), acetaminophen toxicity role, 213, 214
Nuclear runoff assay, transcriptional regulation analysis, 22

OATs, *see* Organic anion transporters, kidney
Organic anion transporters, kidney
   glutathione transport, 322, 323
   tetrachloroethylene and trichloroethylene metabolite transport, 6, 8
13-OXO, *see* Fatty acid glucuronidation

p70 S6 kinase
   chemical inhibitors, 64
   insulin and growth factor signaling, 54
PAS, *see* p-Aminosalicylate
PCR, *see* Polymerase chain reaction
Peroxynitrite, acetaminophen toxicity role, 209, 213, 264, 265
P-glycoprotein
   cytochrome P450 system interactions, 240, 241
   human immunodeficiency virus protease inhibitor transport, 240, 241
Phase I reactions, examples, 46
Phase II reactions, examples, 46
Phosphatidylinositol 3-kinase (PI3K)
   chemical inhibitors, 65
   classes, 53, 54
   function, 50, 51, 54
   insulin receptor signaling, 54
   mitogen-activated protein kinase crosstalk, 57, 58
PI3K, *see* Phosphatidylinositol 3-kinase
PKC, *see* Protein kinase C
Polymerase chain reaction (PCR)
   reverse transcriptase-polymerase chain reaction of human sulfotransferases, 367
   UDP-glucuronosyltransferase gene expression analysis
   primers, 140, 142, 143
   real-time PCR, 141
   semiquantitative real-time PCR, 140, 141
   transcription start site determination using RLM-RACE, 150, 151
Pregnane X receptor (PXR), UDP-glucuronosyltransferase regulation, *see* UDP-glucuronosyltransferase
Probenecid, antibiotic interactions, 233
Protease inhibitors, human immunodeficiency virus
   cytochrome P450 metabolism, 238, 239, 244
   drug–drug interactions, 238, 239, 242–244
   dual protease inhibition, 242, 243
   low-dose boosting, 242, 243
   P-glycoprotein transport, 240, 241
Protein carbonyls
   assay, 264
   oxidative stress marker, 264
Protein kinase C (PKC)
   atypical isoforms in insulin and growth factor signaling, 55
   chemical inhibitors, 64
Protein thiols, drug oxidative stress and depletion, 261, 262

Index   385

Protein tyrosine phosphatase (PTP),
    functions, 58, 59
PTEN, phosphorylative regulation, 61
PTP, *see* Protein tyrosine phosphatase
PXR, *see* Pregnane X receptor

Raf, mitogen-activated protein kinase
    signaling cascade, 56, 57
Ras, mitogen-activated protein kinase
    signaling cascade, 55, 56
Receptor tyrosine kinase (RTK),
    function, 49, 50, 55
Reduced folate carrier (RFC)
    anion sensitivity, 295
    cell studies
        photoaffinity crosslinking, 297
        transfection of transport-impaired
            cells, 297–299
        transport, 296, 297
    history of study, 292, 294
    pH optimum, 294
    sequence homology between human
        and mouse, 302
    stereospecificity, 294, 295
    substrates, 292–294
    tertiary structure, 306
    transmembrane domains
        deletional mutagenesis, 305, 306
        hemagglutinin epitope insertion
            studies, 301
        insertional mutagenesis, 305, 306
        prospects for study, 310, 311
        scanning cysteine accessibility
            mutagenesis studies, 307–310
        scanning glycosylation
            mutagenesis, 301, 302
        site-directed mutagenesis of
            conserved charged residues,
            304, 305
        TMD1 function, 303, 304, 308–310
        TMD3 function, 304
        TMD4 function, 304
        TMD8 function, 304
    topology, 299, 300

Renal organic anion transporters, *see*
    Organic anion transporters,
    kidney
Reverse transcriptase inhibitors
    nonnucleoside inhibitors
        cytochrome P450 metabolism,
            237, 238
        drug–drug interactions, 237, 238
    nucleoside analogs
        activation, 236
        drug–drug interactions, 235–237
        mitochondrial function
            impairment, 237
        MRP4 transport, 235
    nucleotide analogs, drug–drug
        interactions, 237
Reverse transcriptase-polymerase chain
    reaction, *see* Polymerase
    chain reaction
RFC, *see* Reduced folate carrier
RNA interference, *see* Small interfering
    RNA
RTK, *see* Receptor tyrosine kinase

SAAB, *see* Site affinity amplification
    binding
SCAM, *see* Scanning cysteine
    accessibility mutagenesis
Scanning cysteine accessibility
    mutagenesis (SCAM),
    reduced folate carrier
    studies, 307–310
Serine/threonine phosphatases, types
    and functions, 60
Shc, insulin receptor signaling, 52
SHP-2 phosphatase, functions, 58, 59
SiRNA, *see* Small interfering RNA
Site affinity amplification binding
    (SAAB), protein–DNA
    interaction analysis, 33
Site-directed mutagenesis, reduced
    folate carrier studies, 304,
    305
Small interfering RNA (siRNA)

acetaminophen toxicity studies, 218, 219
gene inhibition, 41
protein kinase suppression, 69–71
Southwestern blot, protein–DNA interaction analysis, 26, 27
Stress genes, upregulation in acetaminophen toxicity, 205
Sulfotransferases (SULTs)
   activity assays, 360–364
   functional overview, 341, 342
   human enzymes
      classification, 344–346
      expression systems and purification, 356–359
      SULT1A subfamily
         overview, 345, 347
         SULT1A1, 347, 348
         SULT1A2, 348
         SULT1A3, 349, 350
         SULT1B1, 350, 351
         SULT1C1, 351, 352
         SULT1C2, 351, 352
         SULT1E1, 352, 353
      SULT2 subfamily
         SULT2A1, 353
         SULT2B1, 353–355
         SULT4A1, 355, 356
   immunohistochemistry, 367, 368
   Northern blot, 366
   prospects for study, 368, 369
   reactive electrophilic metabolite generation, 342–344
   reverse transcriptase-polymerase chain reaction, 367
   Western blot, 365
SULTs, see Sulfotransferases

TETRA, see Tetrachloroethylene
Tetrachloroethylene (TETRA)
   N-acetyltransferase detoxification of metabolites, 9, 10
   bioactivation, 4, 5, 11
   carcinogenicity, 4
   flavin-containing monooxygenase metabolism, 11, 13–15
   metabolic oxidation products, 5
   renal metabolism, 4–6, 8–10
   renal organic ion transporter
      handling of metabolites, 6, 8
   toxicity of metabolites, 8, 9
TRI, see Trichloroethylene
Trichloroethylene (TRI)
   N-acetyltransferase detoxification of metabolites, 9, 10
   bioactivation, 4, 5, 11
   carcinogenicity, 4
   flavin-containing monooxygenase metabolism, 11, 13–15
   metabolic oxidation products, 5
   renal metabolism, 4–6, 8–10
   renal organic ion transporter
      handling of metabolites, 6, 8
   toxicity of metabolites, 8, 9

UDP-glucuronosyltransferase (UGT)
   animal studies of regulation
      genetic and pharmacological regulation, 160, 161, 163
      pregnane X receptor activation
         humanized mouse models, 157, 158, 160, 161, 163
         knockout mouse studies, 158
         overview, 157
         transgenic mouse studies, 158–160
      xenobiotic induction, 155, 156
   diabetes effects on expression, 46–48
   fatty acid glucuronidation, see Fatty acid glucuronidation
   functional overview, 113, 114
   physiological relevance of gene regulation
      bilirubin clearance, 163
      steroid hormone homeostasis, 163, 164, 166
   promoter isolation and characterization

DNA footprinting, 152, 153
electrophoretic mobility shift
   assay, 153–155
isolation, 151
overview, 148–150
reporter construct preparation and
   transient transfection, 151,
   152
transcription start site
   determination, 150, 151
regulators, 134, 136
transcriptional regulation studies in
   cells
   activity assays, 146–148
   cell harvesting and subcellular
      fractionation, 145, 146
   cell studies of chemical inducers
      or suppressors, 137, 138
   Northern blot analysis, 141, 145
   nuclear receptor regulation
      plasmids and cloning, 139, 140
      transient transfection, 139
   overview, 133–136, 166
   polymerase chain reaction
      primers, 140, 142, 143
      real-time PCR, 141
      semiquantitative real-time
         PCR, 140, 141
      RNA isolation, 140
      Western blot, 146
UGT, *see* UDP-glucuronosyltransferase
Ultraviolet crosslinking, protein–DNA
   interaction analysis, 25

Western blot
   protein kinases, 61
   sulfotransferases, 365
   UDP-glucuronosyltransferase, 146

Yeast one-hybrid screening, protein–
   DNA interaction analysis,
   27–29